Endoscopic Submucosal Dissection

Norio Fukami

Editor

Endoscopic Submucosal Dissection

Principles and Practice

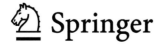 Springer

Editor
Norio Fukami, MD, AGAF, FACG, FASGE
Division of Gastroenterology & Hepatology
University of Colorado Anschutz Medical Campus
Aurora, CO, USA

Videos to this book can be accessed at
http://www.springerimages.com/videos/978-1-4939-2040-2

ISBN 978-1-4939-2040-2   ISBN 978-1-4939-2041-9 (eBook)
DOI 10.1007/978-1-4939-2041-9
Springer New York Heidelberg Dordrecht London

Library of Congress Control Number: 2014955223

Printed on acid-free paper

Springer is part of Springer Science+Business Media (www.springer.com)

Foreword

It was 1996 when I and my colleagues, the Endoscopy Group at the National Cancer Center Hospital, Tokyo, Japan, first developed and used the IT knife in endoscopic submucosal dissection (ESD) for early gastric cancer, and it is unbelievable how fast almost two decades have passed since then. Because surgical treatment, such as esophagectomy, gastrectomy, and colectomy, deteriorate patient condition despite clinical benefit, and because ESD obtains undoubtedly much better quality of life with comparable outcome, ESD has been widely accepted as a standard treatment for early cancer in the gastrointestinal tract and has rapidly spread throughout not only Japan but also many East Asian countries.

We know that doctors in Western countries have seen and experienced not many early-stage cancers or superficial lesions of the GI tract, and because those lesions were not in the majority, they have not provoked physicians' interest. However, I think the situation is changing by a certain degree, and I feel more enthusiasm from Western countries as well.

Successful ESD requires sound surgical skills, aptitude for early tumor detection and accurate assessment and diagnosis of tumor extension and depth, and knowledge about treatment indications. ESD has contributed to the development of more advanced diagnostic procedures using NBI with magnifying endoscopy, and has led to the start of many prospective clinical trials. Furthermore, on the basis of ESD, the endoscopist's work has expanded extensively to cover even peroral endoscopic myotomy (POEM), laparoscopy and endoscopy cooperative surgery (LECS), and endoscopic full-thickness resection (EFTR). Yet, we continue to make ceaseless efforts to push to more new frontiers.

Dr. Fukami, the editor, has worked in both Japan and the USA, and, therefore, he keenly feels the necessity for introduction of all aspects of ESD to Western doctors. Many pioneers and experts of ESD approved of his appeal and contributed to it. I believe this textbook will be a great help to both Eastern and Western endoscopists wanting to create new frontiers. Join us and together let us open up new possibilities for endoscopic therapy.

Hiroyuki Ono, M.D., Ph.D.
Shizuoka Cancer Center
Shizuoka, Japan

Preface

Endoscopic submucosal dissection (ESD) was born in Japan in the 1990s with much enthusiasm to overcome the shortcomings of endoscopic treatment for early gastric cancer. Then, many dedicated physicians explored the expansion of this technique to treat an even wider array of mucosal diseases in the gastrointestinal tract. I was lucky to see the early stages of the ESD procedure in Japan, following its evolution to the established ESD procedure that is now perceived as exceptionally elegant, intricate, and effective in carefully selected patients providing cure from cancer without invasive surgery. ESD has evolved to become a much safer and more capable mucosal resection technique, and has now expanded to treat even submucosal tumors (such as stromal tumors) and also into achalasia treatment (POEM).

ESD spread easily to neighboring countries, for they shared the similar disease prevalence of gastric cancer, but it has taken more time to come to Western countries. Early adaptors of ESD from the Western world learned by hands-on training in Japan or with explant models supervised and trained by ESD experts. Literature on outcome and some techniques is available, but we have limited resources for learning ESD in English.

There was a desperate need for an ESD textbook to teach the much-needed basics for learning and performing ESD, from diagnosis of mucosal disease by evaluation with advanced imaging to understanding the indications and limitations of endoscopic treatment, the actual procedural steps, including tips and tricks, to coping with complications, and how to follow up patients after ESD.

It has been an exceptional privilege, pleasure, and an honor to work with worldwide experts in the field to create this first English textbook for ESD.

I truly hope everyone will enjoy this book full of pearls of wisdom shared by the experts so that they may learn safe and effective ESD. This book is dedicated to help all levels of endoscopists who are eager to learn ESD.

I would like to express my respect and deep appreciation to all the exceptional authors who contributed to this book. As well, my gratitude goes to Jacob Gallay and Andy Kwan, who have been dedicated to the success of this first English ESD textbook.

Norio Fukami, M.D.
University of Colorado
Aurora, CO, USA

Contents

Contributors

Vitor Arantes Department of Surgery, Alfa Institute, School of Medicine, Minas Gerais Federal University, Belo Horizonte, Brazil

Manuel Berzosa Department of Gastroenterology and Hepatology, Mayo Clinic Florida, Jacksonville, FL, USA

Alissa Bults Division of Gastroenterology and Hepatology, University of Colorado Anschutz Medical Campus, Aurora, CO, USA

Amitabh Chak Department of Medicine, Division of Gastroenterology, University Hospitals Case Medical Center, Cleveland, OH, USA

Jun-Hyung Cho Digestive Disease Center, Soonchunhyang University Hospital, Seoul, South Korea

Joo Young Cho Digestive Disease Center, Soonchunhyang University Hospital, Seoul, South Korea

Alberto Herreros de Tejada Department of Gastroenterology, IDIPHIM, Puerta de Hierro University Hospital, Universidad Autónoma de Madrid, Madrid, Spain

Andrés Donoso Department of Surgery, School of Medicine, Pontificia Universidad Católica de Chile, Santiago, Chile

Peter V. Draganov Division of Gastroenterology, Hepatology and Nutrition, University of Florida, Gainesville, FL, USA

Norio Fukami Division of Gastroenterology and Hepatology, University of Colorado Anschutz Medical Campus, Aurora, CO, USA

Mitsuhiro Fujishiro Department of Endoscopy and Endoscopic Surgery, Gastroenterology, The University of Tokyo, Tokyo, Japan

Nicolás González Department of Gastroenterology, Faculty of Medicine, Hospital de Clínicas, Montevideo, Uruguay

Christopher J. Gostout Department of Gastroenterology and Hepatology, Mayo Clinic, Rochester, MN, USA

Takuji Gotoda Department of Gastroenterology and Hepatology, Tokyo Medical University, Tokyo, Japan

Yoshikazu Hayashi Gastroenterology and Endoscopy Center, Jichi Medical University, Shimotsuke, Tochigi, Japan

Haruo Ikeda Digestive Disease Center, Showa University Koto-Toyosu Hospital, Koto-ku, Tokyo, Japan

Masafumi Inomata Department of Gastroenterological and Pediatric Surgery, Oita University Faculty of Medicine, Oita, Japan

Haruhiro Inoue Digestive Disease Center, Showa University Koto-Toyosu Hospital, Koto-ku, Tokyo, Japan

Hiroaki Itoh Digestive Disease Center, Showa University Koto-Toyosu Hospital, Koto-ku, Tokyo, Japan

Mahesh Jayanna Endoscopy Unit, Division of Surgery, Lyell McEwin Hospital, Adelaide, SA, Australia

Chad Kawa Department of Gastroenterology, University Hospitals Case Medical Center, Cleveland, OH, USA

Mitsuhiro Kida Department of Gastroenterology, Kitasato University, Sagamihara, Kanagawa, Japan

Seigo Kitano Department of Surgery, Oita University, Oita, Japan

Bong Min Ko Digestive Disease Center, Soonchunhyang University Hospital, Seoul, South Korea

Kazuhiko Koike Department of Gastroenterology, Graduate School of Medicine, The University of Tokyo, Tokyo, Japan

Anja Landowski Endoscopy Unit, Division of Surgery, Lyell McEwin Hospital, Adelaide, SA, Australia

Hang Lak Lee Department of Gastroenterology, Hanyang University College of Medicine, Seoul, South Korea

Keiko Niimi Department of Endoscopy and Endoscopic Surgery, Gastroenterology, The University of Tokyo, Tokyo, Japan

Satoru Nonaka Endoscopy Division, National Cancer Center Hospital, Tokyo, Japan

Ichiro Oda Endoscopy Division, National Cancer Center Hospital, Tokyo, Japan

Takeshi Ohki Institute of Advanced Biomedical Engineering and Science, Institute of Gastroenterology, Department of Surgery, Tokyo Women's Medical University, Tokyo, Japan

Manabu Onimaru Digestive Disease Center, Showa University Koto-Toyosu Hospital, Koto-ku, Tokyo, Japan

Hiroyuki Ono Division of Endoscopy, Shizuoka Cancer Center, Suntogun, Shizuoka, Japan

Tsuneo Oyama Department of Endoscopy, Advanced Care Center, Saku Central Hospital, Nagano, Japan

Adolfo Parra-Blanco Department of Gastroenterology, School of Medicine, Pontificia Universidad Católica de Chile, Santiago, Chile

Gottumukkala S. Raju Department of Gastroenterology, Hepatology, and Nutrition, The University of Texas MD Anderson Cancer Center, Houston, TX, USA

Yutaka Saito Endoscopy Division, National Cancer Center Hospital, Tokyo, Japan

Esperanza Grace Santi Digestive Disease Center, Showa University Koto-Toyosu Hospital, Koto-ku, Tokyo, Japan

Ray I. Sarmiento Developmental Endoscopy Unit, Mayo Clinic, Rochester, MN, USA

Sang Yong Seol Department of Gastroenterology, Inje University, Busan, South Korea

Hidefumi Shiroshita Department of Gastroenterological and Pediatric Surgery, Oita University Faculty of Medicine, Oita, Japan

Rajvinder Singh Endoscopy Unit, Division of Surgery, Lyell McEwin Hospital, University of Adelaide, Adelaide, SA, Australia

Kazuki Sumiyama Department of Endoscopy, The Jikei University School of Medicine, Tokyo, Japan

Keijiro Sunada Gastroenterology and Endoscopy Center, Jichi Medical University, Shimotsuke, Tochigi, Japan

Hisao Tajiri Division of Gastroenterology and Hepatology, Department of Internal Medicine, The Jikei University School of Medicine, Tokyo, Japan

Department of Endoscopy, The Jikei University School of Medicine, Tokyo, Japan

Manabu Takeuchi Department of Gastroenterology, Niigata University Medical and Dental Hospital, Niigata, Japan

Kohei Takizawa Endoscopy Division, Shizuoka Cancer Center, Shizuoka, Japan

Selvi Thirumurthi Department of Gastroenterology, Hepatology, and Nutrition, The University of Texas MD Anderson Cancer Center, Houston, TX, USA

Takashi Toyonaga Department of Endoscopy, Kobe University Hospital, Kobe, Hyogo, Japan

Michael B. Wallace Department of Gastroenterology and Hepatology, Mayo Clinic Florida, Jacksonville, FL, USA

Naohisa Yahagi Division of Research and Development for Minimally Invasive Treatment, Cancer Center, School of Medicine, Keio University, Shinjuku-ku, Tokyo, Japan

Hironori Yamamoto Gastroenterology and Endoscopy Center, Jichi Medical University, Shimotsuke, Tochigi, Japan

Kazuhiro Yasuda Department of Gastroenterological and Pediatric Surgery, Oita University Faculty of Medicine, Oita, Japan

Shigetaka Yoshinaga Endoscopy Division, National Cancer Center Hospital, Tokyo, Japan

List of Abbreviations

AFI	Autofluorescence imaging
APC	Argon plasma coagulation
BE	Barrett's esophagus
CI	Confidence interval
CLE	Confocal laser endomicroscopy
CO_2	Carbon dioxide
CRC	Colorectal cancer
CRP	C-reactive protein
CRT	Chemoradiation therapy
CT	Computed tomography
D50	50 % Dextrose water
DBE	Double-balloon endoscopy
DW	Dextrose water
EBD	Endoscopic balloon dilation
EDSP	Endoscopic double-snare polypectomy
EDTA	Ethylenediaminetetraacetic acid
EEC	Early esophageal cancer
EFTR	Endoscopic full-thickness resection
EGC	Early gastric cancer
EMR	Endoscopic mucosal resection
EP	Epithelium
EPMR	Endoscopic piecemeal resection
ER	Endoscopic resection
ERHSE	Endoscopic resection with hypertonic saline-epinephrine solution
ESD	Endoscopic submucosal dissection
ESMR-L	Endoscopic submucosal resection with ligation device
ESTD	Endoscopic submucosal tunnel dissection
ETI	Endoscopic triamcinolone injection
EUS	Endoscopic ultrasound
FICE	Fujinon intelligent color enhancement
FNA	Fine-needle aspiration
GEJ	Gastroesophageal junction
GI	Gastrointestinal
GIST	Gastrointestinal stromal tumor
H2RA	H2-receptor antagonist

HA	Hyaluronic acid
HDWLE	High-definition white light endoscopy
HGD	High-grade dysplasia
HPMC	Hydroxypropyl methylcellulose
HS	Hypertonic saline
IPCL	Intrapapillary capillary loop
IRB	Institutional review board
IT	Insulated tip
JES	Japan Esophageal Society
JGES	Japan Gastroenterological Endoscopy Society
KCM	Keratinocyte culture medium
LES	Lower esophageal sphincter
LN	Lymph node
LNM	Lymph node metastasis
LP	Lamina propria
LSS	Light-scattering spectroscopy
LST	Laterally spreading tumor
LST-G	Laterally spreading tumor—granular type
LST-NG	Laterally spreading tumor—non-granular type
M	Mucosa(l)
MC	Methylcellulose
ME	Magnification endoscopy
MGC	Metachronous gastric cancer
MRI	Magnetic resonance imaging
NBI	Narrow-band imaging
NET	Neuroendocrine tumor
NOTES	Natural orifice transluminal endoscopic surgery
NS	Normal saline
OCT	Optical coherence tomography
OR	Odds ratio
OTSC	Over-the-scope clip
POEM	Peroral endoscopic myotomy
POET	Peroral endoscopic tumor resection
PPI	Proton pump inhibitor
PVDF	Polyvinylidene difluoride
SCC	Squamous cell carcinoma
SCMC	Sodium carboxymethylcellulose
SFC	Submucosal fluid cushion
SGN	Synchronous gastric neoplasm
SH	Sodium hyaluronate
SLE	Second-look endoscopy
SM	Submucosa(l)
SMI	Submucosal invasion
ST hood	Small-caliber tip hood
STER	Submucosal tunneling endoscopic resection
TTS	Through-the-scope
US	Ultrasonography

Part I

Introduction

Kazuki Sumiyama and Hisao Tajiri

The Quest for En Bloc Resection

The development of current endoscopic tissue resection (ER) techniques began with polypectomy in the 1960s [1, 2]. Since that time, researchers have been seeking a method to sample larger specimens. Various endoscopic mucosal resection (EMR) techniques were developed in Japan during the 1980s and early 1990s as minimally invasive therapeutic options for small early stage gastric cancers. These EMR techniques included strip biopsy [3], endoscopic resection with local injection of hypertonic saline-epinephrine solution (ERHSE) [4, 5], endoscopic double snare polypectomy (EDSP) [6], and also cap-assisted EMR [7, 8], which promoted international acceptance of EMR. The technology in this field has been steadily evolving and has made ER easier,

K. Sumiyama, M.D., Ph.D. (✉)
Department of Endoscopy, The Jikei University School of Medicine, 3-25-8 Nishi Shinbashi, Mainato-ku, Tokyo 105-8461, Japan
e-mail: kaz_sum@jikei.ac.jp

H. Tajiri, M.D., Ph.D.
Department of Endoscopy, The Jikei University School of Medicine, 3-25-8 Nishi Shinbashi, Mainato-ku, Tokyo 105-8461, Japan

Division of Gastroenterology and Hepatology, Department of Internal Medicine, The Jikei University School of Medicine, 3-25-8 Nishi Shinbashi, Mainato-ku, Tokyo 105-8461, Japan
e-mail: tajiri@jikei.ac.jp

safer, and more reliable. Prior to the development of endoscopic submucosal dissection (ESD), ordinary ER techniques were restricted by resectable specimen size, which was imposed by the caliber of a snare or cap attachment. Therefore, the indication of ER was limited to small lesions less than 2 cm in diameter that were resectable within a single specimen. In fact, the en bloc resection rate of EMR techniques even for small lesions did not reach 70 %, and the resultant incomplete and piecemeal resections could give rise to local recurrence [9–11]. ESD was developed to eliminate the technical limitation of resectable specimen size as a single piece.

During ESD, the diseased mucosa is radically incised from surrounding non-neoplastic tissues with careful, repetitive needle knife dissections that secure the lateral and vertical surgical margins in a step-by-step process. The concept of the en bloc resection during ESD is universally appreciated as a desirable methodology, which respects the principle of surgical excision of neoplastic lesions with "no touch isolation" as far as possible using direct endoscopic inspection. The en bloc tissue sampling technique enables precise histological assessment of the curability of the treatment and optimizes conditions for complete tumor removal compared to piecemeal resection. These advantages have resulted in rapid adoption of the technique and its application in all areas of the gastrointestinal tract. Reimbursement by the National Health Insurance of Japan was initially approved for gastro-duodenal lesions in 2006; it was extended for esophageal lesions in 2008, and eventually for colorectal lesions in 2012. A series of studies mostly from East Asia have demonstrated that the use of ESD increased R0 resection rate and, more importantly, reduced local recurrence rate compared to other ER techniques, regardless of the target organ [5, 12–15].

Development of Instruments for Safer and Easier ESD

ESD is characterized and distinguished by two procedural steps: circumferential mucosal incision and submucosal dissection. Circumferential mucosal incision was originally introduced to ensure that the lateral surgical margins remain intact during treatment in ERHSE, which is one of the snare-based EMR techniques. In ERHSE, the final tissue removal is assisted by tissue countertraction using grasping forceps and a dual working channel scope in the same manner as strip biopsy. During the developmental phase of both the ERHSE and ESD procedures, a traditional safety measure developed for polypectomy was employed that used a simple diathermy needle knife for the mucosal layer incision following saline injection. However, a sharp incision with the naked cutting wire tip of the rudimental needle knife was associated with unacceptably high risks of severe bleeding and perforation. Consequently, ERHSE and ESD were not widely adopted by endoscopists until improvements were made to the instruments that resulted in more sophisticated and safer ESD procedures.

An array of needle knives have been developed with unique tip configurations specifically designed for ESD. ESD knives can be divided into two types, according to the safety measure applied: a blunt tip and a tip-cutting knife. The insulated tip knife, or "IT-knife" was developed by Hosokawa and colleagues and was promoted globally as the optimal therapeutic option [16–18]. The IT-knife (Olympus Medical Systems, Tokyo, Japan) is still commonly used for gastric ESD and is a blunt tipped knife, with a small porcelain hemisphere on the tip of the cutting wire. The hemisphere works as a protector to avoid unintended deep cuts and a pivot to tilt and swing the cutting wire tip to align

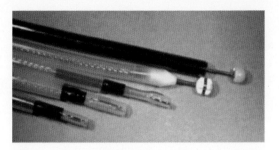

Fig. 1.1 Blunt tip ESD knives. From the *bottom*: IT-knife (Olympus Medical Systems), SAFEKnife V (Fujifilm), Swan Blade (Hoya/Pentax), Mucosectom (Hoya/Pentax)

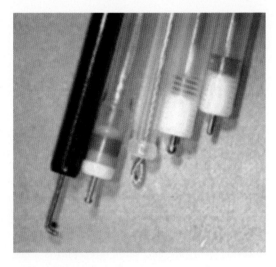

Fig. 1.2 Tip-cutting ESD knives. From the *left*: Hook knife (Olympus Medical Systems), Dual knife (Olympus Medical Systems), Flex knife (Olympus Medical Systems), Flush knife BT and Flush knife (Fujifilm)

the dissection plane to the submucosal layer. It also acts as a stabilizer to arbitrarily control dissection speed. The Mucosasectome (HOYA/PENTAX, Tokyo, Japan) and SAFEKnife (Fujifilm, Tokyo, Japan) are additional examples of the blunt tip knife (Fig. 1.1). The tip-cutting knives allow multi-directionally emitted electrosurgical cautery from both the tip and side of the cutting wire. It is important to apply cautery only under direct endoscopic visualization of the dissection plane for safe tissue dissection using tip-cutting knives. Many tip-cutting knives share the same basic design and function with minor modifications (Fig. 1.2). Typically, they have a thin and short cutting wire exposure from an insulated outer sheath to provide sharp tissue dissection that avoids inadvertent deep tissue damage. They have a thick blunt tip of the outer sheath that acts as a bumper to protect tissues and controls the depth of incision, as well as a bent portion or small disk at the tip of the cutting wire to hook tissues to avoid damaging deeper tissue. Other examples of tip-cutting knives are the Hook knife (Olympus Medical Systems) [19], Flex knife (Olympus Medical Systems) [20], Dual knife (Olympus Medical Systems) [21], Flush knife (Fujifilm) [22], and Hybrid knife (ERBE, Erlangen, Germany) [23] (Fig. 1.2) (Appendix). Optimal electrosurgical generator and cutting current modes are essential for a successful ESD procedure. In particular, the development of the EndoCut mode in ERBE systems alerted users to this fact. Various computerized high-tech electrosurgical generators are commercially available at present. These provide an array of options that automatically modulate cutting and coagulating currents corresponding to tissue resistance. The optimal electrosurgical current may vary according to a number of parameters, including the procedural phase of ESD, the types of knives used, the target tissues, and the operators' preference. Use of the sharp cutting current enables both rapid and accurate dissection of the mucosa, whereas controlled dissection with a coagulating blended current is safer for the dissection of well-vascularized submucosal tissues. Most of the bleeding that occurs during ESD can be immediately controlled by cauterization with hemostatic forceps.

The creation of a submucosal fluid cushion (SFC) is a convenient safety measure to prophylactically avoid inadvertent deep muscularis injury during ER. The procedural simplicity of this measure allows it to be applied universally, regardless of technical variations in the resection, tumor location, or skill level of the operator. Classical saline injection is sufficient for most quick snare-based ER techniques. The creation of a more durable and reliable SFC is desirable for performing more time-consuming ESD procedures safely. The efficacy of various viscous and highly osmotic solutions in producing a long-lasting SFC has been tested. For example, Yamamoto and colleagues introduced hyaluronic acid solution as an injectate for ESD [24–26]. Hyaluronate is widely used in the fields of orthopedics and ophthalmology as a lubricant, and the safety of the drug is ensured with a wealth of clinical data in those fields. The Ministry of Health, Labour and Welfare of Japan approved 0.4 % hyaluronic acid solution as an injectate for ER and it is now commercially available (MUCOUP, Johnson & Johnson, Tokyo, Japan). Because hyaluronate is not readily accessible for the majority of gastroenterologists working outside of Japan, cheaper alternatives such as glycerol, dextrose [27–29], and hydroxypropyl methylcellulose (HPMC) solutions are also used for ESD [30, 31]. Many researchers are still investigating the development of improved needle knives and injectate for submucosal dissection [32–36]. The pathway of ER development clearly demonstrates that the challenges associated with ESD cannot be completely eliminated with a single development, and can be overcome only with a multidisciplinary approach.

Challenges for Globalization and Future Prospects

The efforts of many researchers and technological developers have made ESD both safer and easier, and as a result the ESD technique is now widely practiced in Japan as a first-line therapeutic option for early gastrointestinal neoplasms. The indications of ER could be expanded for larger lesions by ESD. In the extended indications for gastric cancer, there is no limitation on tumor size for differentiated (intestinal type) mucosal cancers without ulceration. An enormous amount of data has been obtained from meticulous histological analysis of ESD specimens following a strict, standardized pathological protocol. These results have indicated that the therapeutic outcomes of ESD for the extended indications of purely differentiated lesions are comparable with those of surgical resection [15, 37]. However, ESD is not yet the global method of choice for ER techniques. The social acceptance of ESD is geographically diverse, and the technique is predominantly practiced in East Asia. ESD requires specialized skills to intuitively manipulate flexible endoscopes and needle knives with unique designs that result in longer operation times. As a result, ESD requires optimal training in selected relatively easy cases to gradually obtain a high level of skill that will permit the safe completion of the procedure for challenging cases such as Barrett's and colonic neoplasms, which are the main indications of ER in the West. In fact, the safety of ESD in Western countries that have a lower prevalence of early gastric cancers and lack the appropriate cases for training is not equivalent to the published data for ESD in Eastern countries [12, 38, 39]. It is difficult to establish the knowledge and skill bases for adequate preoperative assessment of the precise delineation of lesions. These basic attributes are mandatory to achieve a satisfactory outcome from ESD due to the absence of opportunities for screening endoscopies to detect asymptomatic, early cancers in Western countries. Other therapeutic options, including piecemeal resection and even surgical resection, should be considered if overwhelming challenges are encountered during ER.

Various novel, multi-degree-of-freedom therapeutic endoscopes have been developed to enable intuitive performance of complicated surgical procedures with the flexible endoscopic platform. Therapeutic scopes with water-jet capabilities and multi-bending portions are recognized as standard equipment for ESD. The triangulation platform is considered an eventual design of the therapeutic endoscope, which has dual mobile instrumental channels or articulated manipulators at the tip of an endoscope (Fig. 1.3) [40, 41]. These systems provide an operative environment more like laparoscopic surgery rather than ordinary endoscopic intervention. They have been tested with ESD for deflecting the diseased mucosa away from the dissection plane and horizontally swinging a needle knife parallel to the muscularis propria. Ho and colleagues have applied robotics to the triangulation platform and successfully introduced their original master–slave type endoscopic robot to gastric ESD in human patients [42, 43]. At present, all triangulation platforms are still too cumbersome in their current form and need to be miniaturized for use within a narrow GI lumen.

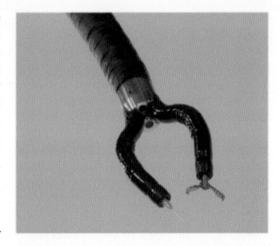

Fig. 1.3 A multi-tasking platform (EndoSAMURAI, Olympus Medical Systems). Reproduction of this image, obtained from Ikeda et al. [40], was permitted by Elsevier

Conclusions

ESD has greatly improved the resectability of early GI neoplasms by ER. The ESD procedure has rapidly increased in sophistication in tandem with instrument developments during the last decade, but there is still room for improvement. In order to truly benefit from the use of ESD, the advantage of en bloc resection should be balanced against the procedural risks. The endoscopists performing ESD must receive appropriate training, and the operative environment should be appropriate for not only the therapeutic procedure but also for preoperative diagnosis and periprocedural management. Recent technological advances, including robotics, may enable the concept of en bloc resection by ESD to be universally accepted in the near future as standard of care for patients with early gastrointestinal neoplastic lesions.

References

1. Niwa H. Improvement of fibrogastroscope for biopsy and application of color television and high frequent currents for endoscopic biopsy (in Japanese). Gastroenterol Endosc. 1968;10:315.
2. Tsuneoka K, Uchida T. Fibergastroscopic polypectomy with snare method and its significance developed in our department: polyp resection and recovery

instruments (in Japanese with English abstract). Gastroenterol Endosc. 1969;11:174–84.

3. Tada M, Shimada M, Murakami F, et al. Development of the strip-off biopsy [in Japanese with English abstract]. Gastroenterol Endosc. 1984;26:833–9.

4. Hirao M, Masuda K, Asanuma T, et al. Endoscopic resection of early gastric cancer and other tumors with local injection of hypertonic saline-epinephrine. Gastrointest Endosc. 1988;34(3):264–9.

5. Kakushima N, Fujishiro M. Endoscopic submucosal dissection for gastrointestinal neoplasms. World J Gastroenterol. 2008;14(19):2962–7.

6. Takekoshi T, Takagi K, Fujii A, et al. Treatment of early gastric cancer by endoscopic double snare polypectomy (EDSP). Gan No Rinsho. 1986;32(10):1185–90.

7. Inoue H, Takeshita K, Hori H, et al. Endoscopic mucosal resection with a cap-fitted panendoscope for esophagus, stomach, and colon mucosal lesions. Gastrointest Endosc. 1993;39(1):58–62.

8. Inoue H, Endo M, Takeshita K, et al. A new simplified technique of endoscopic esophageal mucosal resection using a cap-fitted panendoscope (EMRC). Surg Endosc. 1992;6(5):264–5.

9. Gossner L. The role of endoscopic resection and ablation therapy for early lesions. Best Pract Res Clin Gastroenterol. 2006;20(5):867–76.

10. Sumiyama K, Gostout CJ. Novel techniques and instrumentation for EMR, ESD, and full-thickness endoscopic luminal resection. Gastrointest Endosc Clin N Am. 2007;17(3):471. 85, v–vi.

11. Gotoda T. Endoscopic resection of early gastric cancer. Gastric Cancer. 2007;10(1):1–11.

12. Draganov PV, Gotoda T, Chavalitdhamrong D, et al. Techniques of endoscopic submucosal dissection: application for the Western endoscopist? Gastrointest Endosc. 2013;78(5):677–88.

13. Toyonaga T, Man-i M, East JE, et al. 1,635 Endoscopic submucosal dissection cases in the esophagus, stomach, and colorectum: complication rates and long-term outcomes. Surg Endosc. 2013;27(3):1000–8.

14. Toyonaga T, Man-i M, Chinzei R, et al. Endoscopic treatment for early stage colorectal tumors: the comparison between EMR with small incision, simplified ESD, and ESD using the standard flush knife and the ball tipped flush knife. Acta Chir Iugosl. 2010;57(3):41–6.

15. Tanabe S, Ishido K, Higuchi K, et al. Long-term outcomes of endoscopic submucosal dissection for early gastric cancer: a retrospective comparison with conventional endoscopic resection in a single center. Gastric Cancer. 2014;17:130.

16. Ohkuwa M, Hosokawa K, Boku N, et al. New endoscopic treatment for intramucosal gastric tumors using an insulated-tip diathermic knife. Endoscopy. 2001;33(3):221–6.

17. Ono H, Kondo H, Gotoda T, et al. Endoscopic mucosal resection for treatment of early gastric cancer. Gut. 2001;48(2):225–9.

18. Hosokawa KYS. Recent advances in endoscopic mucosal resection for early gastric cancer [Japanese]. Gan To Kagaku Ryoho. 1998;25:476–83.

19. Oyama T, Tomori A, Hotta K, et al. Endoscopic submucosal dissection of early esophageal cancer. Clin Gastroenterol Hepatol. 2005;3(7 Suppl 1):S67–70.

20. Yahagi N, Fujishiro M, Kakushima N, et al. Endoscopic submucosal dissection for early gastric cancer using the tip of an electrosurgical snare (thin type). Dig Endosc. 2004;16:34–6.

21. Yahagi N, Neuhaus H, Schumacher B, et al. Comparison of standard endoscopic submucosal dissection (ESD) versus an optimized ESD technique for the colon: an animal study. Endoscopy. 2009;41(4):340–5.

22. Toyonaga T, Man-I M, Fujita T, et al. The performance of a novel ball-tipped Flush knife for endoscopic submucosal dissection: a case-control study. Aliment Pharmacol Ther. 2010;32(7):908–15.

23. Neuhaus H, Wirths K, Schenk M, et al. Randomized controlled study of EMR versus endoscopic submucosal dissection with a water-jet hybrid-knife of esophageal lesions in a porcine model. Gastrointest Endosc. 2009;70(1):112–20.

24. Yamamoto H, Yahagi N, Oyama T, et al. Usefulness and safety of 0.4% sodium hyaluronate solution as a submucosal fluid "cushion" in endoscopic resection for gastric neoplasms: a prospective multicenter trial. Gastrointest Endosc. 2008;67(6):830–9.

25. Yamamoto H, Yube T, Isoda N, et al. A novel method of endoscopic mucosal resection using sodium hyaluronate. Gastrointest Endosc. 1999;50(2):251–6.

26. Yamamoto H, Koiwai H, Yube T, et al. A successful single-step endoscopic resection of a 40 millimeter flat-elevated tumor in the rectum: endoscopic mucosal resection using sodium hyaluronate. Gastrointest Endosc. 1999;50(5):701–4.

27. Fujishiro M, Yahagi N, Kashimura K, et al. Tissue damage of different submucosal injection solutions for EMR. Gastrointest Endosc. 2005;62(6):933–42.

28. Fujishiro M, Yahagi N, Kashimura K, et al. Comparison of various submucosal injection solutions for maintaining mucosal elevation during endoscopic mucosal resection. Endoscopy. 2004;36(7):579–83.

29. Fujishiro M, Yahagi N, Kashimura K, et al. Different mixtures of sodium hyaluronate and their ability to create submucosal fluid cushions for endoscopic mucosal resection. Endoscopy. 2004;36(7):584–9.

30. Conio M, Rajan E, Sorbi D, et al. Comparative performance in the porcine esophagus of different solutions used for submucosal injection. Gastrointest Endosc. 2002;56(4):513–6.

31. Feitoza AB, Gostout CJ, Burgart LJ, et al. Hydroxypropyl methylcellulose: a better submucosal fluid cushion for endoscopic mucosal resection. Gastrointest Endosc. 2003;57(1):41–7.

32. Sumiyama K, Gostout CJ, Rajan E, et al. Chemically assisted endoscopic mechanical submucosal dissection by using mesna. Gastrointest Endosc. 2008; 67(3):534–8.

33. Sumiyama K, Tajiri H, Gostout CJ, et al. Chemically assisted submucosal injection facilitates endoscopic submucosal dissection of gastric neoplasms. Endoscopy. 2010;42(8):627–32.

34. Sumiyama K, Toyoizumi H, Ohya TR, et al. A double-blind, block-randomized, placebo-controlled trial to identify the chemical assistance effect of mesna sub-mucosal injection for gastric endoscopic submucosal dissection. Gastrointest Endosc. 2014;79:756.

35. Chandrasekhara V, Sigmon Jr JC, Surti VC, et al. A novel gel provides durable submucosal cushion for endoscopic mucosal resection and endoscopic sub-mucosal dissection. Surg Endosc. 2013;27(8): 3039–42.

36. Khashab MA, Saxena P, Sharaiha RZ, et al. A novel submucosal gel permits simple and efficient gastric endoscopic submucosal dissection. Gastroenterology. 2013;144(3):505–7.

37. Gotoda T, Iwasaki M, Kusano C, et al. Endoscopic resection of early gastric cancer treated by guideline and expanded National Cancer Centre criteria. Br J Surg. 2010;97(6):868–71.

38. Draganov PV, Coman RM, Gotoda T. Training for complex endoscopic procedures: how to incorporate endoscopic submucosal dissection skills in the West? Expert Rev Gastroenterol Hepatol. 2014;8:119.

39. Schumacher B, Charton JP, Nordmann T, et al. Endoscopic submucosal dissection of early gastric neo-plasia with a water jet-assisted knife: a Western, single-center experience. Gastrointest Endosc. 2012;75(6): 1166–74.

40. Ikeda K, Sumiyama K, Tajiri H, et al. Evaluation of a new multitasking platform for endoscopic full-thickness resection. Gastrointest Endosc. 2011;73(1): 117–22.

41. Yonezawa J, Kaise M, Sumiyama K, et al. A novel double-channel therapeutic endoscope ("R-scope") facilitates endoscopic submucosal dissection of super-ficial gastric neoplasms. Endoscopy. 2006;38(10): 1011–5.

42. Ho KY, Phee SJ, Shabbir A, et al. Endoscopic submu-cosal dissection of gastric lesions by using a Master and Slave Transluminal Endoscopic Robot (MASTER). Gastrointest Endosc. 2010;72(3):593–9.

43. Phee SJ, Reddy N, Chiu PW, et al. Robot-assisted endoscopic submucosal dissection is effective in treat-ing patients with early-stage gastric neoplasia. Clin Gastroenterol Hepatol. 2012;10(10):1117–21.

Part II

Indications

Indications of ESD in the Upper Gastrointestinal Tract

2

Hang Lak Lee and Sang Yong Seol

Introduction

Early gastric cancer (EGC) is defined as a gastric cancer that is confined to the mucosa or submucosa of the stomach, irrespective of the presence of regional lymph node metastasis [1, 2]. Endoscopic submucosal dissection (ESD) is a novel endoscopic treatment that enables a clinician to resect early stage gastric cancer in an en bloc fashion [3]. Endoscopic resection is comparable to conventional surgery in many aspects, but it has the advantage of being less invasive and more economical. The absolute and expanded indications of ESD in the upper gastrointestinal tract are introduced in this chapter, and their usefulness, safety and limitations are discussed.

General Concepts for Application of ESD for EGC

Two main factors are considered to determine the application of ESD for each lesion by each operator (Fig. 2.1). The first is the likelihood of lymph

H.L. Lee, M.D. (✉)
Hanyang University College of Medicine,
Hanyang University Hospital, Hangdang dong,
Sungdongu, Seoul, South Korea
e-mail: alwayshang@hanyang.ac.kr

S.Y. Seol, M.D.
Inje University, Busan, South Korea

node metastasis and the second is the technical resectability. The former has been determined by the large numbers of surgically resected cases in each organ before establishment of ESD and the latter may be determined by the applied technique, the expertise of the operator, the location of the lesion, and/or their characteristics. In terms of technical resectability, en bloc resection is more desirable than piecemeal resection for accurate assessment of the appropriateness of the therapy, because the depth of invasion and lymphovascular infiltration of cancer cells cannot be accurately assessed by piecemeal resection [4]. Almost all possible node-negative epithelial neoplasms can be resected en bloc by ESD, when they are treated by very experienced hands.

Absolute and Expanded Indications of ESD for EGC

Currently accepted indications for endoscopic resection of EGC include the resection of small intramucosal EGCs of intestinal histology type. The rationale for this recommendation is based on the knowledge that larger lesions or diffuse histology lesions are more likely to extend into the submucosal layer and thus have a higher risk of lymph node metastasis. In addition, en bloc resection of large lesions was not technically feasible until the ESD procedure was developed. Therefore, at present, the accepted indications for EMR according to the gastric cancer treatment

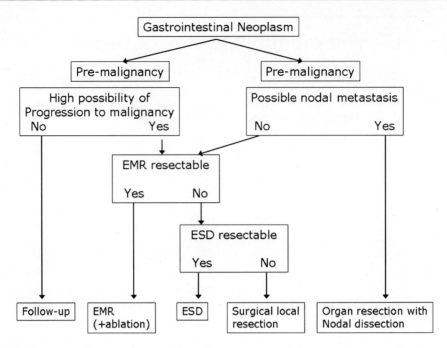

Fig. 2.1 Algorithm for endoscopic submucosal dissection of gastrointestinal neoplasms

Table 2.1 Indications for extension of EMR

Guideline criteria for EMR, ▨ Surgery

	Depth					
	M cancer			SM cancer		
	Ulcer (-)		Ulcer (+)	< SM 1	> SM 1	
	< 20 mm	> 20mm	< 30 mm	> 30 mm	< 30 mm	Any size
Differentiated						
Undifferentiated						

guidelines published in 2001 by the Japanese Gastric Cancer Association are: (1) well-differentiated elevated cancers less than 2 cm in diameter and (2) small (<1 cm) depressed lesions without ulceration. Also, these lesions must be moderately or well-differentiated cancers that are confined to the mucosa and have no lymphatic or vascular involvement [5, 6]. However, it has been observed clinically that the accepted indications for EMR may be too strict, which leads to unnecessary surgery (Table 2.1) [7].

Further studies by Gotoda et al. have defined new criteria for expanding the indications for endoscopic treatment of gastric cancer. Endoscopic submucosal dissection was devel-

oped to dissect directly along the submucosal layer using specialized devices. Preliminary studies have been published on the advantages of ESD over conventional EMR for en bloc removal of larger or ulcerated EGC lesions. Thus, ESD allows for precise histological assessment of the resected specimens, possibly preventing residual disease and local recurrence. Gotoda et al. analyzed more than 5,000 EGC patients who underwent gastrectomy with meticulous D2 level node dissection; they provided important information on the risks of lymph node metastasis, wherein differentiated gastric cancers with no lymphovascular involvement, correlating with a nominal risk of lymph node metastasis, were defined [8].

Table 2.2 Indications for extension of ESD

Guideline for ESD:	■ Expanded indication,	▨ Consider surgery,	▨ Surgery

	Depth					
	M cancer				SM cancer	
	Ulcer (-)		Ulcer (+)		< SM 1	> SM 1
	< 20 mm	> 20mm	< 30 mm	> 30 mm	< 30 mm	Any size
Differentiated						
Undifferentiated						

Thus, they proposed the expanded criteria for endoscopic resection: (1) mucosal cancer without ulceration, irrespective of tumor size; (2) mucosal cancer with an ulcer <3 cm in diameter; and (3) minute (<500 μm from the muscularis mucosa) submucosal invasive cancer <3 cm in size (Table 2.2). However, extending the indications for ESD remains controversial because the long-term outcomes of these procedures have not been fully documented.

Recent Evidence for Expanded Indications of ESD for EGC

Although the absolute indication is applicable only to mucosal cancer, there have been some studies about ESD for submucosal cancer. Of the 145 well-differentiated tumors that had invaded less than 500 μm into the submucosa and were smaller than 30 mm in diameter, none showed evidence of lymph node metastasis, provided that there was no lymphatic or venous invasion. Based on these findings, it was suggested that the criteria for EMR and ESD as local treatment for EGC should be extended [9–13].

According to a recent study of patients who had surgery for EGC at Seoul National University Bundang Hospital [14], of 132 patients with mucosal cancers, 129 met the extended indications for EMR or ESD while three (2.3 %) had lymph node metastasis. Of the 52 submucosal cancer cases that met the extended indications for EMR or ESD, two (4 %) had lymph node metastasis. Differentiated mucosal cancers without ulcer formation did not have lymph node metastasis, irrespective of size. These data suggest that a well-differentiated mucosal cancer of any size without ulceration may be considered as an extended indication for EMR or ESD. However, data from this study showed that 2.8 % of tumors meeting the extended criteria for EMR or ESD had positive lymph nodes, and the authors suggest that if EMR or ESD had been performed in these patients, it would not have been curative.

Regarding the expansion of indications to EGC with undifferentiated histology, the supporting data are continuously being reported. Ye and colleagues reported that EGC with undifferentiated histology has no lymph node involvement, provided that the cancer is smaller than 25 mm and is confined to the mucosa or upper third of the submucosa and has no lymphatic involvement [15]. A similar study for signet ring cell carcinoma was reported by Park et al. [16]; EGC with signet ring cell histology has a high risk for nodal and organ metastases, while smaller cancers of less than 25 mm that are confined to the SM2 layer and have no lymphovascular involvement demonstrated no lymph node involvement.

In another Korean study on the lymph node metastasis of poorly differentiated adenocarcinomas, a retrospective analysis was performed on 234 patients with poorly differentiated EGC who underwent radical gastrectomy with D2 lymph node dissection [17]. Of the 234 lesions with poorly differentiated EGC, half ($n = 116$) showed submucosal invasion in the resection specimen, and 25.9 % (30/116) of those were limited to the upper third (SM1). Of the lesions confined to the mucosa, lymph node metastasis was found in 3.4 % (4/118). With minor submucosal infiltration (SM1), the lymph node metastasis rate was non-existent (0/30). However, with SM2/3 invasion, the lymph node metastasis rate increased sharply to about 30 %. Therefore, poorly differentiated EGC confined to the mucosa or with minimal submucosal infiltration could be considered for curative ESD due to the low risk of lymph node metastasis. Another Korean study [18] focusing on endoscopic resection for undifferentiated-type cancer such as poorly differentiated adenocarcinoma and signet ring cell carcinoma showed interesting results. In this study, a total of 58 lesions with undifferentiated EGC (17 poorly differentiated; 41 signet ring cell) were treated by endoscopic resection. The en bloc and complete resection rates in poorly differentiated cases were 82.4 % and 58.8 %, whereas those in signet ring cell were 85.4 % and 70.7 %, respectively. Interestingly, all of the histologically incomplete resections in poorly differentiated cases were vertical cut end-positive, whereas 83.3 % of these resections in signet ring cell were lateral cut end-positive. The recurrence rate was 5.1 % in complete resection during the follow-up period. Therefore, the authors suggested that endoscopic resection may be a feasible local treatment for undifferentiated EGC if complete resection can be achieved. However, the indication for poorly differentiated cancers is still controversial. Further follow up periods and accumulation of a larger number of cases are still required to clarify this issue.

Yamaguchi et al. reported clinical outcomes of ESD according to indication criteria. A total of 589 EGC lesions were divided into the guideline group and the expanded group [6]. En bloc, complete, and curative resections were achieved in 98.6 % and 93.0 %, 95.1 % and 88.5 %, and 97.1 % and 91.1 % of the guideline and expanded criteria lesions, respectively; the differences between the two groups were significant for all types of resection. The expanded criteria lesions were at significantly higher risk for ESD-associated bleeding and perforation. Overall survival was adequate, irrespective of indication, and the disease-specific survival rates were 100 % in all groups.

Limitations of ESD

However, more aggressive cases have been encountered. Walter et al. reported one case [19] with early gastric cancer that was initially treated by ESD. Esophagogastroduodenoscopy showed a slightly elevated, centrally depressed lesion about 15 mm in diameter with a very small ulceration in the center (type IIa + IIc) and biopsies showed only focal high-grade intraepithelial neoplasia. The resected specimen showed a submucosal infiltration depth of greater than 500 μm. Therefore, the patient underwent gastrectomy. The postoperative stage was pT1 (sm3), pN0 (0/58), cM0, L0, V0, G2 (UICC stage Ia). Three months later, an ultrasound revealed a new mass in the liver, and biopsy showed a rapidly growing metastasis of the gastric adenocarcinoma. This case highlights the risk of affected lymph nodes in early gastric cancer and the consequent risk of metastasis, which increases with greater depth of infiltration into the submucosa.

Another obstacle in EMR and ESD is the presence of micrometastasis [20–24]. Even after curative surgical resection for EGC, the recurrence rate is about 1.7–3.4 %, which could be the result of micrometastasis. According to Cai and colleagues, tumor size, macroscopic type, accompanying ulcers, and depth of invasion are strongly associated with micrometastasis in lymph nodes. Therefore, tumors with suspected submucosal invasion, large size, accompanying ulcers, and undifferentiated histology may have a risk of recurrence owing to micrometastasis, which may indicate the inappropriateness of EMR or ESD.

One more problem should be solved as follows: (1) We cannot be aware of the presence of ulcers before ESD and, as a result, it is very difficult to resect the lesion. We also have to pay attention to the fact that there are some differences in the definition of ulceration among physicians. (2) The way lesion size is measured is also somewhat different among institutions. Therefore, a uniform, standard way for measuring lesion size may become necessary in the future.

Long-Term Follow-Up Data

Long-term follow-up data are needed for the clinical application of the expanded indication. One Japanese study [25] from the National Cancer Center Hospital, involving a total of 1,955 EGC patients enrolled from January 1999 to December 2005, showed that there were no significant differences in the overall 5-year survival rates of the curative resection group, as defined by the expanded criteria, and the non-curative resection group after additional surgery. These data suggest that ESD using the expanded criteria can show excellent long-term outcomes.

Indication of ESD for NETs and GISTs

Neuroendocrine tumors (NETs) can show a broad range of clinical behaviors. In general, NETs are limited to the mucosa or submucosa and less than 11–20 mm in size, demonstrating a low frequency of lymph node and distant metastasis, and thus can be managed with local excision such as ESD or EMR. However, complete histological resection may not always be easy to achieve by using EMR because most gastrointestinal NETs are not confined to the mucosa, but rather, invade the submucosa, which results in frequent involvement of the resection margin. Therefore, ESD must be used for gastrointestinal neuroendocrine tumors. One recent study showed that complete resection was performed in 28 stomach NETs among a total of 29 lesions, and all of them were confined to the submucosa [26].

Gastrointestinal stromal tumors (GISTs) can arise at any location in the gastrointestinal tract. With the rapid advances in endoscopic skill and the development of minimally invasive technologies, there are more choices for treatment of GISTs. Davila et al. first reported endoscopic resection of small superficial GISTs in 2003. According to previous studies, it seems that endoscopic resection is technically feasible and effective for small gastric GISTs. However, with the progress of ESD

techniques, ESD now appears to be an effective treatment for large-sized GISTs in both the esophagus and stomach. Long-term follow-up data about the recurrence or metastasis is required, however.

Indication of ESD in Esophagus and Duodenum

According to the guidelines of the Japanese Esophageal Society for the diagnosis and treatment of esophageal squamous cell carcinoma, endoscopic management of esophageal cancer is principally indicated based on 2 factors: low likelihood of lymph node metastasis and technical resectability of the tumor [27]. Some studies have indicated that high-grade intraepithelial neoplasia, including non-invasive squamous cell carcinoma and intramucosal invasive squamous cell carcinoma limited to the lamina propria without vessel infiltration, have no lymph node metastasis [28, 29]. The location and characteristics of the lesion, and the experiences of the endoscopists, determine the technical resectability.

Superficial duodenal cancers without lymph node metastasis can be cured by endoscopic resection. In 1992, endoscopic mucosal resection of duodenal neoplasia was first described. Technically, duodenal ESD is considered more difficult. The proper muscle layer of the duodenum is very thin and soft. It is even thinner than in the esophagus and colorectum. Therefore, the duodenal wall is more prone to perforation by ESD. Patient selection for ESD in the duodenum should be made cautiously, with consideration of all difficulties and risks. Although there have not been any large long-term follow up studies about duodenal cancers, the indication criteria for gastric ESD can also apply to duodenal lesions. Because surgical resection procedures for duodenal lesions are complicated and invasive, duodenal ESD can be beneficial.

For further discussion of the details regarding indication and technique for ESD in the upper GI tract, please see Chaps. 10, 11, and 13.

Conclusions and Future Prospects

ESD makes it possible to perform complete resection of lesions larger than 20 mm, as well as those with ulceration, regardless of location. There is much clinical data suggesting that ESD may be adequate for both the standard guidelines and the expanded criteria lesions. However, ESD requires highly skilled endoscopists, and a suitable training program is required for permeation of this technique. In the future, long-term follow-up data, newer technology, and more highly developed techniques will be needed to treat EGC according to the expanded indications.

References

1. Carter KJ, Schaffer HA, Ritchie Jr WP. Early gastric cancer. Ann Surg. 1984;199:604–9.
2. Everett SM, Axon AT. Early gastric cancer in Europe. Gut. 1997;41:142–50.
3. Gotoda T, Kondo H, Ono H, Saito Y, Yamaguchi H, Saito D, Yokota T. A new endoscopic mucosal resection procedure using an insulation-tipped electrosurgical knife for rectal flat lesions: report of two cases. Gastrointest Endosc. 1999;50:560–3.
4. Ono H, Kondo H, Gotoda T, Shirao K, Yamaguchi H, Saito D, Hosokawa K, Shimoda T, Yoshida S. Endoscopic mucosal resection for treatment of early gastric cancer. Gut. 2001;48:225–9.
5. Japanese Gastric Cancer Association. Japanese classification of gastric carcinoma. Gastric Cancer. 1998;1:10–24. 2nd English ed.
6. Yamaguchi N, Isomoto H, Fukuda E, Ikeda K, Nishiyama H, Akiyama M, Ozawa E, Ohnita K, Hayashi T, Nakao K, Kohno S, Shikuwa S. Clinical outcomes of endoscopic submucosal dissection for early gastric cancer by indication criteria. Digestion. 2009;80:173–81.
7. Gotoda T. Endoscopic resection of early gastric cancer. Gastric Cancer. 2007;10:1–11.
8. Gotoda T, Yanagisawa A, Sasako M, Ono H, Nakanishi Y, Shimoda T, Kato Y. Incidence of lymph node metastasis from early gastric cancer: estimation with a large number of cases at two large centers. Gastric Cancer. 2000;3:219–25.
9. Yamao T, Shirao K, Ono H, Kondo H, Saito D, Yamaguchi H, Sasako M, Sano T, Ochiai A, Yoshida S. Risk factors for lymph node metastasis from intramucosal gastric carcinoma. Cancer. 1996;77:602–6.
10. Yasuda K, Shiraishi N, Suematsu T, Yamaguchi K, Adachi Y, Kitano S. Rate of detection of lymph node metastasis is correlated with the depth of submucosal

invasion in early stage gastric carcinoma. Cancer. 1999;85:2119–23.
11. Oizumi H, Matsuda T, Fukase K, Furukawa A, Mito S, Takahashi K. Endoscopic resection for early gastric cancer: the accrual procedure and clinical evaluation. Stom Intest. 1991;26:289–300.
12. Gotoda T, Sasako M, Ono H, Katai H, Sano T, Shimoda T. An evaluation of the necessity for gastrectomy with lymph node dissection for patients with submucosal invasive gastric cancer. Br J Surg. 2001;88:444–9.
13. Kim JJ, Lee JH, Jung HY, Lee GH, Cho JY, Ryu CB, Chun HJ, Park JJ, Lee WS, Kim HS, Chung MG, Moon JS, Choi SR, Song GA, Jeong HY, Jee SR, Seol SY, Yoon YB. EMR for early gastric cancer in Korea: a multicenter retrospective study. Gastrointest Endosc. 2007;66:693–700.
14. Jee YS, Hwang SH, Rao J, Park DJ, Kim HH, Lee HJ, Yang HK, Lee KU. Safety of extended endoscopic mucosal resection and endoscopic submucosal dissection following the Japanese Gastric Cancer Association treatment guidelines. Br J Surg. 2009;96:1157–61.
15. Ye BD, Kim SG, Lee JY, Kim JS, Yang HK, Kim WH, Jung HC, Lee KU, Song IS. Predictive factors for lymph node metastasis and endoscopic treatment strategies for undifferentiated early gastric cancer. J Gastroenterol Hepatol. 2008;23:46–50.
16. Park JM, Kim SW, Nam KW, Cho YK, Lee IS, Choi MG, Chung IS, Song KY, Park CH, Jung CK. Is it reasonable to treat early gastric cancer with signet ring cell histology by endoscopic resection? Analysis of factors related to lymph node metastasis. Eur J Gastroenterol Hepatol. 2009;21:1132–5.
17. Park DY, Chung YJ, Chung HY, Yu W, Bae HI, Jeon SW, Cho CM, Tak WY, Kweon YO. Factors related to lymph node metastasis and the feasibility of endoscopic mucosal resection for treating poorly differentiated adenocarcinoma of the stomach. Endoscopy. 2008;40:7–10.
18. Kim JH, Lee YC, Kim H, Song KH, Lee SK, Cheon JH, Kim H, Hyung WJ, Noh SH, Kim CB, Chung JB. Endoscopic resection for undifferentiated early gastric cancer. Gastrointest Endosc. 2009;69:e1–9.
19. Walter B, Probst A, Markl B, Wagner T, Anthuber M, Messmann H. Fulminant metastatic spread in a patient with an early gastric cancer. Endoscopy. 2009;41:907–9.
20. Cai J, Ikeguchi M, Tsujitani S, Maeta M, Kaibara N. Micrometastasis in lymph nodes and microinvasion of the muscularis propria in primary lesion of submucosal gastric cancer. Surgery. 2000;127:32–9.
21. Nakajo A, Natsugoe S, Ishigami S, Matsumoto M, Nakashima S, Hokita S, Baba M, Takao S, Aikou T. Detection and prediction of micrometastasis in the lymph nodes of patients with pN0 gastric cancer. Ann Surg Oncol. 2001;8:158–62.
22. Maehara Y, Oshiro T, Endo K, Baba H, Oda S, Ichiyoshi Y, Kohnoe S, Sugimachi K. Clinical significance of occult micrometastasis in lymph nodes from

patients with early gastric cancer who died of recurrence. Surgery. 1996;119:397–402.

23. Harrison LE, Choe JK, Goldstein M, Meridian A, Kim SH, Clarke K. Prognostic significance of immunohistochemical micrometastasis in node negative gastric cancer patients. J Surg Oncol. 2000;73:153–7.

24. Cai J, Ikeguchi M, Tsujitani S, Maeta M, Liu J, Kaibara N. Significant correlation between micrometastasis in the lymph nodes and reduced expression of E-cadherin in early gastric cancer. Gastric Cancer. 2001;3:66–74.

25. Kusano C, Gotoda T, Iwasaki M. Long-term outcome of ESD for early gastric cancer. Stom Intest. 2008;43: 73–9.

26. Li QL, Zhang YQ, Chen WF, et al. Endoscopic submucosal dissection for foregut neuroendocrine tumors: an initial study. World J Gastroenterol. 2012;18: 5799–806.

27. Kuwano H, Nishinuma Y, Ohtsu A, et al. Guidelines for diagnosis and treatment of carcinoma of the esophagus. April 2007 edition: Part I. Edited by the Japan Esophageal Society. Esophagus. 2008;5:61–73.

28. Natsugoe S, Baba M, Yoshinaka H, et al. Mucosal squamous cell carcinoma of the esophagus: a clinicopathologic study of 30 cases. Oncology. 1998;55:235–41.

29. Tajima Y, Nakanishi Y, Ochiai A, et al. Histopathologic findings predicting lymph node metastasis and prognosis of patients with superficial esophageal carcinomas: analysis of 240 surgically resected tumors. Cancer. 2000;88:1285–93.

Yutaka Saito

Indications for Colorectal ESD

The indications for colorectal ESD are, presently, colorectal cancers (CRC) or adenomas with a large tumor size, 2–5 cm, in which conventional en bloc EMR is predicted to be difficult (Table 3.1) [1]. Endoscopic treatment is local resection without lymph node dissection, and therefore, considered appropriate when the following conditions have been satisfied: a lesion is determined to be well or moderately differentiated; invasion of the submucosal (SM) layer is <1,000 μm; and the lesion is histopathologically negative for both lymphovascular invasion and single cell invasion. These early CRCs are estimated to have an extremely low risk for lymph node metastasis [2]. Early CRC with SM deep invasion should not be treated with EMR or ESD due to an increased risk of lymph node metastasis, which has been reported to range from 6.9 to 22.2 % [2]. Consequently, it is clinically important to accurately diagnose the depth of invasion before treatment. Endoscopic depth diagnosis [3] is clinically based on endoscopic findings of the invasive pit pattern [4, 5] by magnified colonoscopy, or fullness by conventional colonoscopy for superficial type colorectal cancer [3], rather than the non-lifting sign [6].

Indications for Colorectal ESD at Japanese National Cancer Center Hospital (Table 3.2)

Based on previous clinicopathological analyses of laterally spreading tumors (LSTs) [7, 8], LST non-granular type (LST-NG) lesions (Fig. 3.1) have a higher rate of SM invasion, which can be difficult to predict endoscopically. Approximately 30–56 % [9] of LST-NGs have multifocal SM invasion, which is primarily SM superficial (T1a). This is especially difficult to predict before endoscopic treatment. In addition, LST-NGs >20 mm in diameter are quite difficult to resect en bloc by conventional EMR; therefore, these tumors are definite candidates for ESD (Fig. 3.1).

In contrast, LST granular type (LST-G) lesions have a lower rate of SM invasion, which is generally found under the largest nodule or depression. These lesions are easier to predict endoscopically [7, 8]. LST-Gs >20 mm can be treated by elective piecemeal EMR [7] rather than ESD. The area containing the largest nodule should be resected before the rest of the tumor. LST-Gs >30 mm are possible candidates for ESD since such lesions are more difficult to treat by piecemeal EMR (Fig. 3.2). A high SM invasion rate and 25 % rate of multifocal invasion were recently reported [9, 10], compared to other recent series [11, 12].

The endoscopist's skill level and the estimated procedure time of the resection should

Y. Saito, M.D., Ph.D. (✉)
Endoscopy Division, National Cancer Center Hospital,
5-1-1, Tsukiji, Chuo-ku, Tokyo, 104-0045, Japan
e-mail: ytsaito@ncc.go.jp

N. Fukami (ed.), *Endoscopic Submucosal Dissection: Principles and Practice*,
DOI 10.1007/978-1-4939-2041-9_3, © Springer Science+Business Media New York 2015

Table 3.1 Colorectal ESD-applicable lesions proposed by the Colorectal ESD Standardization Implementation Working Group

The conditions indicated for endoscopic en bloc resection are as follows:

1. Lesions for which en bloc resection with snare EMR is difficult to apply
   - LST-NG, particularly LST-NG (PD)
   - Lesions exhibiting a V_I-type pit pattern
   - Cancers with mild submucosal invasion
   - Large depressed-type tumors
   - Large malignant protruded-type lesions[a]
2. Mucosal tumors with submucosal fibrosis[b]
3. Sporadic localized tumors that occur due to chronic inflammation
4. Local residual early cancers after endoscopic resection

[a]Including nodular lesions such as LST-Gs
[b]Due to prolapse caused by biopsy or peristalsis of the lesion
Note: Partially modified from the draft proposed by the Colorectal ESD Standardization Implementation Working Group [16]

also be considered when selecting ESD for large lesions ≥ 5 cm.

0-IIc lesions >20 mm intramucosal tumors with non-lifting sign and large sessile lesions, all of which are difficult to resect en bloc by conventional EMR, are also potential candidates for colorectal ESD.

Treatment of residual and recurrent tumors with ESD can be considered, depending on the circumstances. Such lesions usually involve severe fibrosis; therefore, they are not good candidates unless they are located in the lower rectum where the risk of perforation is very low [13].

Rectal carcinoid tumors measuring less than 1 cm in diameter are not considered an indication for ESD, as they can be treated by endoscopic submucosal resection using a ligation device safely, effectively and easily [14, 15].

Conclusions

Current colorectal ESD indications are large colorectal cancers or adenomas in which conventional en bloc EMR is predicted to be difficult. Because lesions that have submucosal deep invasion should not be treated with ESD, accurate endoscopic diagnosis of depth of invasion is imperative before treatment. Also, an endoscopist's skill level and the estimated procedure time of the resection should be considered when selecting ESD for lesions that are 5 cm or larger in size.

Table 3.2 Indications for Colorectal ESD at the Japanese National Cancer Center Hospital Non-invasive pattern diagnosed by chromo-magnification colonoscopy

	Non-invasive Pattern should be diagnosed by chromomagnification colonoscopy			
Tumor Size (mm)	-10	10-20	20-30	30-
0-IIa, IIc, IIa+IIc (LST-NG)	EMR	EMR	ESD candidate	ESD candidate
0-Is+IIa (LST-G)	EMR	EMR	EMR	Possible ESD candidate
0-Is (Villous)	EMR	EMR	EMR	Possible ESD candidate
Intramucosal tumor with non-lifting sign*	EMR	EMR/ESD	Possible ESD candidate	Possible ESD candidate
Rectal carcinoid tumor	EMR	ESD/Surgery	Surgery	Surgery

1. 0-IIa, IIc, IIa+IIc (laterally spreading tumors non-granular type: LST-NGs) >20 mm
2. 0-Is+IIa (LST granular type: LST-G) >30 mm
3. 0-Is (Villous) >30 mm
4. Intramucosal tumors with non-lifting sign which are difficult to resect *en-bloc* by conventional EMR
5. Rectal carcinoid tumors <1 cm in diameter can be treated by endoscopic submucosal resection using a ligation device (ESMR-L) simply, safely and effectively so not an indication for ESD
*Residual and recurrent tumors can be treated by ESD depending on the circumstances; however, such lesions usually involve severe fibrosis so they are not good candidates except in the lower rectum where the perforation risk is very low

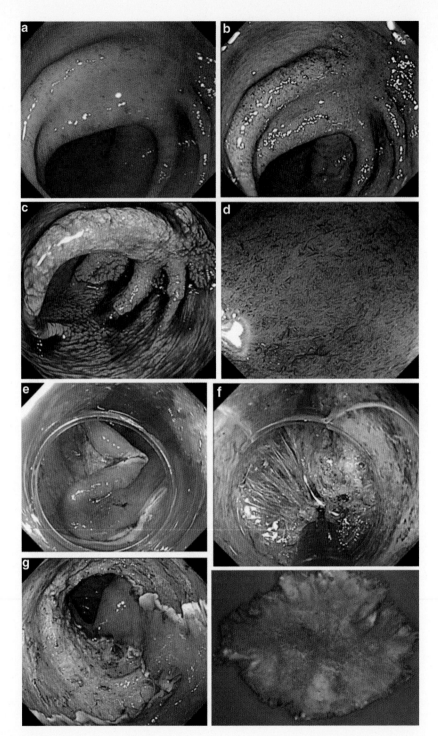

Fig. 3.1 (**a**) A 3/4 circumferential LST-NG was located in the transverse colon. Prominent fold convergences were observed and submucosal invasion was suspected. (**b**) Narrow band imaging (NBI) revealed the margin of this tumor clearly. (**c**) A 0.4 % indigo carmine dye was sprayed on this LST-NG, clearly delineating the margin. (**d**) A 0.05 % crystal violet staining was conducted and the III_s pit pattern was observed on this tumor's surface, despite its large size and prominent fold convergences. A magni-fied colonoscopic diagnosis was III_s (non-invasive) pit pattern and this lesion was diagnosed as intramucosal cancer. (**e**) ESD was started in retroflex position with a pediatric-type colonoscope equipped with a short-type hood. (**f**) An IT-nano knife was used for submucosal dissection. (**g**) Successful en bloc resection was achieved in 140 min without any complication. (**h**) Histopathology revealed a well-differentiated adenocarcinoma with intramucosal depth of invasion, so curative R0 resection was achieved

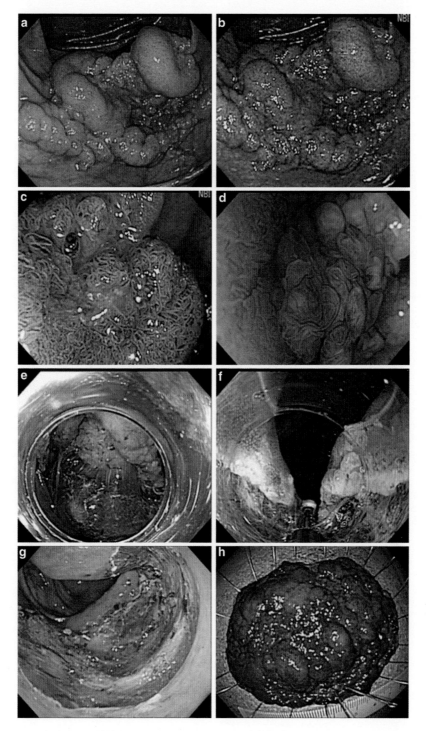

Fig. 3.2 (**a**) A half circumferential LST-G was located in the ascending colon. (**b**) Narrow band imaging (NBI) revealed this tumor's margin clearly. (**c**) Magnified NBI revealed type II or III$_A$ capillary pattern, even on this large nodule, suggesting a lack of submucosal deep invasion. (**d**) A 0.05 % crystal violet staining was conducted and type IV pit pattern was observed. A magnified colonoscopic diagnosis was type IV (non-invasive) pit pattern and confirmed this lesion as intramucosal cancer. (**e**) ESD was started using retroflexion of the pediatric-type colonoscope with short-type ST hood. (**f**) An IT-nano knife was used for submucosal dissection. (**g**) Successful en bloc resection was achieved without complication. (**h**) Histopathology revealed a well-differentiated adenocarcinoma and depth of invasion was intramucosal. Curative R0 resection was achieved

References

1. Saito Y, Kawano H, Takeuchi Y, et al. Current status of colorectal endoscopic submucosal dissection in Japan and other Asian countries: progressing towards technical standardization. Dig Endosc. 2012;24 Suppl 1:67–72.
2. Kitajima K, Fujimori T, Fujii S, et al. Correlations between lymph node metastasis and depth of submucosal invasion in submucosal invasive colorectal carcinoma: a Japanese collaborative study. J Gastroenterol. 2004;39:534–43.
3. Ikehara H, Saito Y, Matsuda T, Uraoka T, Murakami Y. Diagnosis of depth of invasion for early colorectal cancer using magnifying colonoscopy. J Gastroenterol Hepatol. 2010;25(5):905–12.
4. Matsuda T, Fujii T, Saito Y, Nakajima T, Uraoka T, Kobayashi N, Ikehara H, Ikematsu H, Fu KI, Emura F, Ono A, Sano Y, Shimoda T, Fujimori T. Efficacy of the invasive/non-invasive pattern by magnifying chromoendoscopy to estimate the depth of invasion of early colorectal neoplasms. Am J Gastroenterol. 2008; 103(11):2700–6.
5. Fujii T, Hasegawa RT, Saitoh Y, Fleischer D, Saito Y, Sano Y, Kato S. Chromoscopy during colonoscopy. Endoscopy. 2001;33(12):1036–41. Review.
6. Kobayashi N, Saito Y, Sano Y, Uragami N, Michita T, Nasu J, Matsuda T, Fu KI, Fujii T, Fujimori T, Ishikawa T, Saito D. Determining the treatment strategy for colorectal neoplastic lesions: endoscopic assessment or the non-lifting sign for diagnosing invasion depth? Endoscopy. 2007;39(8):701–5.
7. Saito Y, Fujii T, Kondo H, et al. Endoscopic treatment for laterally spreading tumors in the colon. Endoscopy. 2001;33:682–6.
8. Uraoka T, Saito Y, Matsuda T, et al. Endoscopic indications for endoscopic mucosal resection of laterally spreading tumours in the colorectum. Gut. 2006; 55(11):1592–7.
9. Saito Y, Sakamoto T, Fukunaga S, et al. Significance of macroscopic classification of laterally spreading tumors in determining endoscopic treatment strategy. Stom Intest. 2010;45(6):1001–10 (Japanese in English Abst).
10. Kudo S, Kashida H, Tamura T, et al. Colonoscopic diagnosis and management of nonpolypoid early colorectal cancer. World J Surg. 2000;24:1081–90.
11. Terasaki M, Tanaka S, Oka S, et al. Clinical outcomes of endoscopic submucosal dissection and endoscopic mucosal resection for laterally spreading tumors larger than 20 mm. J Gastroenterol Hepatol. 2012; 27(4):734–40.
12. Moss A, Bourke MJ, Williams SJ, et al. Endoscopic mucosal resection outcomes and prediction of submucosal cancer from advanced colonic mucosal neoplasia. Gastroenterology. 2011;140(7):1909–18.
13. Sakamoto T, Saito Y, Matsuda T, et al. Treatment strategy for recurrent or residual colorectal tumors after endoscopic resection. Surg Endosc. 2011;25(1): 255–60.
14. Ono A, Fujii T, Saito Y, et al. Endoscopic submucosal resection of rectal carcinoid tumors with a ligation device. Gastrointest Endosc. 2003;57(4):583–7.
15. Mashimo Y, Matsuda T, Uraoka T, et al. Endoscopic submucosal resection with a ligation device is an effective and safe treatment for carcinoid tumors in the lower rectum. J Gastroenterol Hepatol. 2008;23(2): 218–21.
16. Japan Gastroenterological Endoscopy Society. Colorectal ESD/EMR guidelines. Gastroenterol Endosc. 2014;56:1597–617.

Part III

Pre-procedure Imaging

Role of EUS on Preoperative Staging of Gastric Cancer for ESD

Mitsuhiro Kida

Introduction

Endoscopic ultrasonography (EUS) has assumed an important role in the diagnosis and staging of malignant gastrointestinal and pancreaticobiliary cancers after its development in 1980 [1, 2]. Generally, ultrasonographic endoscopes with 360° radial sector scanners are widely used for diagnosing the local staging of tumors because of their maneuverability, compared to ultrasonographic endoscopes with convex or linear scanners, which are used for performing EUS-guided fine needle aspiration biopsy (EUS-FNA) [3–13]. For gastrointestinal malignancies, endoscopy is usually performed prior to EUS to establish the diagnosis, which should be confirmed by histological examination of the biopsy specimen. Appropriate treatment, such as endoscopic treatment, surgical treatment, or chemotherapy, can be optimally chosen by the staging of tumor with EUS, CT, etc. However, EUS is not useful as a screening method since it takes considerable time to examine the entire upper gastrointestinal tract. Furthermore, endoscopic submucosal dissection (ESD) has been developed and the indications of endoscopic treatment have been expanded.

Clinical demands have ordered increased EUS to determine whether lesions indicate endoscopic treatment or not. That is, we have to definitively diagnose sm1 in order to differentiate sm1 from sm2 invasion.

How to Visualize the Lesion

Methods

There are two scanning methods for diagnosing gastric lesions: the water-filling method and the balloon contact method. In general, the water-filling method is employed for small and flat lesions, such as early gastric cancers, and the balloon contact method is used for large lesions that appear to be advanced gastric cancer. It is difficult to detect early gastric cancers with conventional EUS, because early gastric cancer is detected as an irregularity of the first layer and a slightly thickened stomach wall. Using the balloon contact method, therefore, is sometimes problematic for identification of the irregular first layer of flat lesions and the slightly thickened stomach wall, which is compressed by the balloon. In this situation, a thin ultrasonic probe should be used since it is easier to detect flat lesions with endoscopic guidance.

In the water-filling method, the stomach is rinsed at least one time with about 200 ml of deaerated water and then suctioned up, when mucous and remaining food exists. Generally,

M. Kida, M.D., Ph.D. (✉)
Department of Gastroenterology, Kitasato University,
1-15-1 Kitasato, Sagamihara, Kanagawa
228-8520, Japan
e-mail: m-kida@kitasato-u.ac.jp

N. Fukami (ed.), *Endoscopic Submucosal Dissection: Principles and Practice*, 27
DOI 10.1007/978-1-4939-2041-9_4, © Springer Science+Business Media New York 2015

300–800 ml of deaerated water is flooded into the stomach; the volume of deaerated water should be controlled by keeping the transectional stomach wall including the lesion circular. That is, 300–500 ml of deaerated water is used for stomach body lesions, and 600–800 ml for antrum lesions. However, lesions around the cardia, fornix, and pyloric ring are rather difficult to visualize with the water filling method. When evaluable pictures cannot be obtained, the balloon contact method should be tried along with the water filling method.

In order to obtain clear images, it is important to keep the transducer tip of the ultrasonographic endoscope perpendicular to the lesion. Each transducer has its own focusing point; therefore, the distance between ultrasonographic endoscope and the lesion should optimally be kept at 2–3 cm with a 7.5 MHz transducer and 1–2 cm with a 20 MHz transducer. The distance is controlled by manipulating the angle of the scope, the volume of deaerated water, the positioning of patient from left lateral to prone or supine, and by filling deaerated water to the tip of the balloon.

Instruments

For the staging of gastric cancer, EUS with a radial scanning transducer is generally used due to ease of manipulation and ability to detect lesions. There are three types of EUS; the first is conventional EUS with normal endoscopy and an ultrasonic transducer, the second is with an ultrasonic miniprobe (without endoscopy function), and the third is three-dimensional EUS (3D-EUS), also without endoscopy function [14, 15]. Additionally, there are two scanning types of EUS, which are mechanical radial scanning, such as the GF-UM2000 (Olympus Co., Tokyo), and electronic radial scanning, such as the GF-UE260 (Olympus Co., Tokyo) that is now commercially available around the world. Using electronic scanning is practicable for evaluating blood flow with the additional Doppler function.

Generally, conventional EUS is used for relatively large lesions that appear to be advanced gastric cancer; on the other hand, ultrasonic mini-

probes are used for small and flat lesions. As mentioned above, it is sometimes difficult to detect early gastric cancer with conventional EUS since early gastric cancer is detected as an irregularity of the first layer and a slightly thickened second and sometimes third layer of the stomach wall. In this situation, an ultrasonic miniprobe should be employed since it is best for detecting flat lesions with endoscopic guidance.

Furthermore, 3D-EUS may be useful in cases of flat and small lesions such as early gastric cancers. 3D-EUS was developed in 1994 and the second generation of 3D-EUS was commercialized in 1999 [14, 15], although hand-made 3D-EUS systems were originally tried in 1991 [16]. The 3D-EUS system consists of an image processor, an ultrasound unit, a probe driving unit, and two 3D-EUS scanning ultrasound probes; UM-DG20-25R (20 MHz) and UM-DG12-25R (12 MHz) (Fig. 4.1). While the 3D-EUS probe is sliding in the sheath of the driving unit, its transducer carries out maximal 160° mechanical spiral scanning, like helical computed tomography (Fig. 4.2). Three-dimensional information is obtained from around the probe, then a real-time radial image and a computer-reconstructed linear image displays on the monitor at the same time. Images generated with the system can be reviewed after scanning to select the optimal radial and linear image and to adjust imaging conditions. Using 3D-EUS, a maximum of 160 consecutive radial images can be reviewed, and, therefore, is expected to have higher accuracy for aiding diagnosis of the depth of gastric cancer invasion (Fig. 4.3). It is also possible with 3D-EUS to measure the tumor volume [17, 18].

Indications of EUS for Gastric Cancer

Local Staging

EUS is the most accurate method for local staging of gastric cancer [13, 19–31]. The clinical utility of EUS depends on whether preoperative assessment of local tumor extent will change the

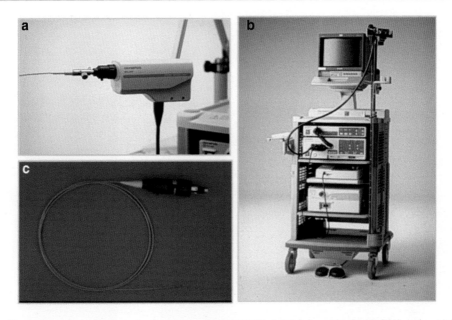

Fig. 4.1 Three-dimensional endoscopic ultrasonography (3D-EUS). (**a**) Driving unit. (**b**) 3D-EUS probe. (**c**) 3D-EUS system

Fig. 4.2 Principle of 3D-EUS

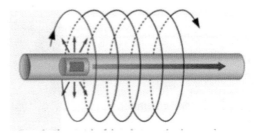

UM–DP20–25R	: 20MHz	Scan	: Mechanical spiral scan
UM–DP12–25R	: 12MHz	Pitch	: 1.0, 0.75, 0.5, 0.35, 0.25mm
Max Diameter	: 2.5mm	Range	: 40, 30, 20, 15mm

choice of therapeutic procedure. That is, several alternatives are now available for the treatment of both early and advanced gastric cancers. Protocols with curative aims offer two possibilities. The first is a choice between conventional surgical resection or local treatment, such as endoscopic submucosal dissection (ESD), endoscopic mucosal resection (EMR), laparoscopic resection, argon plasma coagulation (APC), or photodynamic therapy. According to the Japanese guidelines for gastric cancer treatment [32], the

classical indication of EMR is intramural, well-differentiated adenocarcinoma without ulceration or ulcer scarring, and less than 2 cm in diameter. Furthermore, its indication has been expanded recently as such [33, 34];

1. intramural, well-differentiated adenocarcinoma without ulceration or ulcer scarring, no size limitation,
2. intramural, well-differentiated adenocarcinoma with ulceration or ulcer scarring, less than 3 cm in diameter,

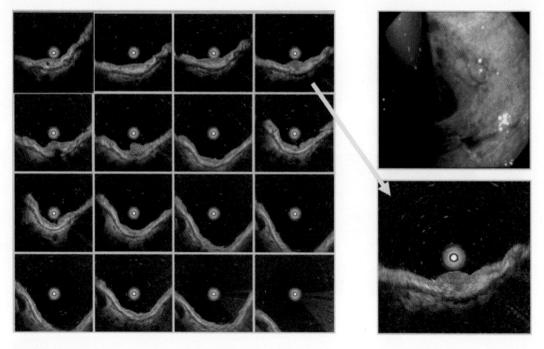

Fig. 4.3 Reviewing function of 3D-EUS 0-IIa, sm (1,250 μm)

3. sm1 (submucosal invasion less than 500 μm), well-differentiated adenocarcinoma, less than 3 cm in diameter, and
4. intramural, poorly differentiated adenocarcinoma, less than 2 cm, without ulceration or scarring.

Those cancers have no likelihood of distant metastasis and can be cured by endoscopic techniques.

The main role of EUS is to choose candidates with those indications. Therefore, we have to differentiate m and sm1 cancers from sm2 (submucosal invasion more than 500 μm).

The second choice is between conventional surgical resection and chemotherapy or radiation therapy. Secondary resection is proposed if there is a significant response with tumor downstaging. If there is no response, treatment is shifted to palliation, which is why it is important to detect whether a T2 or T3 stage tumor is present. Those tumors are curable by surgical resection and, therefore, primary resection is indicated. Tumors of the T4 category without distant metastasis obviously benefit from preoperative chemotherapy. EUS plays a

role in this important decision. The overall accuracy of EUS is superior to CT or MRI, although it is still not completely satisfactory.

Wall Structure and How to Diagnose Gastric Cancer Invasion

All along the digestive tract, the normal wall is visualized as a five-layer structure by EUS, with a 7.5–12 MHz transducer (Fig. 4.4) [35, 36]. From the digestive tract lumen inwards, the first hyperechoic and second hypoechoic layers correspond to the mucosa, the third hyperechoic layer to the submucosa, fourth hypoechoic layer to the muscularis propria, and fifth hyperechoic layer to the subserosa and the serosa of the stomach, respectively.

Using high frequency transducers (12–30 MHz), the gastric wall is detected under optimal conditions as a nine-layer structure (Figs. 4.4 and 4.5). In addition to the normal five layers, there is a border echo of the muscularis mucosae, a hypoechoic muscularis mucosae, a hypoechoic inner muscle, a border echo between the inner and outer muscle layers, and a hypoechoic outer

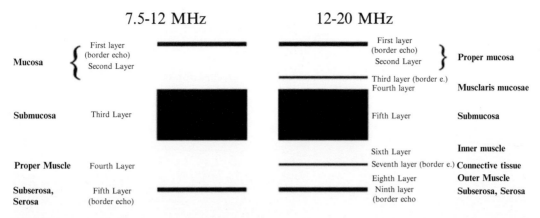

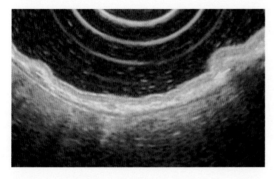

Fig. 4.4 Normal stomach wall by endoscopic ultrasonography

Fig. 4.5 Muscularis mucosae detected by EUS (20 MHz)

muscle [37]. However, the gastric wall is visualized as a seven-layer structure, without components of muscularis mucosae, under usual conditions with high frequency transducers.

T-Staging

The TNM system has been generally used all over the world; however, Japanese classification is mainly used in Japan [32]. All endoluminal shapes of gastric cancer can be visualized with EUS, including protruded, flat, depressed, and ulcerated lesions. The tumor mass itself presents as:

T1: Thickening or tumor infiltration of the mucosal and submucosal layer, leaving the fourth proper muscle layer intact. Discrete flat or depressed early gastric cancers are detected as an irregularity of the first layer and a slight thickening of the second layer. However, histological diagnosis should be done by biopsy as a confirmation of T1 lesions.

T2: Infiltration into the proper muscle layer and the subserosa. Detailed pattern analysis is needed to differentiate subserosal invasion from serosal (see below).

T3: Tumor penetration through the serosa (visceral peritoneum) without invasion of adjacent organs or structure.

T4: Tumor invasion to adjacent structures or organs.

In order to diagnose the depth of gastric cancer invasion, it is usually practical to detect the deepest layer that is destroyed by cancer invasion with EUS. However, it is sometimes problematic to diagnose depressed-type gastric cancers with peptic ulcers or fold convergence since peptic ulcer fibrosis is detected as a hypoechoic area similar to cancer invasion (Fig. 4.6). Although in Western countries early gastric cancers are not happened upon frequently, in Asian countries, especially in Japan, 50–70 % of gastric cancers are at early stage. About 20–30 % of early gastric cancers have ulcerative fibrosis (type 0-IIc+III or 0-IIc+ulcer scar). Therefore a method of pattern analysis capable of distinguishing between cancer invasion and ulcer fibrosis has been introduced in order to evaluate depressed-type gastric cancers (Fig. 4.7) [15, 38], and several pattern analyses have been reported [39, 40].

In order to diagnose the extent of subserosal or serosal invasion, it is first necessary to

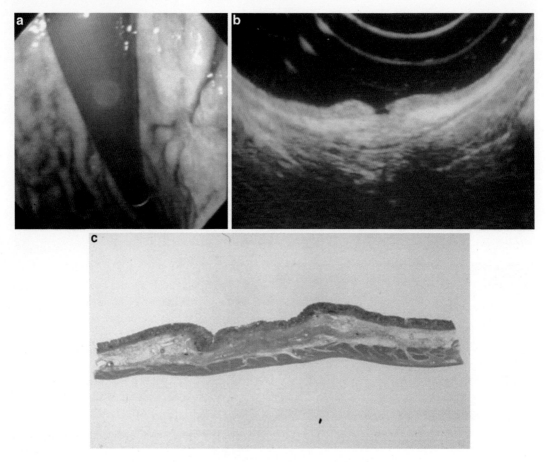

Fig. 4.6 Ulcer fibrosis mimics cancer invasion. 0-IIc + III, mucosal invasion with ulcer fibrosis in the submucosa (**a**) Endoscopic view. (**b**) Endoscopic ultrasound image. (**c**) Histopathological specimen

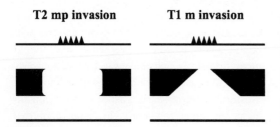

Fig. 4.7 How to differentiate cancer invasion from ulcer fibrosis with EUS (Basic principle) [25, 26]

of the five-layered structure. In the medullary group, a hump on the outer border means that cancer is still limited to the subserosa, and a serrated outer border indicates serosal invasion. In the scirrhous group, an indistinct hump on the outer border indicates serosal invasion, even if it is small, and only a distinct hump of the outer border indicates subserosal invasion.

differentiate between medullary and scirrhous growth, based on their internal pattern (Fig. 4.8). Generally, the medullary pattern has a well-demarcated border and a homogeneous, hypoechoic internal pattern; the scirrhous pattern, on the other hand, has an undefined border, a heterogeneous internal echo, and vestiges

N-Staging

After scanning of the primary lesion, lymph node metastasis is investigated around the primary lesion, lesser curvature, greater curvature, and celiac trunk. The ultrasonographic features of lymph nodes (homogeneous vs. heterogeneous) is found to be the most sensitive parameter for

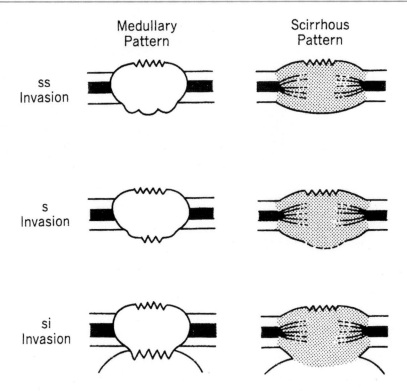

Fig. 4.8   How to differentiate between T2 subserosa, T3 serosa, and T4 si with EUS

Fig. 4.9   How to differentiate malignant from benign lymph node. Malignant lymph node

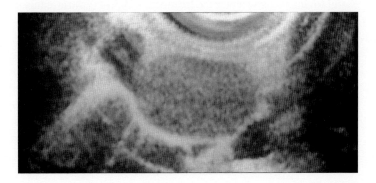

malignant involvement of nodes, followed by border demarcation (sharp vs. fuzzy), shape (round vs. elliptical), and size (>10 mm vs. <10 mm). If all four parameters are present, the positive predictive value is 100 %, whereas central hyperechogenicity is the typical pattern of benign lymph nodes (Figs. 4.9 and 4.10). However, all four of these features are present in only 25 % of malignant lymph nodes and a single feature can independently predict malignancy [14, 41].

Accuracy of EUS

T-staging

After endoscopic and pathological diagnosis, EUS is the most important diagnostic procedure for patients with gastric cancer. Numerous studies have investigated the accuracy of EUS in TNM staging of gastric cancer. According to a recent

Fig. 4.10 How to
differentiate malignant
from benign lymph node.
Benign lymph node

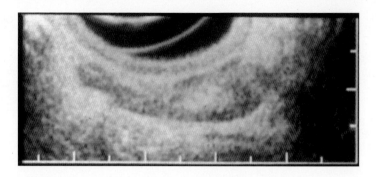

meta-analysis, the diagnostic accuracy of EUS for overall T-staging varied between 56.9 and 87.7 % and the pooled accuracy was 75 % (95 % CI: 57–73 %). The pooled accuracy was 77 % (95 % CI: 70–84 %) for T1, 65 % (95 % CI: 71–80 %) for T2, 85 % (95 % CI: 82–88 %) for T3, and 79 % (95 % CI: 68–90 %) for T4 [31]. These vary with respect to instrumentation, scanning frequency, and location difficulty, such as the cardia, pylorus, or an extremely difficult angle. In general, EUS is the most accurate at differentiating between T3 and T4 lesions, which is useful for choosing whether the treatment should be surgery or chemotherapy.

On the other hand, endoscopic submucosal dissection and endoscopic mucosal resection have been accepted as radical treatment for a certain group of early gastrointestinal cancer because of their less invasiveness, cost effectiveness, and associated shorter hospital stay. However, TNM staging is not enough for preoperative evaluation for ESD and EMR. Using EUS, therefore, it is important to differentiate intramucosal cancers from submucosal ones. Numerous studies have also investigated the accuracy of EUS in staging gastric cancer using the Japanese classification system. The diagnostic accuracy of EUS is summarized as follows: mucosal cancer, 86 % ($n=1,391$), submucosal cancer, 68 % ($n=744$), proper muscle cancer, 65 % ($n=264$), subserosal cancer, 80 % ($n=370$), serosal cancer, 85 % ($n=227$), si (infiltrate to adjacent organ) cancer, 62 % ($n=61$), and totally 79 % ($n=3,442$) [15, 37, 38, 42–48]. EUS is least accurate for submucosal and proper muscle cancers, similar to T2 lesions. The accuracy of si (T4) diagnosis is not

satisfactory because these data are mainly based on surgically resected cases.

Generally, factors that may cause an incorrect diagnosis with EUS are microinvasion, peritumorous inflammation (such as peptic ulcer fibrosis), macroscopic type (such as protruding lesions), and inadequate scanning [15]. Microinvasion may cause understaging, especially if it is very difficult to diagnose sm1 (less than 500 μm vertical invasion to the submucosa) with conventional EUS and an ultrasonic thin probe. If the pattern analysis for depressed-type gastric cancers is not employed, ulcer fibrosis may cause overstaging, according to the depth of ulcer fibrosis [15, 38]. And even if the pattern analysis is employed, it is almost impossible to diagnose between microinvasion such as sm1 and ulcer fibrosis. Protruding lesions introduce an artifact that interrupts the layered structure even if cancer invasion does not exist, and the third layer (sm) commonly protrudes into the lesion. Therefore, it is also difficult to detect narrowing or real interruption due to cancer invasion. Inadequate scanning has been a problem since the earliest days of EUS; that is, it is practically difficult to keep the EUS endoscope in vertical position for relatively small lesions around the cardia, greater curvature of upper body, lesser curvature of angle, and pyloric ring. In fact, there are many factors, such as pulsation, breathing, air bubbles, and mucous, that may cause such an artifact.

In order to perform endoscopic treatment such as EMR and ESD, logically, we have to preoperatively diagnose mucosal and sm1 cancer with high accuracy. There are several reports concerning the pre-procedure evaluation with EUS for ESD and EMR. Kwee et al. did a systematic review of 18 studies, and the sensitivity and specificity of EUS in detecting cancerous extension beyond the mucosa ranged from 18.2 to 100 % (median 87.8 %) and from 34.7 to 100 % (median 80.2 %) [20]. However, we have to differentiate mucosal and sm1 (submucosal invasion less than 500 μm) invasion from sm2 (more invasion) in cases of tumors 3 cm or smaller in diameter, not mucosal from submucosal invasion. Okada et al. reported on this issue and the diagnostic accuracy of EUS in identifying lesions meeting expanded-indication criteria for ESD was 87.8 % (259/295) for differentiated adenocarcinoma 30 mm in diameter or smaller, 43.5 % (10/23) for tumors larger than 30 mm in diameter, and 75 % (42/56) for undifferentiated adenocarcinoma 20 mm in diameter or smaller [21]. Additionally, Mouri et al. concluded the same [22]. As mentioned above, however, conventional EUS has not satisfied the accuracy required for clinical demands. In order to choose candidates for ESD, then, it is feasible to diagnose submucosal invasion more than 500 μm by means of 3D-EUS. According to our data, the diagnostic accuracy of 3D-EUS for diagnosing the depth of gastric cancer invasion is 96 % ($n=325$) for mucosal cancer, 74.6 % ($n=181$) for submucosal, 72 % ($n=25$) for proper muscle, 76 % ($n=25$) for subserosal, 67 % ($n=12$), 0 % ($n=4$) for si (invasion to adjacent organ), and totally 86.3 % ($n=582$) (Table 4.1). Basically, 3D-EUS is a kind of ultrasonic probe, therefore 3D-EUS is suitable for evaluating flat and small lesions such as early gastric cancers, but not for advanced gastric cancers because of poor penetration.

Table 4.1 Accuracy of 3D-EUS for diagnosing gastric cancer invasion

	m	sm	mp	ss	s	si	
T1m (325)	312	11	1	1			96.0
T1sm (181)	41	135	5				74.6
T2mp (25)		6	18	1			72.0
T2ss (25)		3	2	19	1		76.0
T3s (22)	1	1	1	1	18		81.8
T4 si (4)				1	3	0	0
							86.3

Table 4.2 Diagnostic accuracy of 3D-EUS according to the degree of submucosal invasion (0-IIc, IIa + IIc, IIa, I etc.)

Degree of sm inv.	3D-EUS	EUS, USP
≦500 μm	56.7 % (17/30)	12.5 % (2/16)
500<≦1,000	77.8 % (21/27)	50.0 % (14/28)
1,000<≦2,000	86.7 % (26/30)	79.1 % (34/43)
2,000<	91.4 % (32/35)	88.1 % (59/67)
Total	78.7 % (96/122)	70.8 % (109/154)

Table 4.3 Diagnostic accuracy of 3D-EUS according to the degree of submucosal invasion (0-IIc + III, IIc + Uls)

	3D-EUS	EUS, USP
≦500 μm	[80.8 % (21/26)]	[40.0 % (8/20)]
500<≦1,000	54.5 % (6/11)	57.7 % (15/26)
1,000<≦2,000	75.0 % (6/8)	75.6 % (31/41)
2,000<	92.9 % (13/14)	85.2 % (23/27)
Total	78.0 % (46/59)	67.5 % (77/114)

Regarding the degree of submucosal invasion, submucosal invasion more than 500 μm, in cases of early gastric cancers without ulceration or fibrosis, can be detected with an accuracy of more than about 80 %, which is rather satisfactory for choosing candidates for ESD, compared to those of conventional EUS and ultrasonic probes (Table 4.2). Regarding early gastric cancers with ulceration or fibrosis (0-IIc + III, IIc + Uls), the diagnostic accuracy is not satisfactory for clinical demands, even if pattern analysis is employed (Table 4.3). At present, we diagnose those cases as m-sm1 or sm2 invasion; however, those results are not satisfactory because of artifactual ulcer fibrosis, and furthermore, conclusions cannot be drawn in the case of lesions 3 cm or larger in diameter. Whereas the accuracy of 3D-EUS for early gastric cancers without ulceration and fibrosis is clinically satisfactory, especially for lesions 3 cm or smaller in diameter, the accuracy for lesions 3 cm or larger in diameter is not (Table 4.4).

Compared with other diagnostic imaging modalities, computed tomography (CT) and magnetic resonance imaging (MRI) have been the primary method for staging gastric cancer. EUS is superior to CT and MRI in its ability to reveal gastric wall structures, and furthermore, it is almost impossible to detect T1 gastric cancer,

Table 4.4 Accuracy of 3D-EUS for choosing indication of ESD

	m, sm1	sm2	m	sm	Total
IIc + III	93.8 %	88.9 %	85.7 %	71.4 %	87.1 %
	(61/65)	(16/18)	(18/21)	(20/28)	(115/132)
IIc	98.6 %	89.7 %	93.1 %	76.0 %	94.0 %
	(139/141)	(35/39)	(27/29)	(19/25)	(220/234)
IIa + IIc	95.7 %	88.2 %	100 %	87.5 %	92.9 %
	(22/23)	(15/17)	(8/8)	(7/8)	(52/56)
IIa, etc.	100 %	100 %	100 %	50.0 %	98.5 %
	(56/56)	(3/3)	(4/4)	(1/2)	(64/65)
I, etc.	100 %	100 %	100 %	33.3 %	89.5 %
	(12/12)	(3/3)	(1/1)	(1/3)	(17/19)
Total	97.6 %	90.0 %	92.1 %	72.7 %	92.5 %
	(290/297)	(72/80)	(58/63)	(48/66)	(468/506)

except for protruding lesions. However, EUS is not useful for the assessment of distant lymph node and distant metastasis (M). Regarding the accuracy of these modalities, based on the literature, EUS and CT are complementary rather than competitive; EUS is superior in diagnosing the depth of gastric cancer invasion and CT or MRI is preferred for diagnosis of distant metastasis and distant lymph node metastasis.

N-staging

According to a recent meta-analysis [23], the sensitivity and specificity of lymph node metastasis is less accurate than T-staging, varying between 16.7 % and 95.3 % (median, 70.8 %) and 48.4 % and 100 % (median, 84.6 %), compared to 12.2 % and 80 % (median, 39.9 %) and 56.3 % and 100 % (median, 81.8 %) with abdominal ultrasound, 62.5 % and 91.9 % (median, 80 %) and 50 % and 87.9 % (median, 77.8 %) with MDCT, 54.6 % and 85.3 % (median, 68.8 %) and 50 % and 97 % (median, 93.2 %) with MRI, 33.3 % and 64.6 % (median, 34.3 %) and 85.7 % and 97 % (median 93.2 %), respectively. There is a strong correlation between increasing T stage and presence of lymph node metastasis; therefore, concomitant T stage may be suitable for

determining the probability of lymph node metastasis on EUS. If the study sample includes mainly T3 and T4, the accuracy and sensitivity of EUS, abdominal ultrasonography (US), MDCT, MRI, and FDG-PET for diagnosing lymph node metastasis becomes better. Probably, studies with EUS included more early stages, and therefore, we cannot make conclusions on this issue. Anyway, EUS, abdominal US, MDCT, MRI, and FDG-PET cannot reliably be used to confirm or exclude the presence of lymph node metastasis. It is very difficult to detect lymph node metastasis in T1, because only a very small percentage of T1a and about 15 % of T1b have only one or two metastatic lymph nodes. However, the reliable accuracy of EUS for lymph node diagnosis in T1 is of critical importance in evaluating whether local endoscopic treatment of early gastric cancer is suitable or not. Therefore, local endoscopic treatment, such as ESD and EMR, is decided mainly by T-staging in Japan. In general, EUS detects lymph node metastasis around the lesser curvature of the stomach better than that of greater curvature and greater than 3 cm from the stomach, such as the celiac trunk, because EUS has to follow a wide area along the greater curvature and has a maximum depth of penetration approximately 5–7 cm, thus the ability to detect distant metastasis is limited.

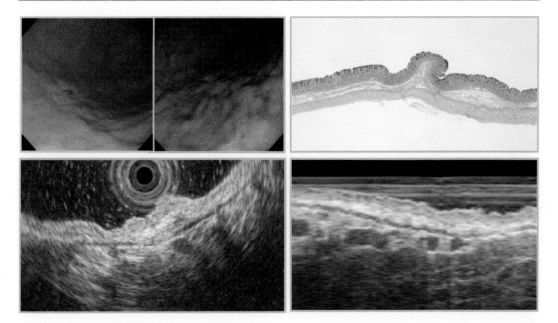

Fig. 4.11 Slightly depressed lesion 0-IIc, T1a

As mentioned above, the criteria for malignant lymph nodes can make them difficult to distinguish from benign lymph nodes. Even benign lymph nodes sometimes have one or two of malignant stigmata. Therefore, when indicated, EUS-FNA is frequently employed.

Case Presentations

Case 1: Gastric Cancer, Mucosal Invasion (Fig. 4.11)

A slightly depressed lesion, so called 0-IIc by Japanese classification, is visualized in the greater curvature of lower body. 3D-EUS reveals this lesion as an irregularity of the first layer and a slight thickening of the second layer, while the third to fifth layers are intact. Therefore, this lesion is diagnosed as intramural cancer. Histology showed that the cancer invasion was limited to the mucosa.

Case 2: Gastric Cancer, Submucosal Cancer (Fig. 4.12)

There is a slightly depressed lesion, so called 0-IIc by Japanese classification, in the posterior wall of angle. 3D-EUS shows this lesion as an irregularity and elevation of the first layer, thickening of the second layer, and slight narrowing of the third layer, which corresponds to submucosal invasion. Histology demonstrated that the cancer invaded the submucosa (807 μm), and it was therefore deemed sm2.

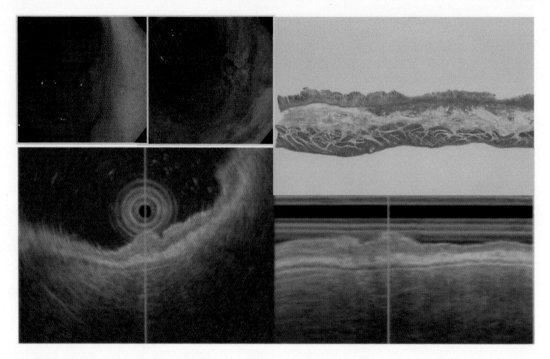

Fig. 4.12 Slightly depressed lesion 0-IIc, T1b sm 807 μm

References

1. DiMagno EP, Buxton JL, et al. Ultrasonic endoscope. Lancet. 1980;1:627–9.
2. Vilmann P, Jacobsen GK, Henriksen FW, et al. Endoscopic ultrasonography with guided fine needle aspiration biopsy in pancreas disease. Gastrointest Endosc. 1992;38(2):172–3.
3. Grimm H, Binmoeller K, Soehendra N. Endosonography-guided drainage of a pancreas pseudocyst. Gastrointest Endosc. 1992;38(2):170.
4. Wiersema MJ, Kochman ML, Cramer HM, et al. Endosonography-guided real-time fine-needle aspiration biopsy. Gastrointest Endosc. 1994;40:700–7.
5. Grees FG, Hawes RH, Savides TJ, et al. Endoscopic ultrasound-guided fine-needle aspiration using linear array and radial scanning endosonography. Gastrointest Endosc. 1997;45:243–50.
6. Willams DB, Sahai AV, Aabakken L, et al. Endoscopic ultrasound guided fine needle aspiration biopsy: a large single centre experience. Gut. 1999;44:720–6.
7. Le Blanc JK, Ciaccia D, Al-Assi MT, et al. Optimal number of EUS-guided fine needle passes to obtain a correct diagnosis. Gastrointest Endosc. 2004;59: 475–81.
8. Savides TJ, Donohue M, Hunt G, et al. EUS-guided FNA diagnostic yield of malignancy in solid pancreatic masses: a benchmark for quality performance measurement. Gastrointest Endosc. 2007;66:277–82.
9. Kida M, Araki M, Miyazawa S, et al. Comparison of diagnostic accuracy of endoscopic ultrasound-guided fine-needle aspiration with 22- and 25-gauge needles in the same patients. J Interv Gastroenterol. 2011;3:102–7.
10. Rong L, Kida M, Yamauchi H, et al. Factors affecting the diagnostic accuracy of endoscopic ultrasonography-guided fine-needle aspiration (EUS-FNA) for upper gastrointestinal submucosal or extraluminal solid mass lesions. Dig Endosc. 2012;24(5):358–63.
11. Polkowski M, Larghi A, Weynand B, et al. Learning, techniques, and complications of endoscopic ultrasound (EUS)-guided sampling in gastroenterology: European Society of Gastrointestinal Endoscopy (ESGE) Technical Guideline. Endoscopy. 2012;44(02):190–206.
12. Kida M, Itoi T. Current status and future perspective of interventional endoscopic ultrasound in Japan. Dig Endosc. 2009;21(Suppl):S50–2.
13. Kida M, Tanabe S, Kokutou M, et al. Staging of gastric cancer with endoscopic ultrasonography and endoscopic mucosal resection. Endoscopy. 1998;30(suppl):A64–8.
14. Kida M. Endoscopic ultrasonography in Japan: present status and standardization. Dig Endosc. 2002; 14(suppl):S24–9.
15. Japan Gastric Cancer Association. Guideline of gastric cancer treatment. Tokyo: Kanehira publ. Co.; 2001.
16. Souquet JC, Valette PJ, Berger F, et al. Contribution of endosonography to the diagnosis of gastric linitis. Gastrointest Endosc. 1988;34:209 (abstr).

17. Andriulli A, Reccina S, De Angelis C, et al. Endoscopic ultrasonographic evaluation of patients with biopsy negative gastric linitis plastica. Gastrointest Endosc. 1990;36:611–5.

18. Caletti G, Ferrari A, Bocus P, et al. Endoscopic ultrasonography in gastric lymphoma. In: Sivak MV (ed), 10th International Symposium on Endoscopic ultrasonography, Cleveland, OH, October 1995, pp. 119–25 (suppl).

19. Lightdale CJ, Botet JF, Kelsen DP, et al. Diagnosis of recurrent upper gastrointestinal cancer at the surgical anastomosis by endoscopic ultrasound. Gastrointest Endosc. 1989;35:407–12.

20. Aibe T, Fuji T, Okita K, et al. A fundamental study of normal layer structure of the gastrointestinal wall visualized by endoscopic ultrasonography. Scand J Gastroenterol. 1986;21(suppl):34–40.

21. Kimmey MB, Martin RW, Haggitt RC, et al. Histologic correlates of gastrointestinal ultrasound images. Gastroenterology. 1989;96:433–41.

22. Yamanaka T. Endosonographic correlation with histology in a layered structure of the gastrointestinal wall. Gastroenterol Endosc. 2001;43:1091–2.

23. Kida M, Saigenji K, Okabe H. Endoscopic ultrasonography in the diagnosis of the depth of gastric cancer invasion. Differential diagnosis between cancerous invasion and fibrosis of the co-existing ulcer. Gastroenterol Endosc. 1989;31:1141–55.

24. Kelly S, Harris KM, Berry E, et al. A systemic review of the staging performance of endoscopic ultrasound in gastro-oesophageal carcinoma. Gut. 2001;49:534–9.

25. Bhandari S, Shim CS, Kim JH, et al. Usefulness of three-dimensional, multidetector row CT (virtual gastroscopy and multiplanar reconstruction) in the evaluation of gastric cancer: a comparison with conventional endoscopy, EUS, and histopathology. Gastrointest Endosc. 2004;59:619–26.

26. Kida M, Kokutou M, Watanabe M, et al. Accuracy of Endoscopic Ultrasonography for diagnosing the depth of early gastric cancer with or without ulcer. Stom Intest. 1999;34:1095–103.

27. De Angelis C, Gindro T, Recchia S, et al. Value and limitations of preoperative endoscopic ultrasonography in predicting stage and respectability of gastric cancer. Gastroenterology. 1994;106:380 (abstr).

28. Dittler HJ, Siewert JR. Role of endoscopic ultrasonography in gastric carcinoma. Endoscopy. 1993;25:224–30.

29. Grimm H, Binmoeller KF, Hamper K, et al. Endosonography for preoperative locoregional staging of esophageal and gastric cancer. Endoscopy. 1993;25:224–30.

30. Ziegler K, Sanft C, Zimmer T, et al. Comparison of computed tomography, endosonography, and intraoperative assessment in TN staging of gastric carcinoma. Gut. 1993;34:604–10.

31. Nattermann C, Galbenu-Grunwald R, Nier H. Endoskopischer ultraschall im TN-staging des magenkarzinims. Ein vergleich mit der computertomographie und der knoventionellen sonographie. Z Gesamte Inn Med. 1993;48:60–4.

32. Caletti G, Ferrari A, Brocchi E, et al. Accuracy of endoscopic ultrasonography in the diagnosis and staging of gastric cancer and lymphoma. Surgery. 1993;113:14–27.

33. Roesch T, Lorenz R, Zenker K, et al. Local staging and assessment of respectability in carcinoma of the esophagus, stomach, and duodenum by endoscopic ultrasonography. Gastrointest Endosc. 1992;38:460–7.

34. Cerizzi A, Botti F, Carrara A, et al. EUS in preoperative staging of gastric cancer. Endoscopy. 1992;24(suppl): 380 (abstr).

35. Akahoshi K, Misawa T, Fujishima H, et al. Preoperative evaluation of gastric cancer by endoscopic ultrasound. Gut. 1991;32:479–82.

36. Botet JF, Lightdale CJ, Zauber AG, et al. Preoperative staging of gastric cancer: comparison of endoscopic US and dynamic CT. Radiology. 1991;181:426–32.

37. Heintz A, Junginger T. Endosonographisches staging von karzinomen in speiserohre und magen. Bildgebung (Imag). 1991;58:4–8.

38. Tio TL, Schouwink MH, Cikot RJ, et al. Preoperative TNM classification of gastric carcinoma by endosonography in comparison with pathological TNM system: a prospective study of 72 cases. Hepatogastroenterology. 1989;36:51–6.

39. Aibe T, Fujimura H, Noguchi T, et al. Endosonographic detection and staging of early gastric cancer. In: Dancygier H, Classen M (editors), Fifth International symposium on EUS, 1989, Munich, Germany, pp. 71–8.

40. Bhutani MS, Hawes RH, Hoffman BJ. A comparison the accuracy of echo features during endoscopic ultrasound (EUS) and EUS-guided fine needle aspiration for diagnosis of malignant lymph node invasion. Gastrointest Endosc. 1997;45:474–9.

41. Catalano MF, Sivak MVJ, Rice T, et al. Endosonographic features predictive of lymph node metastasis. Gastrointest Endosc. 1994;40:442–6.

42. Maluf-Filho F, Dotti CM, Halwan B, et al. An evidence-based consensus statement on the role and application of endosonography in clinical practice. Endoscopy. 2009;41:979–87.

43. Kim GH, Park DY, Kida M, et al. Accuracy of high-frequency catheter-based endoscopic ultrasonography according to the indications for endoscopic treatment of early gastric cancer. J Gastroentrol Hepatol. 2010; 25:506–11.

44. Polkowski M. Endosonographic staging of upper intestinal malignancy. Best Prac Res Clin Gastroenterol. 2009;23:649–61.

45. Cardoso R, Coburn N, Seevaratnam R, et al. A systemic review and meta-analysis of the utility of EUS for preoperative staging for gastric cancer. Gastric Cancer. 2012;15(Suppl):S19–26.

46. Mocelin S, Marchert A, Nitti D. EUS for the staging of gastric cancer: a meta-analysis. GIE. 2011;73:1123–34.

47. Gotoda T, Yanagisawa A, Sasako M, et al. Incidence of lymph node metastasis from early gastric cancer: estimation with a large number of cases at two large centers. Gastric Cancer. 2000;3:219–25.

48. Hirasawa T, Gotoda T, Miyata H, et al. Incidence of lympho node metastasis and feasibility of endoscopic resection undifferentiated type early gastric cancer. Gastric Cancer. 2009;12:148–52.

Advanced Endoscopic Imaging in the Upper Gastrointestinal Tract

Manuel Berzosa and Michael B. Wallace

Introduction

Advanced endoscopic imaging encompasses several methods that enhance visualization of the upper gastrointestinal tract. These techniques are available to assist the advanced endoscopist before, during, and after ESD. There are several different means by which to improve imaging of the mucosa during endoscopy, like dye, optical, and/or electronic technologies (Table 5.1).

Enhanced endoscopic visualization adds valuable information during all stages of ESD. It is important during screening of patients, as it improves detection of lesions [1, 2]. During the treatment phase, it allows better delineation of the margins of the lesion, allowing accurate demarcation of the area to be resected. Some methods can also reveal changes in the mucosal surface and vascular pattern that could help establish the degree of invasion [3]. Therefore, these technologies have become particularly important for helping the endoscopist select the optimal treatment [4]. Finally, during surveillance, these methods can help distinguish between scar tissue and recurrence of or residual lesion [5, 6].

M. Berzosa, M.D. (✉) • M.B. Wallace, M.D., M.P.H., F.A.S.G.E.
Department of Gastroenterology, Mayo Clinic Florida, 4500 San Pablo Road, Jacksonville, FL 32224, USA
e-mail: berzosacorella.manuel@mayo.edu

An endoscopist performing ESD needs to become familiarized with these tools. As these technologies continue to improve our visualization of the mucosa and ongoing research standardizes and validates lesion pattern recognition, it is only a matter of time before they will become standard practice.

Chromoendoscopy

Chromoendoscopy is based on the application of various dye solutions to the mucosa of the gastrointestinal tract, thus enhancing subtle mucosal changes not perceivable by purely optical methods. Several different dye stains are used in the upper GI tract, most of which are absorptive in function (e.g. Lugol's solution, methylene blue, crystal violet, toluidine blue) and require additional time (2–20 min) for staining before interpretation can be carried out. Other agents used work as contrast (e.g. indigo carmine) or reactive agents (e.g. Congo red) [7].

The most widely used classification system was developed by Kudo, and it classifies colonic lesions into seven subtypes [8]. Lesions with advanced, superficially invasive neoplasia are the best candidates for ESD and are termed type V_i (irregular), with highly irregular yet intact pit patterns (Fig. 5.1) [8]. Deeply invasive lesions, which cannot be fully removed by ESD, typically have non-structural, or complete loss of pits. Unfortunately, these patterns typically require

Table 5.1 Advanced endoscopic imaging techniques for the upper gastrointestinal tract

Dye (chromoendoscopy)	Optical	Electronic
Lugol's solution	Magnification endoscopy	Spectrometry
Methylene blue	Narrow band imaging	Optical coherence tomography
Crystal violet	Autofluorescence imaging	Fujinon intelligent color enhancement
Indigo carmine	Endocytoscopy	iScan
Congo red	Confocal endomicroscopy	

magnification and crystal violet staining, which is not widely used in the West.

The use of chromoendoscopy has remained useful in regions with high incidences of squamous cell carcinoma (SCC) of the esophagus. Lugol's solution stains glycogen, which is found within non-keratinized squamous cells, into a dark brown color, allowing delineation of normal epithelium from glycogen-depleted cells (e.g. dysplastic epithelium, SCC, columnar epithelium, or inflammation) [7] (Fig. 5.2).

The dyes most commonly used for chromoendoscopy in Barrett's esophagus (BE) are acetic acid and methylene blue. Acetic acid produces reversible changes on the surface proteins of columnar epithelium, causing transient whitening of the epithelium that usually lasts 2–3 min. This whitening effect is lost faster in dysplastic epithelium compared to the surrounding mucosa, therefore enhancing its identification. Methylene blue is absorbed by BE including dysplastic epithelium, but not by squamous epithelium or gastric-type metaplasia in the lower esophagus. However, the absorption is heterogenous and of a lighter intensity in high-grade dysplasia or adenocarcinoma of the esophagus, allowing differentiation from non-dysplastic BE [9].

In contrast, in areas with high incidence of BE, the use of chromoendoscopy has been declining in favor of virtual chromoendoscopy techniques (e.g. NBI or FICE), which have the advantage of providing mucosal enhancement within seconds by simply pushing a bottom within the endoscope and therefore obviating the need to spray and rinse dye. In fact, a recent meta-analysis evaluating the increased diagnostic yield for the detection of dysplasia or cancer on patients with BE found that both chromoendoscopy and virtual chromoendoscopy equally increased the diagnostic yield for dysplasia [1].

In the stomach, chromoendoscopy has long been used to detect intestinal metaplasia, dysplasia, and early gastric cancer. A combination of methylene blue with Congo red or acetic acid has been found useful for detecting early gastric cancer. In one study, the detection of synchronous lesions increased from 28 % under standard white light endoscopy up to 89 % with a combination of methylene blue and Congo red, as cancerous areas do not stain with either dye [7]. Similarly, others have also found increased early gastric cancer detection with a combination of indigo carmine and acetic acid [10, 11]. In one study, the diagnostic yield almost doubled with a combination of indigo carmine and acetic acid (94 %) versus either one alone (42 % for acetic acid and 52 % for indigo carmine; $p < 0.005$) [10]. In another study, this same combination was able to identify 6 of 39 lesions that were previously missed with standard white light endoscopy and using only indigo carmine [11].

Optical Imaging Technologies

Narrow Band Imaging

Narrow band imaging (NBI) is an optical technique that uses reflected light to visualize the superficial structure and enhances vasculature within the mucosal layer. It selects light within the hemoglobin absorption band, such that blood vessel-rich structures, such as neoplastic lesions, are demonstrated with high contrast relative to their non-neoplastic background.

While conventional white light endoscopy uses the full visible wavelength range (400–700 nm) to produce a red-green-blue image, NBI uses manipulations of the light source (optical) to enhance visualization of the surface. NBI imaging

Type	Schematic	Endoscopic	Description	Suggested Pathology	Ideal Treatment
I	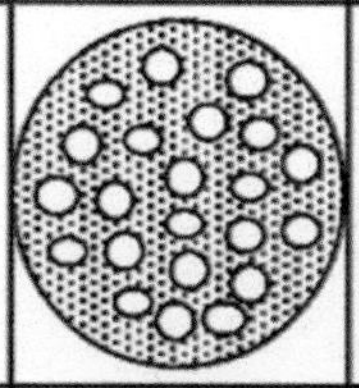	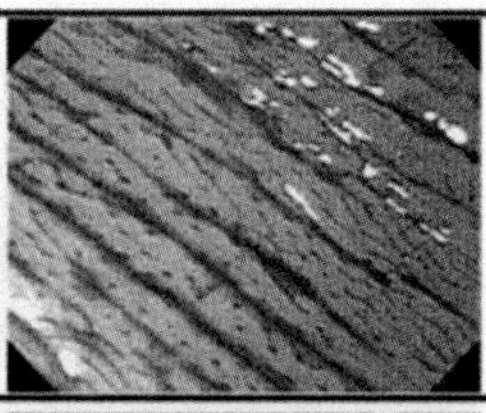	Round pits.	Non-neoplastic.	Endoscopic or none.
II	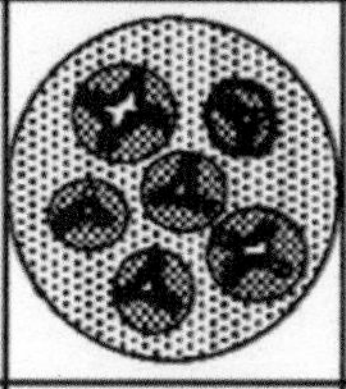	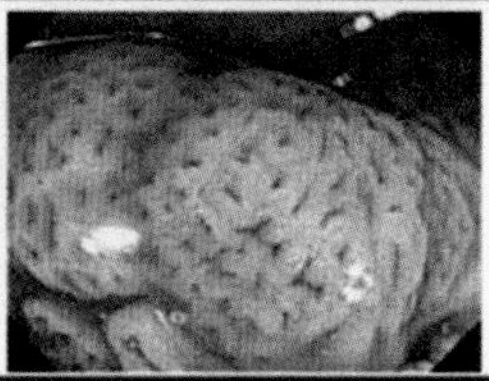	Stellar or papillary pits.	Non-neoplastic.	Endoscopic or none.
IIIs	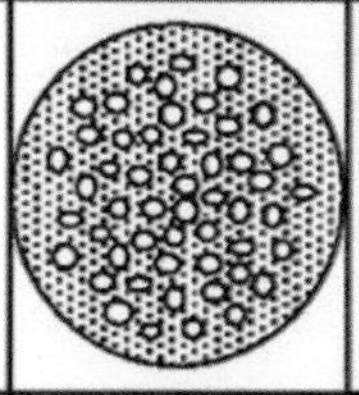	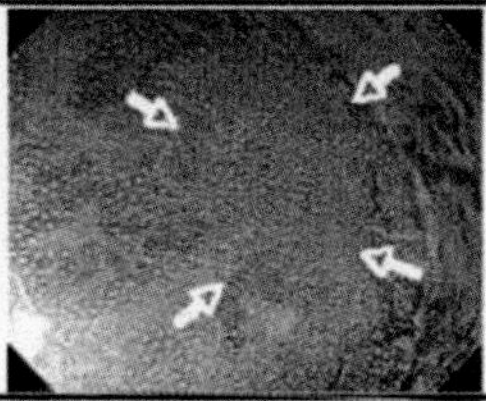	Small tubular or round pits that are smaller than the normal pit	Neoplastic.	Endoscopic.
IIIL	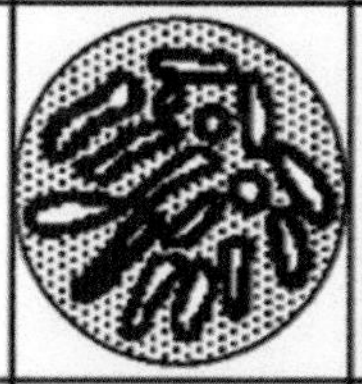	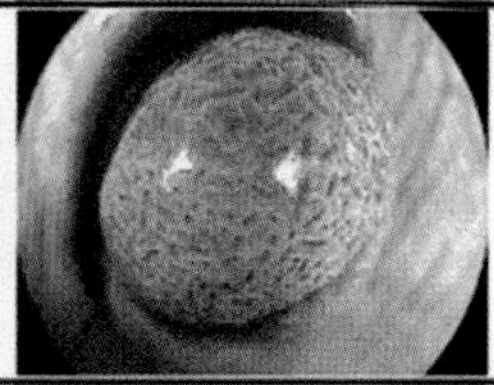	Tubular or roundish pits that are larger than the normal pits.	Neoplastic.	Endoscopic.
IV	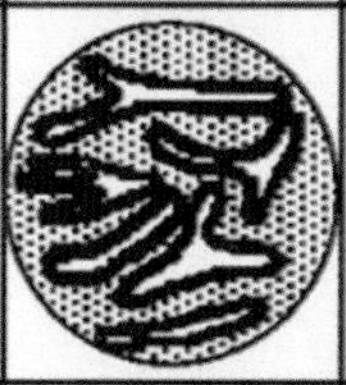	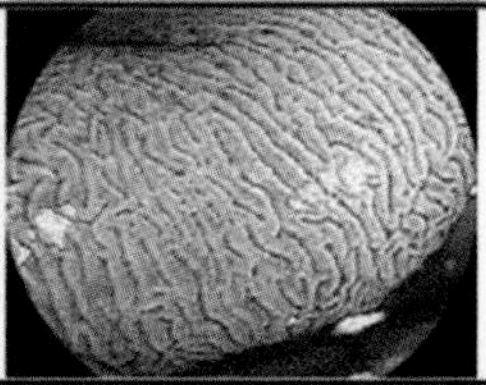	Branch-like or gyrus-like pits.	Neoplastic.	Endoscopic.
VI	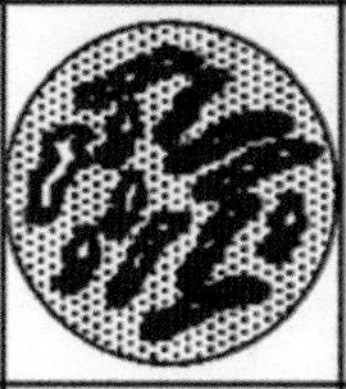	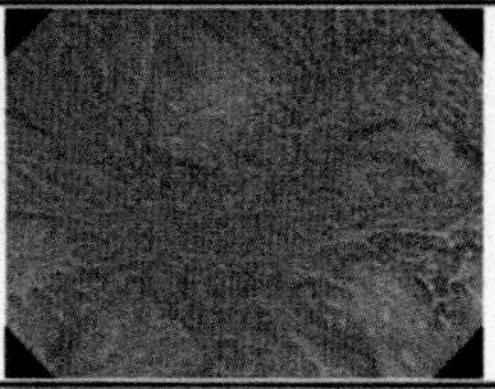	Irregularly arranged pits with type IIIs, IIIL, IV type pit patterns.	Neoplastic (invasive).	Endoscopic or surgical.
VN	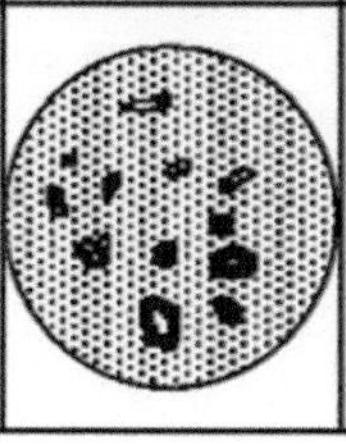	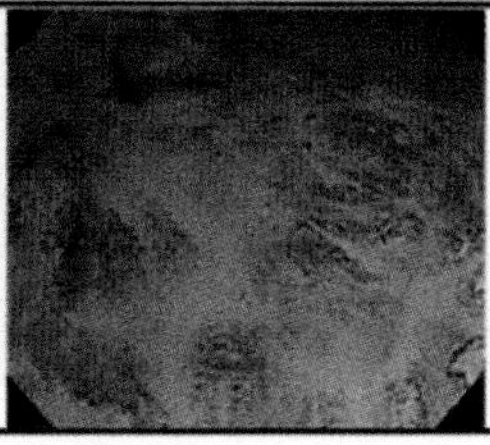	Non-structural pits.	Neoplastic (massive submucosal invasive).	Surgical.

Fig. 5.1   Colonic pit pattern classification. Reproduced with permission, Tanaka GIE 2006;64:604–13

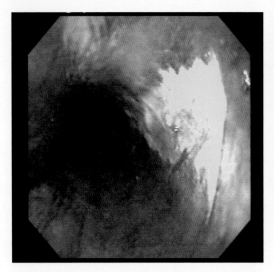

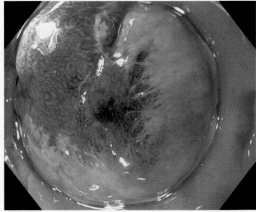

Fig. 5.3 NBI of esophageal nodule in a patient undergoing surveillance for Barrett's esophagus. Note the loss of all pit pattern (Kudo V). Resection specimen revealed T1a adenocarcinoma

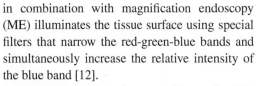

Fig. 5.2 Chromoendoscopy using Lugol's solution to enhance resection margins of an esophageal squamous cell carcinoma (*bright yellow*)

in combination with magnification endoscopy (ME) illuminates the tissue surface using special filters that narrow the red-green-blue bands and simultaneously increase the relative intensity of the blue band [12].

In patients undergoing surveillance for BE, NBI, when compared to standard resolution endoscopy, detected significantly more patients with dysplasia (57 % vs. 43 %) and higher grades of dysplasia (18 % vs. 0 %; $p < 0.001$), but with fewer biopsy samples (mean 4.7 vs. 8.5; $p < 0.001$) [13]. Similarly, when compared to high definition white light endoscopy (HDWLE), NBI detected a higher proportion of areas with dysplasia (30 % vs. 21 %, $p = 0.01$) with fewer biopsies needed per patient (3.6 vs. 7.6, $p < 0.0001$) [14]. Results from a recent meta analysis support the routine use of NBI for detection of dysplasia and neoplasia during BE surveillance [1] (Fig. 5.3).

NBI enhancement of microvascular and microsurface pattern changes in the esophageal and gastric mucosa allows differentiation between early cancer and benign lesions [3, 15]. With the use of ME, NBI has allowed identification of specific vascular patterns in the intrapapillary

capillary loop of the esophagus which helps recognize early SCC [3].

In addition, ME-NBI has been shown as superior to chromoendoscopy (97.4 % vs. 77.8 %; $p = 0.009$) in delineating the margins of early gastric cancer [16] (Fig. 5.4). ME-NBI was able to define the entirety of margins in 72.6 % of the lesions that had unclear margins by chromoendoscopy [17].

Recently, an NBI international consensus for endoscopic (NICE) classification has been developed with regard to distinguishing hyperplastic, neoplastic, and deeply invasive neoplastic lesions to facilitate selection of lesions for ESD with acceptable accuracy and reliability [18] (Fig. 5.5). For predicting deep submucosal invasion, which is a contraindication to ESD, the sensitivity was 91.8 %, specificity 88.3 %, and negative predictive value 91.9 % for lesions predicted with high confidence. However, only half of the lesions could be predicted with high confidence. Most importantly, this classification has only been validated for colonic lesions [18]. In the upper GI tract there are many proposed classifications [15], but there is a lack of standardization between the described patterns and further research is necessary to reach a consensus.

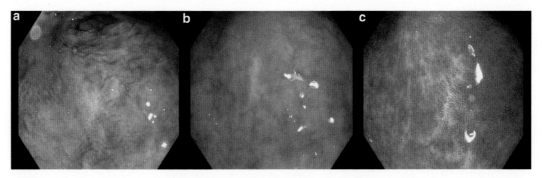

Fig. 5.4 Chromoendoscopy (**a**), HDWLE (**b**), and ME-NBI (**c**) of the same suspicious area found on the lesser curvature of the stomach on a patient with known gastric intestinal metaplasia undergoing surveillance endoscopy

NBI International Colorectal Endoscopic (NICE) Classification*

	Type 1	**Type 2**	**Type 3**
Color	Same or lighter than background	Browner relative to background (verify color arises from vessels)	Brown to dark brown relative to background; sometimes patchy whiter areas
Vessels	None, or isolated lacy vessels coursing across the lesion	Brown vessels surrounding white structures**	Has area(s) of disrupted or missing vessels
Surface Pattern	Dark or white spots of uniform size, or homogeneous absence of pattern	Oval, tubular or branched white structure surrounded by brown vessels**	Amorphous or absent surface pattern
Most likely pathology	**Hyperplastic**	**Adenoma***	**Deep submucosal invasive cancer**
Examples	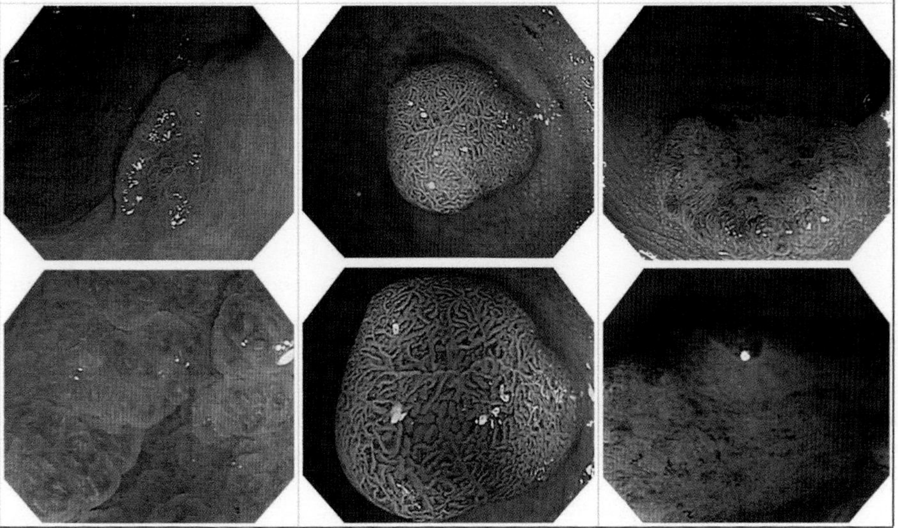		

* Can be applied using colonoscopes with or without optical (zoom) magnification

** These structures (regular or irregular) may represent the pits and the epithelium of the crypt opening.

*** Type 2 consists of Vienna classification types 3, 4 and superficial 5 (all adenomas with either low or high grade dysplasia, or with superficial submucosal carcinoma). The presence of high grade dysplasia or superficial submucosal carcinoma may be suggested by an irregular vessel or surface pattern, and is often associated with atypical morphology (e.g., depressed area).

Fig. 5.5 The NBI international colorectal endoscopic (NICE) classification

Autofluorescence Imaging

Autofluorescence imaging (AFI) is a technique based on the principle that excitation of tissue with light of a shorter wavelength leads to emission of a longer wavelength of light. In the gastrointestinal tract, autofluorescence detects subtle changes in the concentration of specific chemicals in the tissue that have the ability to fluoresce when activated by specific wavelengths of light. Malignant transformation of tissue is associated with emission of relatively longer wavelengths of light (shift from green toward the red end of the spectrum) [12].

However, a recent analysis of data from five prospective clinical trials, encompassing close to 400 patients with BE, found little influence of AFI on the diagnosis of early stage neoplasia or on therapeutic decision making. The authors therefore concluded that AFI has a limited role in routine surveillance or management of patients with BE [19].

AFI has also been assessed for detecting early gastric neoplasia in the stomach [20, 21]. The results of a recent trial suggest that AFI can help detect those patients who are most at risk for developing metachronous lesions after ESD of early gastric cancer (hazard ratio 4.88, CI 95 %: 1.32–18.2, $p=0.018$) by stratifying the patients by the extent of their intestinal metaplasia. However, there are no trials comparing the added benefit of this technology over more readily available advanced imaging modalities (e.g. NBI, HDWLE, CLE).

Endocytoscopy

Endocytoscopy is a novel technology that allows microscopic imaging of the gastrointestinal surface epithelium. Similar to a contact light microscope, it uses a high-power objective lens to project highly magnified (from 400 to 1,400-fold) images onto the charge-coupled device of the scope processor. It allows real-time magnification of the uppermost epithelial layer, allowing cytological and architectural assessment [22]. Methylene blue is commonly used as a contrast agent. Similar to confocal laser endomicroscopy (CLE), there are two systems developed: endoscope and probe-based. However, neither of these systems is currently available for clinical practice. There are limited data on the use of endocytoscopy in the upper GI tract, and most of the reported studies are pilot studies performed for lesion characterization in the esophagus [22, 23].

Confocal Endomicroscopy

Confocal imaging enhancement provides one of the highest resolution imaging of cellular and subcellular tissue within advanced imaging techniques. This confocal laser endomicroscopy (CLE) technology provides real-time in vivo magnification of the mucosa of up to 1,000-fold, allowing histological resolution or so called "virtual biopsies" of the gastrointestinal mucosa during endoscopy. The confocal imaging microscope can be found integrated into a conventional endoscope (eCLE) or as a probe (pCLE) that can be passed through the working channel of any endoscope.

Intravenous and topical contrast agents are used for fluorescence-based contrast-enhanced endomicroscopy. Intravenous fluorescein sodium is the most commonly used contrast agent. It has been proven safe with only rare (1.4 %) and minimal side effects, including nausea/vomiting, transient hypotension without shock, injection site erythema, diffuse rash, and mild epigastric pain [24].

A recent multicenter, randomized, controlled trial demonstrated that a target biopsy strategy by HDWLE and eCLE is superior to standard random biopsy strategy with HDWLE alone by increasing almost threefold the diagnostic yield of neoplasia in flat BE, while reducing the number of biopsies by half and maintaining similar accuracy [2]. Similarly, a combination of HDWLE, NBI and pCLE has proved to increase detection of neoplasia on BE [25] (Fig. 5.6).

In early gastric neoplasia, CLE has been found to have overall superior accuracy for the diagnosis of adenocarcinoma (91.7 % vs. 85.2 %; $p=0.031$) when compared to conventional biopsies after

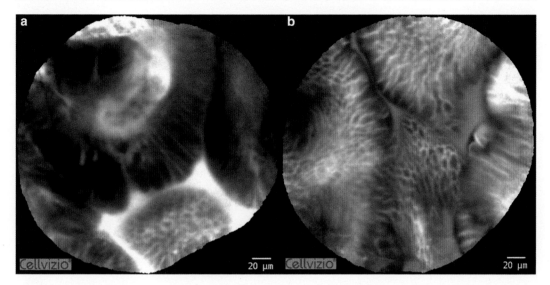

Fig. 5.6 (**a**) CLE of high-grade dysplasia in BE. Note the *dark*, thickened epithelium and dilated irregular vessels. (**b**) CLE of non-dysplastic BE. Note the villiform structure with thin, *grey* epithelium

ESD resection [26]. Therefore, CLE not only allows real-time virtual biopsies but can also reduce sampling error.

Electronic Imaging Technologies

Spectroscopy

Light-scattering spectroscopy (LSS) is a novel technique that uses the variation in scattered light across a full spectrum to obtain information about the number and the size of nuclei of the epithelial cell layer. Epithelial cell nuclei are the primary targets of reflected light that is single or multiple scattered (absorbed, re-emitted, or shifted to a different wavelength) before it is collected back into the probe [12, 27].

Spectroscopy can be an accurate method for the detection of dysplasia in Barrett's esophagus [28, 29]. LSS has been shown to have a sensitivity and specificity of 90 % for the detection of dysplasia [29]. Further research has suggested that this technology can be further used, in screening, to improve the accuracy of other advanced imaging modalities in the detection of dysplasia in Barrett's esophagus [30].

Optical Coherence Tomography

Optical coherence tomography (OCT) is an innovative wide-field imaging technique that allows high-resolution cross-sectional imaging of the mucosa, up to the level of low power microscopy. This technology is similar to ultrasound, but instead of processing acoustic signals it processes the path length of reflected light into an image [27].

A recent device has been approved for use in the United States (volumetric laser endomicroscopy; Ninepoint Medical, Cambridge, Mass) that provides resolution to 10 μm and imaging depth down to 3 mm scanning over a 6 cm length of esophagus over a period of 90 s [27]. This imaging modality is a great breakthrough technology, although more data and controlled studies are warranted for validation (Fig. 5.7).

FICE and iScan

Based on the same physical principles as NBI, both Fujinon (Flexible spectral imaging color enhancement (FICE)) and Pentax Corporation (iScan) have developed computed spectral

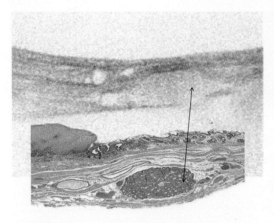

Fig. 5.7 Volumetric laser endomicroscopy with matching surgical resection showing BE with high-grade dysplasia and a large submucosal gland

estimation technology that is not dependent on optical filters within the light source of the videoendoscope to enhance certain wavelengths. Instead, these technologies take an ordinary white light endoscopic image from the video processor and arithmetically process the reflected photons to reconstitute virtual images, by increasing the relative intensity of narrowed blue light to a maximum and by decreasing narrowed red and green light to a minimum [31]. This leads to enhancement of the tissue microvasculature as a result of the differential optical absorption of light by hemoglobin in the mucosa.

Results of several studies using these alternative methods of virtual chromoendoscopy (VC) appear to be similar to those described for NBI in both esophageal and gastric cancer. However, no head-to-head studies have compared the available VC technologies (NBI vs. FICE vs. iScan).

Applications in Clinical Practice

While there have been major advancements in both technical development and assessment of advanced technologies for upper GI lesions, there are few guidelines as to how to integrate these systems into practice. A general concept has emerged of using "red-flag" imaging methods to enhance detection of early neoplasia, followed by

highly focused and magnified images to confirm, classify, and guide therapy. A practical example is Barrett's esophagus, where virtual chromoendoscopy, particularly NBI, is widely used to detect early neoplasia based on irregular vascular and surface patterns. This is followed by close inspection using magnification, confocal, or simply highly-targeted inspection. Based on the common macroscopic shape (Paris) and surface (NICE or Kudo) classification systems, albeit adapted to the upper GI tract, a decision can be made to biopsy, resect by EMR or ESD (early neoplasia), or refer to surgery (deeply invasive neoplasia).

Conclusions

The advanced endoscopist performing ESD has to become familiarized with the wide array of imaging alternatives available to enhance visualization of the upper GI tract. These modalities can aid the endoscopist at each stage of ESD. They can improve patient selection, can facilitate curative resection by improving margin demarcation, and even assist in identification of new lesions or even recurrence during surveillance. Some modalities, like chromoendoscopy and, more recently, virtual chromoendoscopy, have been widely adapted by most advanced endoscopists. However, newer technologies are being developed and might even substitute the need for biopsy. Therefore, the advanced endoscopist should be ready to incorporate, and most likely even combine, these new technologies to improve outcomes on their ESD practice.

References

1. Qumseya BJ, Wang H, Badie N, et al. Advanced imaging technologies increase detection of dysplasia and neoplasia in patients with Barrett's esophagus: a meta-analysis and systematic review. Clin Gastroenterol Hepatol. 2013;11:1562–70.e1-2.
2. Canto MI, Anandasabapathy S, Brugge W, et al. In vivo endomicroscopy improves detection of Barrett's esophagus-related neoplasia: a multicenter international randomized controlled trial (with video). Gastrointest Endosc. 2014;79:211–21.
3. Jang JY. The usefulness of magnifying endoscopy and narrow-band imaging in measuring the depth of

invasion before endoscopic submucosal dissection. Clin Endosc. 2012;45:379–85.

4. Kaltenbach T, Sano Y, Friedland S, Soetikno R. American Gastroenterological Association (AGA) Institute technology assessment on image-enhanced endoscopy. Gastroenterology. 2008;134:327–40.

5. Capelle LG, Haringsma J, de Vries AC, et al. Narrow band imaging for the detection of gastric intestinal metaplasia and dysplasia during surveillance endoscopy. Dig Dis Sci. 2010;55:3442–8.

6. Shahid MW, Buchner AM, Coron E, et al. Diagnostic accuracy of probe-based confocal laser endomicroscopy in detecting residual colorectal neoplasia after EMR: a prospective study. Gastrointest Endosc. 2012;75:525–33.

7. Wong Kee Song LM, Adler DG, Chand B, et al. Chromoendoscopy. Gastrointest Endosc. 2007;66:639–49.

8. Tanaka S, Kaltenbach T, Chayama K, Soetikno R. High-magnification colonoscopy (with videos). Gastrointest Endosc. 2006;64:604–13.

9. Saxena P, Canto MI. Red flag imaging techniques in Barrett's esophagus. Gastrointest Endosc Clin N Am. 2013;23:535–47.

10. Sakai Y, Eto R, Kasanuki J, et al. Chromoendoscopy with indigo carmine dye added to acetic acid in the diagnosis of gastric neoplasia: a prospective comparative study. Gastrointest Endosc. 2008;68:635–41.

11. Yamashita H, Kitayama J, Ishigami H, et al. Endoscopic instillation of indigo carmine dye with acetic acid enables the visualization of distinct margin of superficial gastric lesion; Usefulness in endoscopic treatment and diagnosis of gastric cancer. Dig Liver Dis. 2007;39:389–91.

12. Buchner AM, Wallace MB. Future expectations in digestive endoscopy: competition with other novel imaging techniques. Best Pract Res Clin Gastroenterol. 2008;22:971–87.

13. Wolfsen HC, Crook JE, Krishna M, et al. Prospective, controlled tandem endoscopy study of narrow band imaging for dysplasia detection in Barrett's Esophagus. Gastroenterology. 2008;135:24–31.

14. Sharma P, Hawes RH, Bansal A, et al. Standard endoscopy with random biopsies versus narrow band imaging targeted biopsies in Barrett's oesophagus: a prospective, international, randomised controlled trial. Gut. 2013;62:15–21.

15. Li HY, Ge ZZ, Fujishiro M, Li XB. Current clinical applications of magnifying endoscopy with narrow band imaging in the stomach. Diagn Ther Endosc. 2012;2012:271914.

16. Kiyotoki S, Nishikawa J, Satake M, et al. Usefulness of magnifying endoscopy with narrow-band imaging for determining gastric tumor margin. J Gastroenterol Hepatol. 2010;25:1636–41.

17. Nagahama T, Yao K, Maki S, et al. Usefulness of magnifying endoscopy with narrow-band imaging for determining the horizontal extent of early gastric cancer when there is an unclear margin by chromoendoscopy (with video). Gastrointest Endosc. 2011;74:1259–67.

18. Hayashi N, Tanaka S, Hewett DG, et al. Endoscopic prediction of deep submucosal invasive carcinoma: validation of the narrow-band imaging international colorectal endoscopic (NICE) classification. Gastrointest Endosc. 2013;78:625–32.

19. Boerwinkel DF, Holz JA, Kara MA, et al. Effects of autofluorescence imaging on detection and treatment of early neoplasia in patients with Barrett's esophagus. Clin Gastroenterol Hepatol. 2014;12:774.

20. Hanaoka N, Uedo N, Shiotani A, et al. Autofluorescence imaging for predicting development of metachronous gastric cancer after Helicobacter pylori eradication. J Gastroenterol Hepatol. 2010;25:1844–9.

21. Kato M, Uedo N, Ishihara R, et al. Analysis of the color patterns of early gastric cancer using an autofluorescence imaging video endoscopy system. Gastric Cancer. 2009;12:219–24.

22. Goetz M, Malek NP, Kiesslich R. Microscopic imaging in endoscopy: endomicroscopy and endocytoscopy. Nat Rev Gastroenterol Hepatol. 2014;11:11–8.

23. Kumagai Y, Kawada K, Yamazaki S, et al. Endocytoscopic observation for esophageal squamous cell carcinoma: can biopsy histology be omitted? Dis Esophagus. 2009;22:505–12.

24. Wallace MB, Meining A, Canto MI, et al. The safety of intravenous fluorescein for confocal laser endomicroscopy in the gastrointestinal tract. Aliment Pharmacol Ther. 2010;31:548–52.

25. Sharma P, Meining AR, Coron E, et al. Real-time increased detection of neoplastic tissue in Barrett's esophagus with probe-based confocal laser endomicroscopy: final results of an international multicenter, prospective, randomized, controlled trial. Gastrointest Endosc. 2011;74:465–72.

26. Jeon SR, Cho WY, Jin SY, Cheon YK, Choi SR, Cho JY. Optical biopsies by confocal endomicroscopy prevent additive endoscopic biopsies before endoscopic submucosal dissection in gastric epithelial neoplasias: a prospective, comparative study. Gastrointest Endosc. 2011;74:772–80.

27. ASGE Technology Committee. Enhanced imaging in the GI tract: spectroscopy and optical coherence tomography. Gastrointest Endosc. 2013;78:568–73.

28. Georgakoudi I, Jacobson BC, Van Dam J, et al. Fluorescence, reflectance, and light-scattering spectroscopy for evaluating dysplasia in patients with Barrett's esophagus. Gastroenterology. 2001;120:1620–9.

29. Wallace MB, Perelman LT, Backman V, et al. Endoscopic detection of dysplasia in patients with Barrett's esophagus using light-scattering spectroscopy. Gastroenterology. 2000;119:677–82.

30. Douplik A, Zanati S, Saiko G, et al. Diffuse reflectance spectroscopy in Barrett's Esophagus: developing a large field-of-view screening method discriminating dysplasia from metaplasia. J Biophotonics. 2014;7:304.

31. Pohl J, Nguyen-Tat M, Pech O, May A, Rabenstein T, Ell C. Computed virtual chromoendoscopy for classification of small colorectal lesions: a prospective comparative study. Am J Gastroenterol. 2008;103:562–9.

Advanced Endoscopic Imaging in the Lower GI Tract

Rajvinder Singh, Anja Landowski, and Mahesh Jayanna

Introduction

Gastrointestinal cancers are often preceded by a curable, non-invasive, premalignant stage that may progress asymptomatically. The transformation process begins with the formation of atypical cells in the epithelium, directly above the basal membrane. Early screening may enable detection of anomalies at very early stages before neoplasia permeates into the deeper submucosal layer and beyond. Morphological characteristics of the mucosa can then be interrogated to obtain further information, which may aid the endoscopist in deciding whether to proceed with endoscopic biopsies or resection.

Detection

Most newer electronic image enhancing modalities perform no better than white light endoscopy in the detection of colorectal neoplasia (Table 6.1). There is simply no substitute for good bowel preparation and a meticulous withdrawal technique, ensuring clear views are maintained to enable careful interrogation of mucosal folds.

R. Singh, M.B.B.S., F.R.A.C.P., F.R.C.P. (✉)
Lyell McEwin Hospital, Haydown Road,
Elizabeth Vale 5112, SA, Australia

University of Adelaide, Adelaide, SA, Australia

A. Landowski, M.D. • M. Jayanna, M.D.
Lyell McEwin Hospital,
Haydown Road, Elizabeth Vale 5112, SA, Australia

Characterization

Lesions which are detected should be interrogated further to gain additional information should be studied further to gain valuable information. Ideally, this is performed in a methodical manner, initially with a "wide field" overview of the lesion where the Paris classification and granularity are assessed, followed by a closer or "micro" or "magnified" view where the vascular patterns are visualised, with some of the electronic chromoendoscopy techniques. If further information is needed and where possible, the Kudo's pit pattern is assessed. In vivo classification of polyps using advanced imaging is important for two reasons: (1) the significant cost of histological examination of all polyps, particularly small low-risk lesions, has prompted consideration of a "diagnose, resect, and discard" strategy which could be cost effective, and (2) accurately differentiating invasive from non-invasive cancers may enable clinical decisions to be made in real time, thereby immediately guiding therapy.

Lesion Assessment with Wide Field View

Paris Japanese Classification
The Paris Japanese classification system is especially important not only for standardization but also because it allows prediction of submucosal invasion risk [9].

N. Fukami (ed.), *Endoscopic Submucosal Dissection: Principles and Practice*,
DOI 10.1007/978-1-4939-2041-9_6, © Springer Science+Business Media New York 2015

Table 6.1 Image enhanced endoscopy in detecting colorectal polyp

Author	Year	Technology	# of pts	Design	Result
Rex [1]	2007	NBI	434	RCT	–
Inoue [2]	2008	NBI	243	RCT	–
Adler [3]	2008	NBI	401	RCT	–
Matsuda [4]	2008	AFI	167	Random, Tandem	+
Pohl [5]	2008	FICE	764	RCT	–
Kaltenbach [6]	2008	NBI	276	Random, Tandem	–
Van Den Broek [7]	2009	AFI	100	Random, Tandem	–
Adler [8]	2009	NBI	1,256	RCT	–

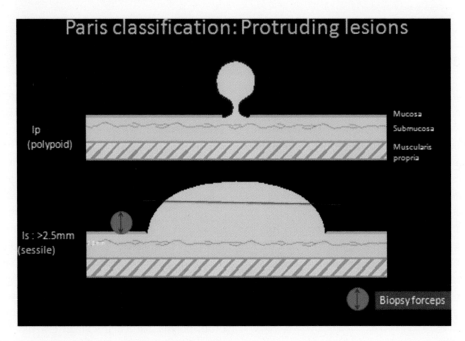

Fig. 6.1 Paris Japanese classification for protruding lesion

Polyps can be divided into:

1. Protruding lesions (Fig. 6.1)
   (a) Ip (peduncalated)
   (b) Is (sessile): >2.5 mm* from base of polyp (surrounding mucosa)
2. Flat lesions (Fig. 6.2)
   (a) IIa: Slightly elevated (<2.5 mm*)
   (b) IIb: True flat lesion
   (c) IIc: Mildly depressed lesion

*The 2.5 mm limit is used to differentiate sessile (Is) from flat (0-IIa) lesions and approximates the diameter of a closed biopsy forceps.

Flat colorectal lesions account for up to half of all colorectal polyps, while depressed lesions occur less frequently and account for about 1–3 % of all polyps (Table 6.2). The prevalence of high-grade dysplasia (HGD) or invasive cancer, however, increases as lesions become depressed (Paris IIc). Up to 59 % of all Paris type IIc lesions harbor HGD or submucosal invasion (SMI) (Table 6.3).

Large colorectal lesions (measuring >20 mm in size) are relatively infrequent and may account for up to 4 % of all polyps (Table 6.4). The size of the lesion does not appear to matter when lesions are assessed for SMI, though. Moss and colleagues prospectively assessed colorectal LSTs in a large cohort of Australian patients; SMI was detected in 33/514 (6.4 %) polyps. The mean size of these pol-

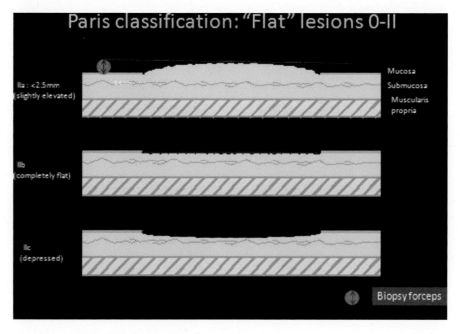

Fig. 6.2 Paris Japanese classification for flat lesions

Table 6.2 Percentage of flat-depressed colorectal lesions

Author	No. of adenomas	% of flat lesions
Jaramillo [10]	261	42
Rembacken [11]	321	36
Saitoh [12]	136	40
Rex [1]	785	56
Okuno [13]	66,670	1.9
Togashi [14]	5,408	2.8
Soetikno [15]	1,535	1.2
Tsuda [15]	973	1.4

yps was 35.3 mm, in comparison to 35.6 mm when no SMI was detected ($p=0.87$) [18].

Granularity

Flat lesions >20 mm should be further evaluated based on the granularity of the surface. They can be divided into granular (G), non-granular (NG), or a mixed pattern which contains both morphologies. The surface of G lesions appears ragged and almost polypoid ("lumpy bumpy"), whereas NG lesions have a smooth, elevated, and almost seamless surface. Lesion which are

non granular and depressed has the highest role of SMI (upto 54×) compared to granular, flat, non-depressed lesions [18].

Lesions Assessment on Closer "Micro" View

Kudo's Pit Pattern

The introduction of Kudo's pit pattern (KPP) led to a paradigm shift of how colorectal polyps are assessed [19]. Pit pattern visualization has enabled polyp histology to be predicted in real time. Some of the dyes used during evaluation include:

1. Indigo carmine (0.2 %), which is a surface contrast agent
2. Methylene blue (4–5 %), which is absorbed actively into the mucosa
3. Crystal violet (0.2 %), which is an absorptive dye that is generally used in exceptional cases where KPP type V needs to be defined further

The pit pattern of lesions are best visualized using high definition scopes with either digital or

Table 6.3 Prevalence of HGD and SMI in colorectal polyps according to Paris Japanese classification

	HGD			SMI		
Author	Ip	IIa/b	IIc	Ip	IIa	IIc
Rembacken [11]	7.4 %	12.8 %	25 %	0.9 %	1.7 %	50 %
Soetikno [15]	0.5 %	3.5 %	225	0.5 %	1.0 %	11 %
Tsuda [16]	7.3 %	12.8 %	35.7 %	–	–	–
Hurlstone [17]	12 %	15.4 %	59 %	–	–	–

Table 6.4 Comparison of Paris Japanese classification and size

	Total	≤5 mm	6–10 mm	11–19 mm	≥20 mm
Polypoid (Is, Ip)	14,814	47.6 %	37.7 %	12.6 %	2.1 %
Flat (IIa, IIb)	10,363	73.1 %	13.9 %	9.0 %	4.0 %
Flat-depressed (IIc)	585	45.0 %	29.4 %	21.7 %	3.9 %
Total	24,862	14,892	7,190	2,919	761

Adapted from Kudo SE, Lambert R, Allen J et al. Nonpolypoid neoplastic lesions of the colorectal mucosa. Gastrointest Endosc 2008; 4: Suppl 3

Table 6.5 Comparison of various endoscopic techniques in predicting colorectal neoplasia

Technique	#Studies	#Polyps	Sensitivity	Specificity	Area under ROC
Standard	8	1,493	71.3	81.4	0.80
Chromoendoscopy	11	3,097	88.6	85.0	0.87
Magnification	4	1,108	81.5	79.7	0.87
Magnification +Chromo	21	21,446	97.1	74.3	0.95
Magnification +NBI	10	1,016	88.5	80.0	0.91

Adapted from Subramaniam V, Mannath J, Ragunath K et al. Gastrointest Endosc Vol. 69, Issue 5, Page AB277

optical magnification (80–115×) [20]. The different types of pits can be summarized as follows:

1. Type I: Pits appears round—normal colonic mucosa
2. Type II: Pits appear star or "onion skin" like—hyperplastic polyps
3. Type III$_L$ or III$_S$: Elongated or small round pits, respectively—tubular adenomas
4. Type IV: Cerebreform pits—tubular, villous or tubulovillous
5. Type V$_I$: Irregular (I) asymmetrical pits indicating malignancy confined to the mucosa (suitable for endoscopic resection)

Type V$_N$: Pit patterns disappear, non-structured (N) or "structure-less"—advanced or signifying invasive cancer (avoid endoscopic resection, surgery recommended)

A systematic review looked at more than 50 studies comparing the accuracy of standard white light endoscopy, chromoendoscopy, white light endoscopy with magnification, chromoendoscopy with magnification, and narrow band imaging (NBI) with magnification in the prediction of colorectal polyp histology (Table 6.5) [21]. The authors found that chromoendoscopy and virtual chromoendoscopy (NBI), both with optical magnification, were the most effective methods for predicting polyp histology resulting in an area under the ROC of more than 0.90.

Electronic Chromoendoscopy

Some of the electronic chromoendoscopy technologies that are now widely available include NBI (Olympus), I-scan (Pentax) or the Flexible spectral Imaging Color enhancement (FICE, Fujinon). All these imaging modalities assist in defining the microvascular architecture in colorectal polyps [22–24]. There have been numerous classifications utilized which at times can be confusing. These are based on the presence or absence of superficial meshed capillary vessels, which will be explained here in more detail.

Sano Classification

The Sano classification system is based on inspection of the microvascular architecture on the surface of polyps [25]. The microvascular architecture (capillary pattern) was classified into *I*, *II*, *IIIA*, or *IIIB*. *Type I* pattern is characterized by meshed capillary vessels being visually unidentifiable, and is mostly observed in hyperplastic polyps. *Type II*, mostly observed in adenomas, is characterized by meshed capillary vessels that are clearly visualized and surrounds mucosal glands. *Type III*, mostly observed in carcinomas, is characterized by meshed capillary vessels, which shows features of branching, irregularity and occasionally avascularity. *Type III* is divided into two subtypes: *Type IIIA* that is characterized by high microvessel density with lack of uniformity, and *Type IIIB* that is characterized by the presence of avascular areas. *Type IIIB* is observed in deep submucosal-invasive carcinomas [26].

In a preliminary feasibility study using the Sano classification system, the sensitivity (Sn), specificity (Sp), positive (PPV), and negative predictive values (NPV) in differentiating neoplastic from non-neoplastic lesions with high confidence was 98 %, 89 %, 93 %, and 97 %, respectively, whilst the Sn, Sp, PPV, and NPV in predicting endoscopic resectability (*Type II/IIIa* vs. *Type I/IIIb*) was 100 %, 90 %, 93 % and 100 %, respectively [27]. The interobserver agreement between assessors (*k* value) was also substantial at 0.89.

Hiroshima Classification

The Hiroshima classification system is based on both the surface pattern and the microvasculature of colorectal lesions [28]. These features are classified as *Types A*, *B* and *C*, on the basis of both their surface pattern and microvascular architecture.

Lesions are classified as *Type A* when microvessels are not visible or are extremely opaque, *Type B* when a regular surface pattern or a regular meshed capillary network is observed, or as *Type C* when an irregular surface pattern with no particular structure is observed. *Type C* is comprised of three subtypes (*C1*, *C2* and *C3*), according to the surface pattern and the detailed magnifying NBI depiction of microvessel diameter, degree of irregularity, and microvessel distribution. Lesions are classified as *Type C1* when the microvessel network is irregular, when the surface pattern is somewhat non-distinct, and when microvessel diameter or distribution is uniform (mostly in intramucosal or superficial submucosal invasion); *Type C2* when the microvessel network is irregular and the surface pattern is irregular because of increased microvessel intensity around the pits, and vessel diameter or distribution is not uniform; and the *Type C3* pattern when the surface pattern is not clear, microvessels are thick, or vessel distribution is not uniform with avascular areas being visualized. *Type C2* and *C3* patterns signify invasive cancers.

Showa Classification

The Showa classification is based on the evaluation of the microvascular architecture [29]. This classification does not use the symbols such as type I or type A for categorization. The evaluated data are categorized according to the findings of vessel changes and classified into six categories: *normal*, *faint*, *network*, *dense*, *irregular*, and *sparse* pattern.

The *faint* pattern is characterized by an inability to identify microvessels surrounding the gland, and is mostly observed in hyperplastic polyps. The *network* pattern is characterized by regular meshed microvessels surrounding glands, and is observed in tubular adenomas. The *dense* pattern is characterized by thick and dense microvessels surrounding glands, and is observed in villous/tubulovillous adenomas and intramucosal carcinomas (though mostly in villous/tubulovillous adenoma). The *irregular* pattern is characterized by microvessels that are irregular, have large calibers, and are highly tortuous; whilst the *sparse* pattern is characterized by avascular areas due to underlying desmoplastic reactions. Both patterns can be observed in deep SM-invasive carcinomas.

NICE Classification

The NICE classification was established by an international cooperative group (Colon Tumor NBI Interest Group—CTNIG) including Japanese, American, French, and British endoscopists in an effort to unify the above classifications [30, 31]. It is based on the evaluation of the following three characteristics: color, vessel, and surface pattern. The NICE classification has been advocated to be user friendly with both conventional or magnified views. It consists of three patterns.

Type 1 is characterized by the color being the same or lighter than the background, no or isolated lacy vessels, and a surface pattern which is dark or has white spots of uniform size, or even a homogeneous absence of pattern. This pattern is typically seen in hyperplastic lesions. *Type 2* is characterized by the color being browner relative to the background, a lesion demonstrating thick brown vessels surrounding white structures with a surface pattern being oval, tubular or branched white structures surrounded by the vessels described above (adenomas). *Type 3* is characterized by the color being brown to dark brown relative to the background; markedly distorted or missing vessels, and areas showing distortion or absence of surface pattern. *Type 3* is considered an index for deeply SM-invasive carcinoma. Although more simplistic, this classification, unfortunately, does not address sessile serrated adenomas/polyps.

Currently, there are no comparative data looking at the diagnostic accuracy amongst all of these classifications. It is therefore difficult to objectively comment on the advantage of each of these classifications, although it may be prudent to adopt any one of them while assessing colonic neoplasia.

Conclusions

Advanced endoscopic imaging and a step-by-step methodological approach as described above can often aid in the characterization of colorectal polyps before a decision is made to proceed with endoscopic resection. This includes looking at the lesion from afar, where the gross morphology and granularity is determined, followed by assessing the vasculature, and when in doubt, the pit pattern. This sequential method of assessment will enable a calculated and precise decision to be made in real time as to whether endoscopic resection can be performed safely and adequately.

References

1. Rex DK, Helbig CC. High yields of small and flat adenomas with high definition colonoscopes using either white light or narrow band imaging. Gastroenterology. 2007;133:42–7.
2. Inoue T, Murano M, Murano N, et al. Comparative study of conventional and pan colonic narrow band imaging system in the detection of neoplastic colonic polyps: a randomised controlled trial. J Gastroenterol. 2008;43(1):45–50.
3. Adler A, Pohl H, Papanikolaou I, et al. A prospective study on Narrow Band Imaging versus conventional colonoscopy for adenoma detection: does NBI induce a learning effect? Gut. 2008;57(1):59–64.
4. Matsuda T, Saito Y, Fu KL, et al. Does Autofluorescence imaging videoendoscopy system improve the colonoscopic polyp detection rate? A pilot study. Am J Gastroenterol. 2008;103(8):1926–32.
5. Pohl J, Lotterer E, Balzer C, et al. Computed virtual colonoscopy versus standard colonoscopy with targeted indigo carmine chromoendoscopy: a randomised multicentre trial. Gut. 2009;58(1):73–8.
6. Kaltenbach T, Friedland S, Soetikno R, et al. A randomised tandem colonoscopy trial of narrow band imaging versus white light examination to compare neoplasia miss rates. Gut. 2008;57(10):1406–12.
7. Adler A, Aschenbeck J, Yenerim T, et al. Narrowband versus white-light high definition television endoscopic imaging for screening colonoscopy: a prospective randomised trial. Gastroenterology. 2009;136(2):410–6.
8. van den Broek FJ, van Soest EJ, Naber AH, et al. Combining autofluorescence imaging and narrowband imaging for the differentiation of adenomas from non-neoplastic colonic polyps among experienced and non-experienced endoscopists. Am J Gastroenterol. 2009;104(6):1498–507.
9. Endoscopic Classification Review Group. Update on the Paris Classification of superficial neoplastic lesions in the digestive tract. Endoscopy. 2005;37:570–8.
10. Jaramillo E, Watanabe M, Slezak P, et al. Flat neoplastic lesions of the colon and rectum detected by high-resolution video endoscopy and chromoscopy. Gastrointest Endosc. 1995;42:114–22.

11. Rembacken BJ, Fujii T, Cairns A, et al. Flat and depressed colonic neoplasms: a prospective study of 1000 colonoscopies in the UK. Lancet. 2000;355:1211–4.

12. Saitoh Y, Waxman I, West AB, et al. Prevalence and distinctive biologic features of flat colorectal adenomas in a North American population. Gastroenterology. 2001;120:1657–65.

13. Okuno T, Sano Y, Ohkura Y, et al. Incidence and clinicopathological characteristics of depressed type lesions: base line findings of multicenter retrospective cohort study [in Japanese]. Ear Color Cancer. 2004;8:21–7.

14. Togashi K, Konishi F, Koinuma K, et al. Flat and depressed lesions of the colon and rectum: pathogenesis and clinical management. Ann Acad Med Singapore. 2003;32:152–8.

15. Soetikno RM, Kaltenbach T, Rouse RV, et al. Prevalence of nonpolypoid (flat and depressed) colorectal neoplasms in asymptomatic and symptomatic adults. JAMA. 2008;299:1027–35.

16. Tsuda S, Veress B, Toth E, et al. Flat and depressed colorectal tumours in a southern Swedish population: a prospective chromoendoscopic and histopathological study. Gut. 2002;51:550–5.

17. Hurlstone DP, Cross SS, Adam I, et al. A prospective clinicopathological and endoscopic evaluation of flat and depressed colorectal lesions in the United Kingdom. Am J Gastroenterol. 2003;98:2543–9.

18. Moss A, Bourke MJ, Williams SJ, Hourigan L, Brown G, Tam W, Singh R, et al. Endoscopic mucosal resection outcomes and prediction of submucosal cancer from advanced colonic mucosa. Gastroenterology. 2011;140:1909–18.

19. Kudo S, Hirota S, Nakajima T, et al. Colorectal tumours and pit patterns. J Clin Pathol. 1994;47:880–5.

20. Singh R, Owen V, Shonde A, et al. White light endoscopy, narrow band imaging and chromoendoscopy with magnification in diagnosing colorectal neoplasia. World J Gastrointest Endosc. 2009;1(1):45–50.

21. Subramaniam V, Mannath J, Ragunath K, et al. Utility of Kudo Pit Pattern for Distinguishing adenomatous from non adenomatous colonic lesions in vivo: meta-analysis of different endoscopic techniques. Gastrointest Endosc. 2009;69(5):AB277.

22. Singh R, Kaye PV, Ragunath K. Distinction between neoplastic and non neoplastic colorectal polyps utilizing Narrow Band Imaging with magnification: a novel technique to increase the efficacy of colorectal cancer screening? Scand J Gastroenterol. 2008;43(3):380–1.

23. Hoffman A, Kagel C, Goetz M, Tresch A, Mudter J, Biesterfeld S, Galle PR, Neurath MF, Kiesslich R. Recognition and characterization of small colonic neoplasia with high-definition colonoscopy using i-Scan is as precise as Chromoendoscopy. Dig Liver Dis. 2010;42:45–50.

24. Togashi K, Osawa H, Koinuma K, Hayashi Y, Miyata T, Sunada K, Nokubi M, Horie H, Yamamoto H. A comparison of conventional endoscopy, Chromoendoscopy, and the optimal-band imaging system for the differentiation of neoplastic and non-neoplastic colonic polyps. Gastrointest Endosc. 2009;69:734–41.

25. Uraoka T, Saito Y, Ikematsu H, et al. Sano's capillary pattern classification for narrow-band imaging of early colorectal lesions. Dig Endosc. 2011;23 Suppl 1:112–5.

26. Ikematsu H, Matsuda T, Emura F, Saito Y, Uraoka T, Fu KI, Kaneko K, Ochiai A, Fujimori T, Sano Y. Efficacy of capillary pattern type IIIA/IIIB by magnifying narrow band imaging for estimating depth of invasion of early colorectal neoplasms. BMC Gastroenterol. 2010;10:33.

27. Singh R, Nordeen N, Mei SL, et al. West meets East: preliminary results of Narrow band Imaging with optical magnification in the diagnosis of colorectal lesions: a multicentre Australian study using the modified Sano's classification. Dig Endosc. 2011;23 Suppl 1:126–30.

28. Oka S, Tanaka S, Takata S, et al. Clinical usefulness of narrow band imaging magnifying classification for colorectal tumors based on both surface pattern and microvessel features. Dig Endosc. 2011;23 Suppl 1:101–5.

29. Wada Y, Kudo SE, Misawa M, et al. Vascular pattern classification of colorectal lesions with narrow band imaging magnifying endoscopy. Dig Endosc. 2011;23 Suppl 1:106–11.

30. Hewett DG, Kaltenbach T, Sano Y, et al. Validation of simple classification system for endoscopic diagnosis of small colorectal polyps using narrow band imaging. Gastroenterology. 2012;143(3):599–607.

31. Tanaka S, Sano Y. Aim to unify the narrow band imaging (NBI) magnifying classification for colorectal tumors: current status in Japan from a summary of consensus symposium in the 79th annual meeting at the Japan Gastroenterological Endoscopy Society. Dig Endosc. 2011;23 suppl 1:131–9.

Part IV

Procedure

Injection Material for ESD: Eastern Perspective

Keiko Niimi, Mitsuhiro Fujishiro,
and Kazuhiko Koike

Introduction

To carry out safe ESD, selecting the proper injection solution to be used prior to mucosal incision is very important. Two main aspects concerning submucosal fluid cushions (SFC) have to be considered: lifting ability and tissue damage. It is necessary to create a prominent and long-lasting mucosal elevation. The duration of lesion lifting is crucial for successful results. Physiologic saline solution dissipates quickly when injected into the submucosal layer, with the consequent rapid disappearance of the mucosal elevation; whereas viscous solutions, such as sodium hyaluronate (SH), methylcellulose (MC), and fibrinogen mixtures, create a long-lasting submucosal cushion because of their viscosity. The more viscous a solution for submucosal injection is, the longer the submucosal fluid cushion lasts. Various solutions for submucosal injection, such as glycerin mixtures, sodium

hyaluronate, and normal saline (NS), have been used in Japan. Although hypertonic fluids may be better for creating higher lift and obtaining effective hemostasis, because of high osmolality, potential tissue damage must be considered. By taking into account the advantages and disadvantages of each injection solution for each specific situation, performance of successful ESD is possible.

Tissue Damage

ESD is a local resection without removal of any lymph nodes. It is necessary to make a histological evaluation and determine whether the lesion's resection was curative. Tissue damage has to be considered, firstly, because the purpose of endoscopic resection is to confirm the nature of a lesion by histology. If the submucosal injection solution has properties that can damage the resected specimen, it may be difficult to make a precise histological diagnosis of the targeted lesion. Furthermore, tissue damage of the muscle layer may result in delayed bleeding or perforation, especially in those cases occurring in the thinner gut wall, such as the esophagus or the large and small intestines.

In the 2000s, normal saline (NS), hypertonic saline (HS), 20 and 50 % dextrose water (DW), 10 % glycerin and 5 % fructose in a normal saline solution (Glyceol), and sodium hyaluronate (SH) were widely used as common submucosal injection solutions in Japanese clinical practice.

K. Niimi, M.D., Ph.D. (✉) • M. Fujishiro, M.D., Ph.D.
Department of Endoscopy and Endoscopic Surgery,
Graduate School of Medicine, The University of Tokyo
7-3-1, Hongo, Bunkyo-ku, Tokyo 113-8655, Japan

Department of Gastroenterology, Graduate School
of Medicine, The University of Tokyo,
7-3-1, Hongo, Bunkyo-ku, Tokyo 113-8655, Japan
e-mail: k-niimi@umin.ac.jp

K. Koike, M.D., Ph.D.
Department of Gastroenterology, Graduate School
of Medicine, The University of Tokyo,
7-3-1, Hongo, Bunkyo-ku, Tokyo 113-8655, Japan

N. Fukami (ed.), *Endoscopic Submucosal Dissection: Principles and Practice*,
DOI 10.1007/978-1-4939-2041-9_7, © Springer Science+Business Media New York 2015

In a previous study [1], there were no apparent mucosal changes seen endoscopically by NS, Glyceol, and SH solutions. Hypertonic solutions, except Glyceol, can have greater or lesser degrees of tissue damage. Mucosal erosion and shallow ulceration were formed a day after injection and were persistent a week after injection of HS, 20 and 50 % DW. Moreover, neither NS, Glyceol, nor SH solutions caused any apparent tissue damage as seen by histology. In HS and 20 % DW, acute mucosal erosion with degradation of epithelial glands and congestion of capillary blood vessels was observed on the day of injection, and was persistent as mucosal erosion with fibrosis of the submucosal layer a week after injection. With 50 % DW, not only mucosal damage but also muscle damage emerged on the day of injection, and ulceration extending to the submucosal layer was formed a week after injection. Therefore, NS, Glyceol, and SH solutions are most desirable when taking tissue damage into consideration.

Mucosal Lifting Duration

The most effective and simplest way to prevent complications, especially perforation, is to maintain a thick submucosal layer with sufficient SFC. A long-lasting SFC is beneficial for performance of ESD. Moreover, the application of an adequate SFC into the submucosa is essential to prevent not only perforation during ESD but also cautery effect on specimens.

In our previous study [2], the elevation created by SH solution was significantly greater than that produced by NS, HS, or 20 % DW. There were no significant differences among the other solutions, although NS tended to produce less elevation than the three hypertonic solutions, and Glyceol tended to produce greater elevation than the other hypertonic solutions. Moreover, when assessed over time, SH solution maintained a greater degree of elevation than the others at all times. Hypertonic solutions maintained an intermediate degree of mucosal elevation between those achieved by NS and SH. No differences were evident between the three hypertonic solutions, although Glyceol

tended to maintain a greater mucosal elevation until 10 min after injection. The elevation produced by NS was less than that of the three hypertonic solutions at all times, but there was no significant difference. Therefore, SH is desirable considering mucosal lifting ability.

Characteristics of Various Solutions

Normal Saline Solution (NS, 0.9 % NaCl)

Normal saline solution is an isotonic solution that is commonly used for SFC. It does not cause any apparent tissue damage as seen by histology. However, NS diffuses quickly when injected into the submucosa with the consequent rapid disappearance of mucosal elevation. Low elevation makes treatment difficult, and burning of the muscularis propria can cause perforation. NS has been widely used for endoscopic mucosal resection (EMR) using high-frequency snares. However, NS might not be the right choice for ESD, which is a much more time-consuming procedure than EMR.

Hypertonic Saline (HS, 3.75 % NaCl)

Hypertonic saline solution is longer lasting compared to NS, but still insufficient for long operations. An expedited approach to the targeted area and repeated injection for extensive resection are required. Moreover, HS may cause mucosal damage because of its high osmolarity. Thus, HS might not be proper for ESD.

Dextrose Water (DW)

Tissue damage and lesion-lifting ability differ according to the concentration of DW. Isotonicity with extracellular fluid is obtained by using a 5 % solution.

In our previous study [1], at 5 and 10 % DW, there were no apparent mucosal changes seen by endoscopy. Mucosal erosion and shallow ulceration were formed a day after injection and were persistent a week after injection of 20, 30, 40, and 50 % DW. Moreover, neither 5 nor 10 % DW caused any apparent tissue damage, as seen by histology. With 15 % DW, slight degradation of epithelial glands with mild congestion of capillary blood vessels in the superficial mucosal layer was observed on the day of injection, whereas there was no tissue damage a week after injection. With 20 % DW, acute mucosal erosion with degradation of epithelial glands and congestion of capillary blood vessels was observed on the day of injection, and these damages were persistent as mucosal erosion with fibrosis of the submucosal layer a week after injection. With 30, 40, and 50 % DW, not only damage of the mucosa but also the muscle emerged on the day of injection, and ulceration extending to the submucosal layer was apparent a week after injection. Therefore, 15 % dextrose may cause mucosal damage, although 5 and 10 % DW solutions do not cause any apparent tissue damage as seen by histology. Therefore, concentrations lower than 15 % DW, which has an osmotic pressure three times higher than extracellular fluid, are recommended for submucosal injection with respect to tolerable tissue damage. However, in the same way as HS, DW is still insufficient for longer operations. An expedited approach to the target area and repeated injection for extensive resection are required. Thus, DW might not be proper for ESD.

Glyceol (10 % Glycerin and 5 % Fructose in a Normal Saline Solution)

Glycerin is a hypertonic solution that is widely used in Japan for the treatment of intracranial hypertension as an intravenous drip infusion. It is speculated that Glyceol does not cause any apparent tissue damage because glycerin can pass freely through the cell membrane, since the osmotic pressure difference between the inside and outside of the cell membrane is only generated by the addition of non-destructive 5 % fructose. On the contrary, because the osmotic pressure of Glyceol is approximately seven times higher than extracellular fluid, Glyceol has the ability to produce sufficient submucosal cushion [2]. Also, the cost of Glyceol is less expensive than SH. Considering both cost and benefit, Glyceol is good to use for ESD, however, Glyceol has yet to be approved by the Japanese health insurance system as an injection solution for endoscopic treatment.

Sodium Hyaluronate (SH) (Mucoup; an 800 kDa Preparation)

Sodium hyaluronate is an isotonic solution. It is a thick substance with high viscosity that is widely found in human connective tissues and body fluids. SH is physicochemically water-retentive and viscoelastic, and is thus clinically used as a safe intra-articular injection preparation or as an auxiliary compound in cataract surgery. SH maintains mucosal elevation better than other solutions. Because it is highly viscoelastic, even at concentrations up to 1 %, SH does not increase osmotic pressure and is not antigenic or toxic in humans. Only minor adverse effects have been reported in clinical use [3–5]. There is seemingly only one disadvantage to SH solutions, though it is crucial, and that is the high cost.

Mucoup (800 kDa preparation; Johnson & Johnson, Tokyo, Japan or Seikagaku Corporation, Tokyo, Japan) is a 0.4 % SH solution that was approved by the Japanese Health Insurance System as an injection solution for EMR in the stomach and colon in 2007. It costs 7,700 yen for 20 ml in Japan, compared to 61 yen for 20 ml of NS. SH is very useful for ESD, considering ease of handling, mucosal elevation duration and high protrusion ability [6]. Moreover, when considering cost effectiveness, a mixture of SH and glycerin or NS might be better for ESD in clinical practice [7–9]. We recommend a 0.2 % hyaluronic acid solution (twofold diluted Mucoup® with normal saline) or a 0.1 % hyaluronic acid solution (fourfold diluted Mucoup® with Glyceol), according to availability, as the basic injection solutions for normal lesions. When there is a need for increased mucosal elevation, we recommend an undiluted solution of 0.4 % hyaluronic acid preparation.

Methylcellulose (MC)

Hydroxypropyl methylcellulose (HPMC) and sodium carboxymethylcellulose (SCMC) are available cellulose derivatives. HPMC, which is used as an aid for certain ophthalmic operations such as cataract removal, lens implantation, artificial tears, and as a matrix for controlled drug release, has viscoelastic characteristics similar to SH. In contrast to SH, HPMC is readily available, inexpensive, and a viscous material that, when diluted, provides a dependably long-lasting submucosal fluid cushion [10]. In the United States, HPMC has been used as the standard SFC for EMR in clinical practice.

SCMC is a water-soluble polymer derived from cellulose. It is widely used in food, cosmetics, and pharmaceuticals, and is commonly known as a cellulose gum with high viscosity when dissolved in water. A submucosal injection of SCMC solution has been used to dissect the mucosal layer from the muscular layer without complications such as massive bleeding or perforation. Submucosal injection of SCMC dissects most of the mucosal layer from the muscular layer, with no connective tissue of the submucosal layer. Because a SCMC solution with a viscosity above 200 mPa does not diffuse after injection into the submucosal layer, injection of a viscous SCMC solution into the submucosal layer dissects the mucosal layer from the muscular layer bluntly by the mechanical pressure of expansion [11]. Thus, ESD with submucosal injection of a viscous SCMC solution appears to be a safe and technically efficient method for dissection. SCMC is neither a primary irritant nor a sensitizing agent, and it is neither antigenic nor toxic to human beings [12, 13]. However, injection of viscous solutions through a 21-gauge needle is difficult, so development of a special injection needle is necessary.

Although MC is a suitable alternative for SH, there is some concern for use in humans, especially in Japan, as such a non-mammalian product may be antigenic in humans.

Proper SFC Use Depending on the Situation

Many different injection solutions have been invented for use in ESD, as the technique has progressed so quickly. Each SFC has advantages and disadvantages, as shown in Table 7.1. Although SH is expensive compared to other injection solutions, it is one of the best injection solutions available because it creates higher mucosal elevation and obtains such elevation for long periods. It is important for us to use SFCs based on the specific situation, such as which devices are being used, which organ, specific location and characteristics of lesions, and experiences of operators.

Locations

Any tissue damage to the muscle layer may result in delayed bleeding or perforation, especially in the case of the thin gut wall. Enough mucosal lifting is necessary to perform ESD safely, especially where the gut wall is thinner. The walls of the esophagus and colon are thinner than that of the stomach. Thus, SH is suitable for injection in

Table 7.1 Comparison of various injection solutions

		Osmolarity rate	PH	Tissue damage	Mucosal lifting ability	Cost	Hemostatic effect
Carious solutions	HS	4	4.5–8.0	+	+	Cheap	+
	20 % DW	4	3.5–6.5	+	+	Cheap	+
	50 % DW	10	3.5–6.5	++	++	Cheap	++
Non-carious solutions	NS	1	4.5–8.0	–	–	Cheap	–
	Glyceol	7.0	3.0–6.0	–	++	Cheap	++
	SH	1–1.2	7.0–8.0	–	+++	Expensive	–

the esophagus and colon. For the stomach, SH is desirable, especially in the upper third of the stomach, whereas Glyceol, which is a hypertonic solution that causes less tissue damage, might be permissible throughout.

Lesions

Submucosal fibrosis, which usually results from inflammation or tumor invasion, makes it more difficult to lift tumor tissue from the muscle layer. This in turn lengthens procedure time, creating a greater risk for complications such as perforation, and reduces the success rate of complete en bloc resection. Submucosal injection with NS may not achieve adequate lifting in cases with submucosal fibrosis; however, SH may be a good choice in cases with submucosal fibrosis because it does not cause tissue damage, and because of its high viscosity it has the ability to maintain submucosal lifting.

Operators

A relationship between complete resection and the experience of the endoscopist has been reported [6]. Even less experienced endoscopists could achieve a high rate of complete resection using SH injection for EMR, similar to skilled endoscopists. It takes a long time for less experienced endoscopists to perform ESD. When using a short-lasting injection solution, it is necessary to work fast after submucosal injection or to inject frequently in order to complete ESD. SH is effective for maintaining a long duration of mucosal elevation. Thus, less-experienced endoscopists should use SH for ESD, as this facilitates sustained mucosal elevation and definitive en bloc resection and prevents perforation.

Conclusion

Injection materials for ESD have been discussed in terms of an Eastern perspective. Among available solutions, sodium hyaluronate may be the best SFC with regards to minimal tissue damage and lesion-lifting ability. If the cost of SH solution is unacceptable, Glyceol is more readily available and may be a practical alternative too. However, attention needs to be given to the potential tissue damage caused by such hypertonic solutions. A combination of high-molecular-weight SH and Glyceol is ideal for submucosal injection, with acceptable cost, considering the viscoelasticity and hypertonicity of SH for creating sufficient lesion-lifting effects without causing tissue damage.

References

1. Fujishiro M, Yahagi N, Kashimura K, Matsuura T, Nakamura M, Kakushima N, Kodashima S, Ono S, Kobayashi K, Hashimoto T, Yamamichi N, Tateishi A, Shimizu Y, Oka M, Ichinose M, Omata M. Tissue damage of different submucosal injection solutions for EMR. Gastrointest Endosc. 2005;62:933–42.
2. Fujishiro M, Yahagi N, Kashimura K, Mizushima Y, Oka M, Enomoto S, Kakushima N, Kobayashi K, Hashimoto T, Iguchi M, Shimizu Y, Ichinose M, Omata M. Comparison of various submucosal injection solutions for maintaining mucosal elevation during endoscopic mucosal resection. Endoscopy. 2004; 36:579–83.
3. Hirasaki S, Kozu T, Yamamoto H, Sano Y, Yahagi N, Oyama T, Shimoda T, Sugano K, Tajiri H, Takekoshi T, Saito D. Usefulness and safety of 0.4% sodium hyaluronate solution as a submucosal fluid "cushion" for endoscopic resection of colorectal mucosal neoplasms: a prospective multi-center open-label trial. BMC Gastroenterol. 2009;9:1.
4. Yamamoto H, Yahagi N, Oyama T, Gotoda T, Doi T, Hirasaki S, Shimoda T, Sugano K, Tajiri H, Takekoshi T, Saito D. Usefulness and safety of 0.4% sodium hyaluronate solution as a submucosal fluid "cushion" in endoscopic resection for gastric neoplasms: a prospective multicenter trial. Gastrointest Endosc. 2008; 67(6):830–9.
5. Yamamoto H, Yube T, Isoda N, Sato Y, Sekine Y, Higashizawa T, Ido K, Kimura K, Kanai N. A novel method of endoscopic mucosal resection using sodium hyaluronate. Gastrointest Endosc. 1999;50(2): 251–6.
6. Onaya J, Yoshioka Z, Zuinen R, Hoshino J, Minamisawa Y, Takahashi T, Yamamoto H. Evaluation of hyaluronan as an endoscopic submucosal injectant. Endosc Diges. 2008;20:242–8.
7. Fujishiro M, Yahagi N, Kashimura K, Mizushima Y, Oka M, Matsuura T, Enomoto S, Kakushima N, Imagawa A, Kobayashi K, Hashimoto T, Iguchi M, Shimizu Y, Ichinose M, Omata M. Different mixtures

of sodium hyaluronate and their ability to create submucosal fluid cushions for endoscopic mucosal resection. Endoscopy. 2004;36(7):584–9.

8. Fujishiro M, Yahagi N, Nakamura M, Kakushima N, Kodashima S, Ono S, Kobayashi K, Hashimoto T, Yamamichi N, Tateishi A, Shimizu Y, Oka M, Ogura K, Kawabe T, Ichinose M, Omata M. Successful outcomes of a novel endoscopic treatment for GI tumors: endoscopic submucosal dissection with a mixture of high-molecular-weight hyaluronic acid, glycerin, and sugar. Gastrointest Endosc. 2006; 63(2):243–9.

9. Yoshida N, Naito Y, Inada Y, Kugai M, Yagi N, Inoue K, Okuda T, Hasegawa D, Kanemasa K, Kyoichi K, Matsuyama K, Ando T, Takemura T, Shimizu S, Wakabayashi N, Yanagisawa A, Yoshikawa T. Multicenter study of endoscopic mucosal resection using 0.13 % hyaluronic acid solution of colorectal polyps less than 20 mm in size. Int J Colorectal Dis. 2013;28:985–91.

10. Feitoza AB, Gostout CJ, Burgart LJ, Burkert A, Herman LJ, Rajan E. Hydroxypropyl methylcellulose: a better submucosal fluid cushion for endoscopic mucosal resection. Gastrointest Endosc. 2003;57:41–7.

11. Yamasaki M, Kume K, Yoshikawa I, Otsuki M. A novel method of endoscopic submucosal dissection with blunt abrasion by submucosal injection of sodium carboxymethylcellulose: an animal preliminary study. Gastrointest Endosc. 2006;64(6):958–65.

12. Burns JW, Colt MJ, Burgees LS, Skinner KC. Preclinical evaluation of Seprafilm bioresorbable membrane. Eur J Surg Suppl. 1997;577:40–8.

13. Fredericks CM, Kotry I, Holtz G, Askalani AH, Serour GI. Adhesion prevention in the rabbit with sodium carboxymethylcellulose solutions. Am J Obstet Gynecol. 1986;155(3):667–70.

Submucosal Fluid Cushion Injection Fluid: Western Perspective

8

Christopher J. Gostout and Ray I. Sarmiento

Ode to the SFC

Oh, were I to see, an SFC
Through toil and drudgery
That would brighten sun, moon and star
For anyone to perform EMR
I would sing its praise
And shout for joy
That we found
The ideal toy

by Christopher J. Gostout [1]

Introduction

In 1984, Tada et al. introduced endoscopic mucosal resection, a flexible endoscopic technique allowing removal of superficial gastrointestinal neoplasms using a two-channel scope with a grasper and snare after injection of fluid into the submucosa of flat or depressed lesions. ESD subsequently evolved from one of the early EMR techniques, EHRSE (endoscopic resection after local injection of a solution of hypertonic saline-epinephrine) [2]. ESD became the treatment of choice for neoplasia confined to the mucosa or submucosa, but only in Asian countries. It has been slow to become adopted in the West for a variety of reasons, including a lack of both ideal target disease and readily available training [3, 4].

In 2008, The American Society of Gastrointestinal Endoscopy (ASGE) published a Technology Status Report on EMR and ESD; a summary of results by Japanese endoscopists involving 1,832 patients that reported a complete resection rate of 73.9 % and a combined complication rate of 1.9 % (1.4 % to bleeding and 0.5 % to perforation). The ASGE report identified the common submucosal injection solutions in use [5]. In the ode above, from a 2004 editorial by Gostout on the subject of the submucosal fluid cushion (SFC), as with the ASGE Technology Report in 2008, the ideal SFC material has not been identified. There are subsequent publications comparing different injection materials for EMR and ESD in both animal laboratory and clinical settings. These publications may represent a quest by the western endoscopist to avoid, or at least minimize, adverse outcomes associated

C.J. Gostout, M.D., F.A.S.G.E. (✉)
R.I. Sarmiento, M.D.
Gastroenterology and Hepatology, Mayo Clinic,
200 First St. SW, Rochester, MN 55905, USA
e-mail: gostout.christopher@mayo.edu

with mucosal resection and, especially, ESD. This chapter will address the current SFC solutions in use, including:

- normal saline
- saline with 1:10,000 epinephrine
- 50 % dextrose
- hyaluronic acid
- Glyceol
- 10 % glycerin
- 0.83 % hydroxypropyl methylcellulose
- mesna (sodium 2-mercaptoethane sulfonate)

The SFC has key mechanical and visual functions (Table 8.1). It acts as an expansile barrier between the mucosa and the muscularis propria to limit thermal injury to the muscularis propria, which may lead to bleeding from eroded vessels and with full thickness muscle injury and perforation. It separates tissue planes and, by doing so, allows visual identification of the mucosa, fibroareolar connective tissue, blood vessels, and the muscular layer, guiding the mucosal excision process and further reducing the adverse events of bleeding and perforation.

The Mayo Clinic Developmental Endoscopy Unit (DEU) has been active in SFC research. Initial efforts at testing solutions resulted in the recognition that the ex vivo animal model was unreliable to assess solution performance. The ex vivo model can often be useful for preliminary testing of concepts, materials and methods, but fluid performances in unperfused tissue cannot be reliably translated to clinical application. Conio, Rajan et al., in 2002 [6], compared five injection solutions in an in vivo porcine model. The fluids compared were: saline, saline with 1:10,000 epinephrine, 50 % dextrose (D50), rooster comb-derived hyaluronic acid, and 10 % glycerin. Glyceol, at that time, was only commercially available in Japan (Chugai Pharmaceutical Co.) and consisted of 10 % glycerin and 5 % fructose in normal saline. All the test solutions had indigo carmine dye added and were injected into the distal esophagus at room temperature. The elapsed time for the subcutaneous bleb to disappear was measured. The disappearance time for normal saline (median of 2.4 min) was significantly shorter than the other solutions, except normal saline with epinephrine, which correlates with clinical observations.

Table 8.1 The ideal SFC fluid

Ideal SFC solution characteristics	SFC solution should be: [5, 10, 14]
Cost	Inexpensive
Clarity	Transparent enough to help identify submucosal structures
Local and systemic toxicity	Non-toxic
Availability	Readily in bulk
Storage	At room temperature and no need for refrigeration while in transport
Handling	Does not require mixing with other solutions other than dilution, can be sterilized without degrading
Viscosity	Fluid outside of the body
Ease of injection	Easily injected through a standard sclerotherapy needle
Length of stay in the submucosal space	Entire duration of the EMR/ESD, or long enough to keep the number of re-injections low
Electroconductivity	Almost impenetrable, does not conduct electricity well
Additional ideal local tissue effects	Promotes ulcer healing, hemostatic, ability to separate tissue planes, softens connective tissue to facilitate blunt dissection, no char artifact after electrocauterization

D50 and 10 % glycerin dissipated 2 min later than normal saline. Hyaluronic acid had a median of 22.1 min, making it significantly longer lasting than all the other solutions. Long before ESD was conceptualized, this paper was intended to identify the most suitable SFC solution for EMR and piecemeal polypectomy. As a result of this study, D50 became the SFC solution of choice in our clinical practice in Rochester, Minnesota until the next discovery.

Later that same year, Feitoza, Gostout et al. [7], published a report on the use of another submucosal fluid cushion for EMR, hydroxypropyl methylcellulose (HPMC). The group already saw the value of a long-lasting SFC to facilitate lengthy EMR and polypectomy procedures. The prohibitive cost, lack of availability, and lack of regulatory approval of hyaluronic acid prompted them to look for an alternative SFC injectate [8]. One day in the DEU animal lab, a surgical lubricant was tried in an injectable dilute form and proved to offer an astounding SFC. Unfortunately, all the commercially available formulations of surgical lubricants are made of multiple ingredients and not approved for injection. The most significant component of these was identified as methylcellulose. HPMC is commonly used as an ophthalmic solution during anterior chamber operations. This formulation of methylcellulose was chosen due to its viscoelastic properties and approved for injection. In contrast to HA, HPMC was inexpensive and readily available in a generic 2.5 % solution commonly sold as eye drops. This feasibility study was done to observe the safety, durability and tissue response to submucosally injected HPMC. Results showed that HPMC stayed in the submucosal space up to 45 min and induced minimal tissue reaction on histopathology. A diluted solution of 0.83 % of HPMC can be easily injected into the esophageal wall to create a long-lasting SFC at low cost.

By the year 2004, Rajan and most of the Apollo 8 group published a report on Widespread EMR (WEMR) of the distal esophagus in a porcine model [9]. The SFC used was 0.83 % HPMC. There was no procedure-related complication. It emphasized the importance of a long-lasting protective SFC in prolonged procedures. The SFC fluid duration was approximately 35 min.

In 2007, Sumiyama and Gostout published on novel techniques for WEMR and ESD [10]. It was noted that in the Mayo Clinic, HPMC had replaced D50 and was clinically used as the SFC solution of choice, in contrast to HA, due to cost effectiveness and ease of storage and handling. ESD was just being described in Japan during this period and the SFC solution of choice used in Japan was hyaluronic acid.

The DEU also originally reported the concept of using the submucosa as a working space for endoscopic intervention. Converting the submucosa into a tunnel can offer safe entry into sterile spaces such as the peritoneal cavity and mediastinum. Off-set entry from the lumen, passage through a submucosal space or tunnel, and a myotomy distal exit prevents peritoneal soiling, by allowing the overlying mucosa to serve as a sealant flap (submucosal endoscopy with mucosal flap or SEMF). Early experience used high pressure carbon dioxide injection supplemented with careful electrosurgical dissection to tunnel relatively easily. The concept of submucosal endoscopy, originally referred to as the Submucosal Inside Out Project (SIOP) [10], was actually initiated to simplify mucosal resection as a more expedient alternative to EMR and ESD that might enable more endoscopists to perform widespread mucosal resection (Fig. 8.1). With this approach, mucosal disease is first undermined by a submucosal free space. The endoscope and endoscopic devices within this space are directed toward the lumen away from the muscularis propria, thereby reducing full thickness injury by this reversed direction of intervention. Submucosal endoscopy with mucosal flap (SEMF) and submucosal endoscopy with mucosal resection (SEMR) have evolved into many practical uses, specifically in natural orifice transluminal endoscopic surgery (NOTES), per-oral endoscopic myotomy (POEM) and endoscopic full thickness resection (EFTR). Both submucosal techniques fundamentally require a reliable SFC for initiation [11].

Whether one is performing traditional EMR, or ESD, or SEMF or SEMR, the SFC is critical. Work in the DEU was directed at trying to identify an adjunctive material to the SFC solution that could further facilitate all these procedures. Sumiyama, Gostout, and Rajan published a report on chemically assisted endoscopic submucosal dissection using mesna [12]. Mesna is a thiol compound, sodium-2-mercaptoethanesulfonate, originally developed to define surgical planes. Mesna is a mucolytic solution whose action is to disrupt disulfide bonds, making mucus less viscous and connective tissues weaker. Mesna significantly ($p > 0.05$) reduced tissue resistance to balloon-catheter insertion in submucosal dissection. Mesna was added to 0.83 % HPMC and was compared to HPMC alone.

En bloc resection may be of more value in North America to remove advanced colorectal polyps, especially large sessile or laterally spreading lesions. The most common procedure in sessile polyps >2 cm is piecemeal resection which carries a significant risk of residual adenoma and repetitive endoscopies. Traditional

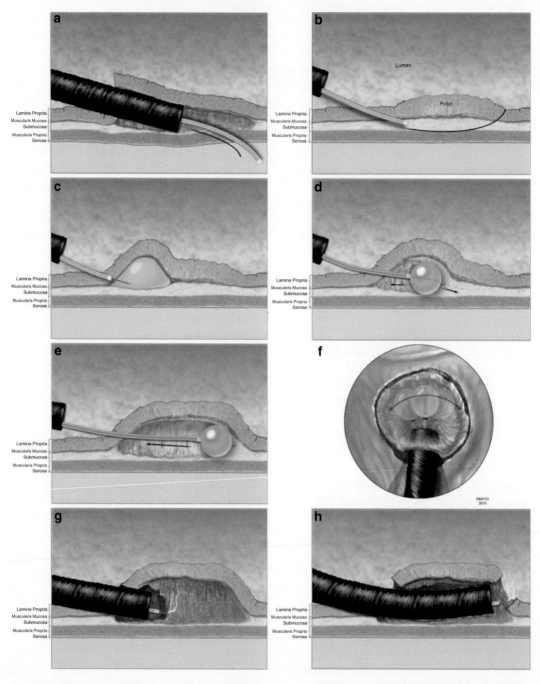

Fig. 8.1 Submucosal inside out project (SIOP)—concept of submucosal endoscopy: (**a**) A submucosal tunnel can allow safe access to body cavities. (**b**) Submucosal tunneling can undermine overlying mucosal disease for en bloc excision. (**c**) Submucosal endoscopy is dependent on the SFC. (**d**) Hybrid ESD can be performed using blunt balloon dissection in lieu of conventional electrosurgical cutting. (**e**) Blunt balloon tunneling undermines overlying mucosal disease completely. (**f**) Blunt balloon dissection is extended beyond the tunnel to completely undermine overlying mucosal disease and is dependent on an isolating circumferential excision. (**g**) In hybrid ESD, conventional electrosurgical excision is combined with balloon dissection. (**h**) In hybrid ESD, the combination of balloon dissection and electrosurgical excision is carried out to the excised margins of the lesion for an en bloc removal

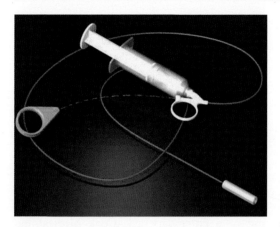

Fig. 8.2 SuMO Balloon

ESD is more challenging in the colon, with a greater risk of bleeding and perforation compared to piecemeal resection. ESD is time-consuming, sub-optimally reimbursed, and requires advanced endoscopic skills. SEMR allows large diameter resections; in the rectum of a porcine model, up to 8 cm. This hybrid ESD procedure is heavily reliant on a robust submucosal fluid cushion to allow isolation of the mucosal disease and facilitate the balloon dissection unique to this method. In the initial reported animal study, the combination of HPMC 0.83 % and mesna was used. The SEMR method was compared to traditional ESD performed by a Japanese expert in ESD, and was found to be less technically demanding than the traditional ESD procedure with a shorter learning curve. SEMR or hybrid ESD could open the opportunity for more endoscopists to perform en bloc resection of ESD proportions.

In 2013, an off shoot of SIOP, primary mechanical submucosal balloon dissection, was advanced by Dobashi, Sumiyama and colleagues. An engineered balloon dissector or the SuMO (Apollo Endosurgery, Austin TX, USA) was used to cleave submucosal fibrosis in an ulcerated lesion in a porcine model (Fig. 8.2). Submucosal fibrosis clinically presents a situation which frustrates the ability to create an effective SFC [13].

In 2007, Shastri from Germany, and, in 2012, Al-Taie from Brazil [14, 15] both published ex vivo experiences with SFC solutions that included components of blood, comparing normal saline, different concentrations of hyaluronic acid, dextrose water, hydroxyethyl starch (HES), 6 % glycerol, whole blood, plasma and serum. Whole blood provided an SFC that was significantly more durable than the other solutions and equivalent to sodium hyaluronate. Although blood gave superior height and duration to the SFC, there were several issues, as blood has many drawbacks. It could hamper the endoscopists view due to dark discoloration; resultant thermal (char) artifacts may also impair vision; premature coagulation can impair injection. As previously mentioned, one must be cautious about SFC performance in this work, as non-perfused ex vivo models were used.

Clinical SFC Investigation

Varadarajulu et al. used 50 % dextrose for 55 polypectomies in 50 patients [16]. Dextrose 50 % was superior to normal saline in ensuring an en bloc resection rate of 82 % vs. 44 % for NS ($p > 0.01$). The SFCs persisted after completion of the polypectomy in 96 % of patients. There was no difference in complication rates or rates of complete resection between the two solutions. Bacani et al. compared HPMC to normal saline [17]. Adverse events (bleeding, perforation, and unplanned hospital admission due to pain or decreased Hgb level < 10 g/dl) were observed in 5/67 (8 %) HPMC patients, compared to 1/22 (5 %) saline patients. HPMC became the exclusive lifting agent in Mayo Clinic Jacksonville as a result of this 2003 publication. HPMC (Gonak, Akron Inc. Buffalo Grove, IL) was prepared as follows: HPMC 15 cm^3 + 60 cm^3 normal saline + 1 cm^3 1:10,000 epinephrine and 2–3 cm^3 of indigo carmine (Fig. 8.3). At Mayo Clinic Rochester, the standardized HPMC solution derived from animal studies is: 15 cm^3 of HPMC + 85 cm^3 of normal saline + 1 cm^3 1:1,000 epinephrine and 1 cm^3 of 0.8 % indigo carmine.

Fasoulas et al. from Greece, in 2011 [18], performed a blinded study comparing HES, a volume

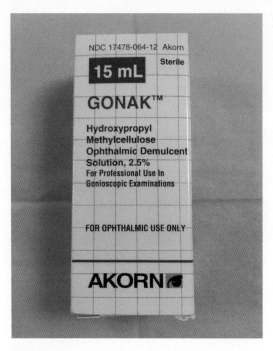

Fig. 8.3 Gonak ophthalmic solution, undiluted, prior to preparation

model, done by Neuhaus et al. in 2009, demonstrated that the hydrodissection method allowed resection of more mucosa than standard cap EMR [20]. Clinical application of this method, coined as the "STEP (selective tissue elevation by pressure) procedure" was first published by Belle et al. in 2011, involving 70 mucosal resections of flat colon polyps in 59 patients. Lesions up to 80 mm (mean of 27 mm) were resected with a complete resection rate of 91 % (64/70 lesions) [21–24].

In 2013, John's Hopkins reported a preliminary experience with an extreme SFC, reporting use of a proprietary gel (Cook Medical Inc, Winston-Salem, NC). A "starter," small amount of saline SFC was required for the gel to then be pressure injected. It is described as a hydraulic dissection of the submucosa due to the high viscosity gel, which requires a 19-gauge EUS needle with a pressure injector. The authors felt the gel added efficiency and decreased procedure time for applications such as ESD [25, 26].

expander commonly used in hypovolemic shock, vs. normal saline. In 49 patients, HES+epinephrine had a longer (18.5 min; 14–25 min range) SFC duration compared with NS+epinephrine (11.6 min; 9.6–13.6 min range). The number of re-injections was lower in HES. Adverse events involved 4 out of 24 patients in the HES+epinephrine group and 6 out of 24 in NS+epinephrine. Adverse events included one macroperforation, two post polypectomy syndrome cases, and one delayed bleed in the HES+E group. Intraprocedural bleeding was encountered in six NS+E group patients but all were resolved with endoscopic intervention. Histologic evaluation demonstrated no difference between the two groups.

In 2010, Fernandez-Esparrach et al. reported an experience using on-demand pressure injected saline (Erbejet, ERBE, Tubingen, Germany) [19]. The injection catheter also contained a needle knife, thereby eliminating catheter exchanges. This system allowed saline to function as well as the more viscous SFC solutions mentioned thus far. A randomized trial comparing EMR vs. ESD using the water-jet hybrid-knife in an animal

Conclusions

The benefits of en bloc resection and complete histopathology are paramount for effective management of neoplasia. Methods that enable en bloc excision, such as EMR, ESD, and hybrid ESD using blunt balloon dissection, can have a long-term favorable economic impact by reducing the need for repetitive follow-up procedures and propel patients into more desirable surveillance with longer intervals between interventions. These techniques are all highly dependent on the SFC, for which there is a diverse opinion set on a preferred solution. Active research has been done "through toil and drudgery" to find the ideal SFC solution. At present, based upon the published literature, it would appear to be 0.83 % hydroxypropyl methylcellulose.

References

1. Gostout CJ. Ode to the submucosal fluid cushion. Endoscopy. 2004;36(7):638–9.

2. Mokenmuller K, Wilcox CM, Munoz-Navas M (editors). Interventional and therapeutic gastrointestinal endoscopy. Front Gastrointest Res. Basel Krager, 2010; 27:156–68.
3. Othman MO, Wallace MB. Endoscopic mucosal resection (EMR) and endoscopic submucosal dissection (ESD) in 2011, a Western perspective. Clin Res Hepatol Gastroenterol. 2011;35:288–94.
4. Neuhaus H. Endoscopic mucosal resection and endoscopic submucosal dissection in the West – too many concerns and caveats? Endoscopy. 2010;42:859–61.
5. ASGE Technology Status Evaluation Report. Endoscopic mucosal resection and endoscopic submucosal dissection. Gastrointest Endosc. 2008;68(1):11–8.
6. Conio M, Rajan E, et al. Comparative performance in the porcine esophagus of different solutions used for submucosal injection. Gastrointest Endosc. 2002;56(4):513–6.
7. Feitoza AB, Gostout CJ, et al. Hydroxypropyl methylcellulose: a better submucosal fluid cushion for endoscopic mucosal resection. Gastrointest Endosc. 2003;57(1):41–7.
8. Farrel JJ. Submucosal fluid cushion and EMR: who rules the roost? Gastrointest Endosc. 2008;67(6):840–2.
9. Rajan E, Gostout CJ, et al. Widespread EMR: a new technique for removal of large areas of mucosa. Gastrointest Endosc. 2004;60(4):623–7.
10. Sumiyama K, Gostout CJ. Novel techniques and instrumentation for EMR, ESD, and full-thickness endoscopic luminal resection. Gastrointest Endosc Clin N Am. 2007;17:471–85.
11. Gostout CJ, Knipshield MA. Submucosal endoscopy with mucosal resection: a hybrid endoscopic submucosal dissection in the porcine rectum and distal colon. Gastrointest Endosc. 2012;76(4):829–34.
12. Sumiyama K, Gostout CJ, et al. Chemically assisted endoscopic mechanical submucosal dissection by using mesna. Gastrointest Endosc. 2008;67(3):534–8.
13. Dobashi A, Sumiyama K, Gostout CJ, et al. Can mechanical balloon dissection be applied to cleave fibrotic submucosal tissues? A pilot study in a porcine model. Endoscopy. 2013;45:661–6.
14. Al-Taie OH, Bauer Y, et al. Efficacy of submucosal injection of different solutions inclusive blood components on mucosa elevation for endoscopic resection. Clin Exp Gastroenterol. 2012;5:43–8.
15. Shastri YM, Kriener S, et al. Autologous blood as a submucosal fluid cushion for endoscopic mucosal

therapies: results of an ex vivo study. Scand J Gastroenterol. 2007;42:1369–75.
16. Varadarajulu S, Tamhane A, Slaughter RL. Evaluation of dextrose 50 % as a medium for injection-assisted polypectomy. Endoscopy. 2006;38(9):907–12.
17. Bacani CJ, Woodward TA, et al. The safety and efficacy in humans of endoscopic mucosal resection with hydroxypropyl methylcellulose as compared with normal saline. Surg Endosc. 2008;22:2401–6.
18. Fasoulas K, Lazaraki G, et al. Endoscopic mucosal resection of giant laterally spreading tumors with submucosal injection of hydroxyethyl starch: comparative study with normal saline solution. Surg Laparosc Endosc Percutan Tech. 2012;22(3):272–8.
19. Fernandez-Esparrach G, Matthes EL, et al. A novel device for endoscopic submucosal dissection that combines water-jet submucosal hydrodissection and elevation with electrocautery: initial experience in a porcine model. Gastrointest Endosc. 2010;71(3):615–8.
20. Neuhaus H, Withs K, et al. Randomized controlled study of EMR versus endoscopic submucosal dissection with a water-jet hybrid-knife of esophageal lesions in a porcine model. Gastrointest Endosc. 2009;70(1):112–20.
21. Kahler GF, Sold M, et al. Selective tissue elevation by pressure injection [STEP] facilitates endoscopic mucosal resection [EMR]. Surg Technol Int. 2007;16:107–12.
22. Lingenfelder T, Fischer K, et al. Combination of water-jet dissection and needle-knife as a hybrid knife simplifies endoscopic submucosal dissection. Surg Endosc. 2009;23:1531–5.
23. Lepilliez V, Robles-Medrana C, et al. Water-jet dissector for endoscopic submucosal dissection in an animal study: outcomes of the continuous and pulsed modes. Surg Endosc. 2013;27:2921.
24. Belle S, Collet PH, et al. Selective tissue elevation by pressure for endoscopic mucosal resection of colorectal adenoma: first clinical trial. Surg Endosc. 2012;26:343–9.
25. Khashab MA, Saxena P, et al. A novel submucosal gel permits simple and efficient gastric endoscopic submucosal dissection. Gastroenterology. 2013;144:505–7.
26. Khashab MA, Sharaiha RZ, et al. Novel technique of auto-tunneling during peroral endoscopic myotomy (with video). Gastrointest Endosc. 2013;77(1):119–22.

Electrocautery for ESD

9

Norio Fukami and Alissa Bults

Introduction

The electrosurgical unit (ESU) is an essential tool in endoscopic treatment. It creates the necessary electrosurgical current to create thermal energy in the target tissue delivered by endoscopic devices (e.g. snare, probes, and forceps). The current is an alternating current at high frequency (more than 100,000 Hz) to avoid neuromuscular response. Endoscopic submucosal dissection is a surgical procedure performed with endoscopy and endoscopic accessory devices, and electrocautery plays a key role in this procedure for effective tissue cutting and coagulation. Recent advancements in ESUs have tremendously helped the ESD procedure by reducing intra-procedural bleeding and helping with precise tissue cutting and dissection, especially when negative margins are concerned for tumor resection. In this chapter, ESUs and their various modes are explained, in order to understand the theoretical basics and to benefit by help with selecting the appropriate mode for each step of ESD.

Electronic supplementary material: Supplementary material is available in the online version of this chapter at 10.1007/978-1-4939-2041-9_9. Videos can also be accessed at http://www.springerimages.com/videos/978-1-4939-2040-2.

N. Fukami, M.D., A.G.A.F., F.A.C.G., F.A.S.G.E. (✉)
A. Bults, M.S.
Division of Gastroenterology & Hepatology,
University of Colorado Anschutz Medical Campus,
Aurora, CO 80045, USA
e-mail: norio.fukami@ucdenver.edu

Current Mode

Major current forms created by the ESU are "cut," "coagulation," and "blended" current [1, 2].

Cut

Cut current is produced by a continuous alternating current that creates a continuous flow of electrons that, when used with high current density, creates a steam barrier of vaporization and precise dissection (Fig. 9.1). At least 200 Volts peak (Vp) is necessary to electrosurgically dissect or cut. This high current density creates energy within the tissue, causing a rapid increase in tissue temperature. Intracellular water boils rapidly and vaporizes, thus resulting in explosion of cells. This response creates electrosurgical cutting of tissue, and the temperature does not increase significantly in response. Therefore, only minimum coagulation effect, also referred to as thermal spread, is created.

Coag

In general, coagulation current is produced by intermittent bursts of higher voltage alternating current (Fig. 9.2). The effect is a slower increase in temperature that induces the dehydration and denaturation of tissue without bursting cells

Cutting current

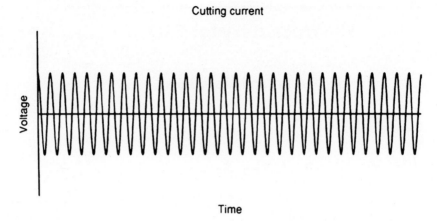

Fig. 9.1 Cutting current

Coagulation current

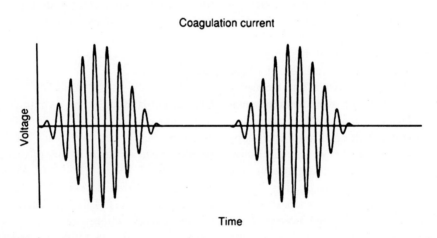

Fig. 9.2 Coagulation current

(desiccation). This response creates a coagulation effect, with some cutting properties depending on the voltage, duty cycle (see Blend section), etc. Coagulation waveforms generally use voltages of approximately 1,000 Vp with very little current flow (relative to cut).

Two "specific termed" coagulation waveforms are: SOFT COAG, a voltage-controlled waveform of less than 200 Vp, which is used to create "pure coagulation without cutting;" and SPRAY COAG, a high voltage (4,000 Vp) current used more often in tunneling procedures other than ESD. These modes will be discussed later.

Blend

Blend current is created by changing the voltage and modifying the on and off ratio (duty cycle) of the current (Fig. 9.3). Duty cycle is the current on and current off percentage, as modulated by the ESU. The less duty cycles, the more coagulation the effect assumes. A pure cut current typically uses a 100 % duty cycle (current is always on); on the other hand, pure coagulation current typically uses a 6 % duty cycle (current is on only 6 % of the time and is off 94 % of the time). Various ESUs create a variety of voltage and duty

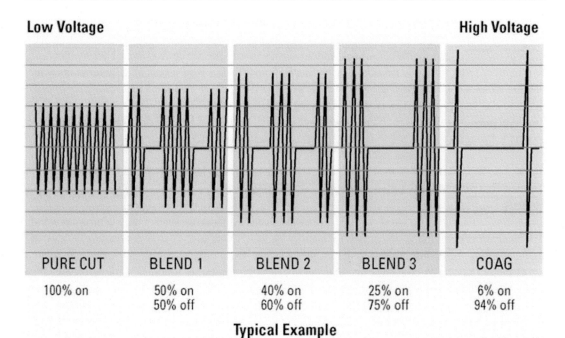

Low Voltage   **High Voltage**

PURE CUT	BLEND 1	BLEND 2	BLEND 3	COAG
100% on	50% on 50% off	40% on 60% off	25% on 75% off	6% on 94% off

Typical Example

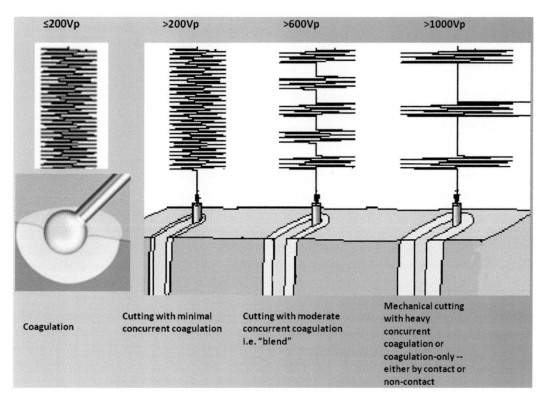

≤200Vp   >200Vp   >600Vp   >1000Vp

Coagulation | Cutting with minimal concurrent coagulation | Cutting with moderate concurrent coagulation i.e. "blend" | Mechanical cutting with heavy concurrent coagulation or coagulation-only -- either by contact or non-contact

Fig. 9.3 Cut to coagulation wave form (courtesy of ERBE)

cycles to provide the effect desired by the operator (physician), depending on the targeted tissue. It is prudent to understand the basis of the blend current in order to be able to expect the tissue effect created by the ESU. Review articles have summarized the variety of ESUs as well as having provided the properties of cut, blend, and coagulation [1, 2].

Tissue Response and Expected Result

Tissue effect is determined not only by the ESU output. During the endoscopic procedure a variety of factors have to be taken into account. As in Ohm's law, voltage and resistance determine current. Factors important to consider for ESD are tissue resistance, current density, and contact time (application time), in addition to ESU output mode.

Tissue Resistance

Variable tissue has different tissue resistance; notably, high resistance is noted for adipose tissue or, for ESD-related issues, is created in the submucosa by fibrosis from previous biopsy or attempt at resection. Furthermore, as tissue dehydrates during application of electrocautery, or if it has less water content (e.g. fibrosis), tissue resistance increases and coagulation effect becomes more prominent than cutting effect even with the same ESU output, or more voltage is needed to create the same effect.

Current Density

Current density is the amount of current that goes through a standardized area. Current density is an important factor affecting desired effect. When target tissue goals are electrosurgical cutting, higher current density results in better cutting effect, regardless of waveform. The output should be adjusted to the expected current density created by the device and operator on the target tissue.

Contact Surface: Device

If the contact surface is small (e.g. cutting with the tip of a needle knife), current density becomes higher than it would be with a larger contact surface (e.g. cutting with the whole length of needle knife such as IT knife or a snare); therefore, it cuts the tissue more effectively without much coagulation effect.

Contact Surface: Amount of Tissue Targeted

The amount of tissue targeted is also important. Even with the same device, such as the Hook knife (Olympus, USA), for example, and the same ESU output, use of the long arm portion results in a larger amount of tissue contact than using only the L-shaped tip. The cutting effect is reduced, thereby creating more coagulation effect and sometimes causing a charring effect. Further, when the intent is to "cut" or "vaporize" target tissue, and a delay occurs due to low current density (or under powered), then even more—often unrecognized—thermal insult occurs.

Contact Time (Application Time): Speed of Device Movement and Duration of Application

Speed of movement of the ESD knife and application duration (foot step "on" time) determines the amount of current applied to the targeted tissue. Faster movement of an ESD knife often results in the gathering of more tissue, resulting in low current density and less cutting effect, and alternatively resulting in more thermal insult than cutting through the tissue. Slower, steady movement of an ESD knife with shorter bursts of "on" time generally creates a more controlled electrocautery application to target tissue; however, static application of electrocautery current often results in a tissue char effect that is usually not desired. Control of the movement speed of the ESD knife and directional tension on the tissue are, therefore, very important.

Understanding this concept is exceptionally helpful during ESD procedures since the operator can modify the current density freely to achieve the desired effect (e.g. cutting fibrous tissue without char, coagulating the vessels prior to cutting through, cutting with forced coagulation without char) by modifying the device, the amount of tissue to target, and the speed of device movement.

Computerized ESUs

We have seen tremendous advancement of ESUs recently. Addition of computer software within the ESUs has made the control of blend current more sophisticated. A variety of output modes have been created for ease of desired tissue response. The most widely used ESUs for ESD procedures are the ICC™ and VIO™ systems (ERBE, USA). The recently released Olympus ESG system has output modes with same or similar names (e.g. ForcedCoag, SoftCoag, and Pulse Cut), but are not all based upon the same generator algorithms. It is important to understand the technological outputs associated with any generator, as well as the rationale for choosing "what" and "when." Other notable modes are SWIFT COAG®, DRY CUT™, and Spray coagulation [3]. Here, each mode is discussed based on ERBE ESU.

ENDO CUT (similar for Pulse Cut) (Video 9.1)

ENDO CUT™ uses a patented spark generation and recognition algorithm that calculates in real-time when a spark is present based on circuit variables. Spark needed for cutting is produced to initiate the cutting phase and it is maintained for the preset length of time (determined by a selection of Duration) (Fig. 9.4a, b—yellow bar: duration is its width). This cutting phase alternates with coagulation current (Fig. 9.4a, c—blue bar). Coagulation effect is determined by a selection of Effect. Effect is set as follows: no coagulation with 1, soft-type coagulation with 2, and forced-type coagulation with 3 and 4 (4 provides more coagulation effect) (Fig. 9.4c). Cut-coagulation cycle repeats at the preset length of time determined by a selection of Interval as long as the foot pedal is depressed (Fig. 9.4d). For example, 400 milliseconds (ms) between the cycles for Interval 1, 880 ms for Interval 4, and 1,840 ms for interval 10. (NOTE: ENDO CUT is primarily a cutting mode whereby microelectric arcing occurs rapidly within 5 ms, and the cutting spark time occurs in ranges of 2–24 ms. Coagulation effect to tissue during ENDO CUT is minimal relative to the other modes discussed herein, or when the operator taps the footswitch.)

ENDO CUT I and Q differ by controlled voltage adjusting for the type of device (I for needle type device and Q for snare device) but other parameters remain the same. ENDO CUT is primarily used for mucosal incision, and often the mode of choice for dissecting fibrotic tissue within the submucosal layer.

Forced Coagulation (Videos 9.2 and 9.3)

FORCED COAG mode is a basic coagulation mode and uses approximately 1,000 Vp. Effect controls coagulation effect. Increasing Effect in increments of 1 enhances coagulation effect, and thus hemostasis, by increasing voltage to strengthen thermal insult. Wattage (Watt) is setting for the maximally allowed energy delivered to the tissue (same for all the other described modes below). FORCED can be used for submucosal dissection, especially helpful in more vascular anatomy, when a good lift is present. It must be noted that higher voltage can lead to more prominent thermal damage of the submucosal layer during dissection, which may obscure the deep margin on pathological evaluation.

Soft Coagulation (Video 9.4)

SOFT COAG is a pure coagulation mode primarily used for hemostasis with hemostatic forceps and for marking the lesion with a knife. ESU uses less than 200 Vp so that it does not allow any cutting effect or carbonization. As target tissue dehydrates and proteins denature (coagulate), impedance rises and current falls off when voltage is constant. The result is virtually non-stick and very homogenous and controlled application of energy for tissue coagulation.

Effect controls the power applied; however, it should be understood that the higher the effect,

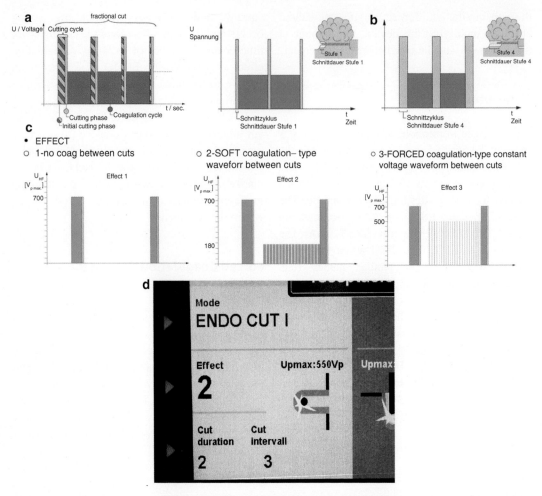

Fig. 9.4 (**a**) ENDO CUT Mode (courtesy of ERBE). (**b**) ENDO CUT: Duration 1 vs. 4 (courtesy of ERBE). (**c**) ENDO CUT: Effect 1–3 (courtesy of ERBE). (**d**) ENDO CUT mode setting panel (VIO300D)

the shallower the depth of heat injury becomes. This is a result (in general) of the lower Effect setting causing a slower rise in impedance and a "longer" current flow until power drops to near zero (application time); thus, the tissue effect at lower effect settings is deeper and more intense.

Swift Coagulation

SWIFT COAG is a coagulation mode with enhanced cutting property and uses 850–1,050 Vp from Effect 2–4 (Fig. 9.5a). It is less hemostatic than FORCED COAG and more hemostatic with less cutting than DRY CUT (see below). It can be used like FORCED COAG for pinpoint hemosta-

sis of vessels during submucosal dissection, but can create a "divot" or cut during coagulation. This mode is preferentially used for submucosal dissection with certain knives.

Dry Cut

DRY CUT is a cutting mode with enhanced coagulation property (increased concurrent hemostasis relative to ENDO CUT, but algorithm is very different). DRY CUT uses 600–800 Vp from Effect 2–4 (Fig. 9.5b). DRY CUT is used when precise submucosal dissection is needed and also is used for mucosal incision when bleeding is more frequent, but the increased thermal effect should be

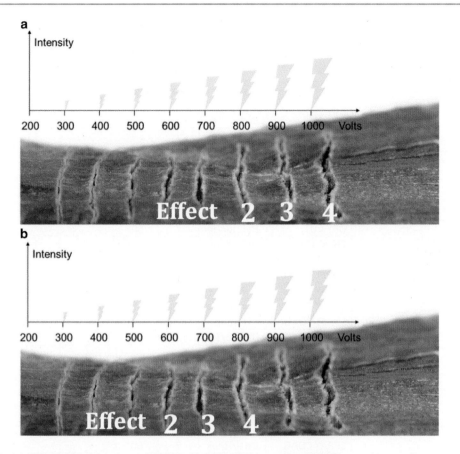

Fig. 9.5 (**a**) SWIFT COAG (courtesy of ERBE). (**b**) DRY CUT (courtesy of ERBE)

taken into account in order to proactively reduce deep thermal injury, limiting the application time and to cut with wider margin to protect specimen for proper pathological assessment.

Spray Coagulation (Video 9.5)

SPRAY COAG is a continuous very high voltage (4,000 Vp max) mode at low duty cycle as FORCED COAG (approximately 6 %). This creates significant arcing to the nearby tissue, similar to Argon Plasma Coagulation, and this is used primarily for non-contact coagulation; however, this mode is preferentially used during Per-Oral Endoscopic Myotomy (POEM) procedure, taking advantage of its widespread hemostatic property on nearby tissue and the ease of submucosal tunneling with non-contact submucosal dissection.

Specific Mode for Steps of ESD and Difficult Situations

For your reference, a table is attached to show a variety of settings used with different knives at different stages of ESD (Table 9.1). These are not firmly set or officially recommended settings and should be considered as a starting point to be modified according to the knife, anatomical location, tissue characteristics and vascularity, and the technique.

Mucosal Incision

Mucosal incision is frequently performed with ENDO CUT. Some prefer DRY CUT or SWIFT COAG depending on the knife and anatomical location.

Table 9.1 Reference list of electrosurgical settings used at various expert ESD centers

	Mode	Tool	Effect	Watts	Duration	Interval
Marking	SOFT COAG	Tip Knife	4-5	20-50		
Mucosal incision	DRY CUT	IT Nano/Tip	3	80		
	ENDO CUT	Tip Knife	3		1-3	1
	ENDO CUT	IT-2 Knife	3		2-3	1
	ENDO CUT	IT Knife	2		2	2
	ENDO CUT	Dual, Hook	3		2	2
	SPRAY COAG (esophagus)	Dual, Hook	2	60		
Submucosal dissection	DRY CUT	Hybrid/Tip	2	50		
	ENDO CUT	Hybrid/Tip	3		2	1
	ENDO CUT	Dual, Hook	3		2	2
	FORCED COAG	Hybrid/Tip	2	35-50		
	SPRAY COAG	Hook	2	60		
	SPRAY COAG	Hybrid/Tip	1	35-50		
	SWIFT COAG	IT Knife	4/5	100		
	SWIFT COAG	ITnano/Tip	2	40		
Hemostasis	Bipolar soft	Bipolar forceps	4	25		
	FORCED COAG	Hybrid/Tip	2	35-50		
	FORCED COAG	ITnano/Tip	2	40		
	SOFT COAG	Coagrasper	5	80		
	SOFT COAG	forceps	5	40		
	SPRAY COAG	Dual/Hook	2	60		

All settings listed are for ERBE ESU VIO300D. (This is a reference and is not meant to be recommended settings)

Submucosal Dissection

FORCED COAG is used with adequate needle movement (manipulation) to avoid carbonization. SWIFT COAG or DRY CUT is becoming more popular with better cutting capability especially in less vascular tissue. These modes are not exclusive to one area and can be switched actively depending on the vascularity and tissue response, in order to achieve best dissection (smooth cutting of tissue without hemorrhage).

Coagulating Vessels (Pre-coagulation, Coagulation of Bleeding Site)

If the vessels are smaller in caliber (often quoted as "less than 1 mm"), then FORCED COAG, DRY CUT, or SWIFT COAG application with ESD knife is efficient. It is important to slow the movement of the knife to maximize the current flow and application of energy to seal the vessels, especially with DRY CUT and SWIFT COAG, which have more cutting property. If the vessels are larger, then proactive coagulation with hemostatic forceps using SOFT COAG is strongly advised prior to cutting the tissue in this area. SOFT COAG application with knife is often inadequate for vessels and is not advised. Once bleeding occurs, then identification of the bleeding site and pinpoint coagulation with grasping hemostatic forceps using SOFT COAG is the most effective method. The SOFT COAG mode can be applied and is effective even underwater.

Special Situations: Fibrosis, Vascular-Rich Structures, POEM

Fibrotic tissue does have less water and easily dehydrates to create carbonization. Therefore, application of coagulation current is often counter-productive. Cut current is recommended with careful and stepwise dissection (small area to be dissected at one time). ENDO CUT is most suitable and powerful, but DRY CUT can also be used where less dense fibrosis is seen.

Vascular-rich structures are seen especially with cancerous lesions. Multiple small to larger vessels interlace within the submucosal fibers. In this case, more coagulation is needed to avoid bleeding in the cutting plane. FORCED COAG is the preferred mode; however, this leads to carbonization frequently. More cutting property is desired to avoid dense carbonization, and therefore, SWIFT COAG or DRY CUT is more effective. If bleeding still occurs with dissection, increase in Effect (Voltage) and/or Watt (allowable energy) is to be tried. Pre-coagulation with forceps and SOFT COAG with subsequent use of ENDO CUT mode may be a good alternative.

During POEM, submucosal dissection is rather easily performed because of less vasculature seen within the normal submucosal tissue. Myotomy is performed with SPRAY COAG, but it is of utmost importance to pull the circular muscle away from longitudinal muscle prior to cutting with SPRAY COAG since this is a constant high voltage mode. It has the benefit of less bleeding during myotomy (muscle has large vascular supply, thus has tendency to bleed upon myotomy). ENDO CUT can also be used with a higher Effect setting.

Conclusions

We have seen a dramatic advancement in endoscopic tissue resection during recent decades. Effective tissue dissection is greatly aided by better and smarter ESUs; however, it is our responsibility to understand the output from ESUs to achieve desired effects on tissue and to perform ESD smoothly and safely.

It is likely that preferred electrocautery modes will evolve along with the modification of equipment, technique, and further advancement of ESUs. There is no one right answer for proper settings and no one right ESU, but there is one right outcome—safe and successful ESD procedure.

Acknowledgement The authors deeply thank John Day, ERBE USA, who shared his vast knowledge and deep insight on electrosurgical units and their function, and target tissue response, and kindly shared many diagrams for better understanding.

References

1. Morris ML, Tucker RD, Baron TH, Song LM. Electrosurgery in gastrointestinal endoscopy: principles to practice. Am J Gastroenterol. 2009;104(6):1563–74.
2. Committee AT, Tokar JL, Barth BA, et al. Electrosurgical generators. Gastrointest Endosc. 2013;78(2):197–208.
3. Morita Y. Electrocautery for ESD: settings of the electrical surgical unit VIO300D. Gastrointest Endosc Clin N Am. 2014;24(2):183–9.

Endoscopic Submucosal Dissection for Superficial Esophageal Cancer

10

Tsuneo Oyama

Introduction

Esophageal endoscopic mucosal resection (EMR) was developed in the late 1980s, and it quickly became widely accepted as the premiere treatment for superficial esophageal cancers [1–4]. However, there were limitations regarding resectable size, and precise resection was impossible. Piecemeal resection was performed for larger lesions, but local recurrence rates after piecemeal EMR were high [5]. Therefore, a novel endoscopic treatment, endoscopic submucosal dissection (ESD), was developed to resolve such disadvantages of EMR [6–10]. Ten years have passed since esophageal ESD was established, and now, specially designed equipment is available to help make esophageal ESD safer and easier.

Indications

The indication of ESD for esophageal cancer is superficial cancer without lymph node metastasis (LNM).

Squamous Cell Carcinoma

According to the guidelines of the Japanese esophageal society, indications for endoscopic resection are T1a cancers limited to the epithelium or lamina propria. Because such cancers are extremely rarely associated with lymph node metastasis, endoscopic resection is a sufficient treatment for these lesions. Lesions reaching the muscularis mucosae or slightly infiltrating the submucosa (up to 200 μm) are also amenable to mucosal resection, but the incidence of LNM is about 15 %. Therefore, cross-sectional imaging or endoscopic ultrasound should be performed to stage the LNM before ESD.

T1a lesions infiltrating the muscularis mucosa or T1b lesions confined to the upper third of the submucosal, without LNM, represent relative indications. Furthermore, 50 % of lesions invading deeper (more than 200 μm) into the submucosa (T1b) are associated with metastasis, and even superficial carcinomas should be treated in the same manner as advanced carcinomas (carcinomas exceeding the muscularis propria).

Adenocarcinoma

According to the guidelines of the Japanese esophageal association, the indication of ESD for esophageal adenocarcinoma is T1a cancers infiltrating the lamina propria or the muscularis mucosa superficially. Additionally, T1a cancers

T. Oyama, M.D., Ph.D. (✉)
Department of Endoscopy, Saku Central Hospital
Advanced Care Center, 3400-28 Nakagomi,
Saku, Nagano 385-0051, Japan
e-mail: oyama@coral.ocn.ne.jp

N. Fukami (ed.), *Endoscopic Submucosal Dissection: Principles and Practice*,
DOI 10.1007/978-1-4939-2041-9_10, © Springer Science+Business Media New York 2015

reaching deep muscularis mucosa are relative indication. Recently, in a meta-analysis of LNM for esophageal adenocarcinoma, 70 relevant reports were identified that included 1,874 patients who had esophagectomy performed for HGD or intramucosal carcinoma in Barrett's esophagus. Lymph node metastases were found in 26 patients (1.39 %; 95 % CI 0.86–0.92) [11]. No metastases were found in the 524 patients who had a final pathology diagnosis of HGD, whereas 26 (1.93 %; 95 % CI 1.19–2.66) of the 1,350 patients with a final pathology diagnosis of intramucosal carcinoma had positive lymph nodes [11]. Therefore, all subtypes of T1a lesions could be the indication for ESD of esophageal adenocarcinomas since esophagectomy has a mortality rate that often exceeds 2 %.

Mucosal resection covering three-fourth of the entire circumference is likely to be associated with postoperative cicatricial stenosis; therefore, sufficient explanation should be given to the patient prior to the procedure and preventive measures must be taken. In cases of superficially enlarged carcinoma, deep infiltration may occur in multiple areas, necessitating careful diagnosis of the depth of invasion.

Tools and Techniques

Endoknives

Many endoknives have been developed for ESD. The basic knives are the Hook knife (KD-620LR, Olympus, Tokyo) and the Dual knife (KD-650, Olympus, Tokyo). The insulated tip (IT) knife is widely used for gastric ESD, but is not suitable for esophageal ESD because of the increased perforation rate. Recently, however, the IT-nano (KD-612, Olympus, Tokyo) was developed for colonic and esophageal ESD. The size of the insulation tip is smaller than that of the usual IT knife, and good maneuverability in narrow space is now obtainable. However, the risk of perforation is relatively higher, and therefore hyaluronic acid is recommended for the submucosal injection.

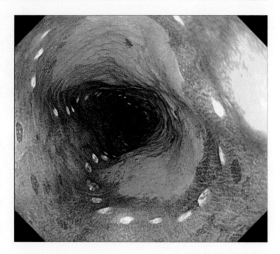

Fig. 10.1 The tip of the ESD knife is retracted within the sheath, and a mark is placed when the tip of the knife comes into contact with the mucosa

The Flush knife (Fujinon, Tokyo) is a unique device that incorporates a water flush function. It is useful for additional injection during submucosal dissection. And, even more recently, scissor-like knives such as the Clutch cutter (Fujinon, Tokyo) and the SB knife (Sumitomo Bakelite, Tokyo) have been developed. The cutting speed is slow, but they are easy for beginners to use.

Marking

The lateral extension of squamous cell carcinoma (SCC) can be visualized easily after 0.75–1 % iodine dye spray chromoendoscopy. Marks should be placed 2–3 mm away from the edge of the unstained area that represents the cancer. The esophageal wall is thinner than that of the stomach, and so perforation can occur during marking if a needle knife is used. Hook and Dual knives are useful devices for placing the marks safely. The tips of both knives can be retracted within the sheath, and a mark can be placed when the tip of knife is contacted with the mucosa and coagulated by soft coagulation (Effect 4, 20 W) (Fig. 10.1).

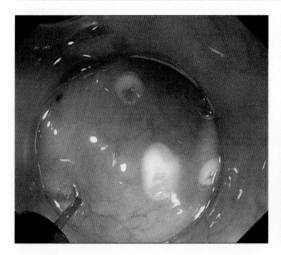

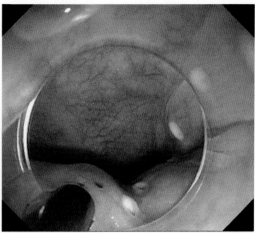

Fig. 10.2 The back side of the Hook Knife is placed so as to make contact with the mucosa, after submucosal injection of the fluid cushion, and a mucosal defect is made using the Endocut I mode

Fig. 10.4 The Hook Knife's arm is used for vertical mucosal incision. The knife is directed toward the lumen and then inserted into the submucosal. The mucosa is then elevated toward the lumen with the knife's arm, and then the mucosa is cut

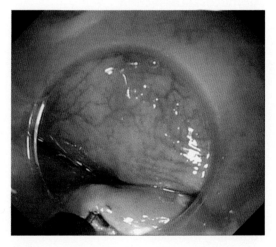

Fig. 10.3 The tip of the Hook Knife is inserted into the submucosal layer. The knife is used to hook and cut the mucosa

Mucosal Incision

The strategy for mucosal incision is dependent upon the endoknife type. When a Dual or Hook knife is used, basically the mucosal incision is performed from the oral side. At first, the back-side of the hook knife is contacted with the mucosa, and a hole is made by Endocut I mode (Effect 3) (Fig. 10.2). After that, the tip of the hook knife is inserted into the submucosal layer, and the mucosa is hooked and cut with the hook part of the knife (Fig. 10.3). This is an important part of the process in order to prevent perforation. The arm part of the hook knife is used for longitudinal mucosal incision. The direction of the Hook knife is turned toward the esophageal lumen, and the knife is inserted into the submucosal layer by sliding the back side. Then the mucosa is captured by the arm part of the knife (Fig. 10.4), and, finally, the mucosa is cut with a combination of Spray coagulation (Effect 2, 60 W) and Endocut mode (Effect 3, duration 2, and interval 2). It is important in order to prevent bleeding during mucosal incision. The submucosal vessels cannot always be observed by endoscopy. Sometimes they are cut unexpectedly, and bleeding occurs during mucosal incision. Initial spray coagulation can coagulate submucosal vessels, and so such unexpected bleeding can be prevented with initial spray coagulation.

A deeper cut of submucosal fibers is performed after mucosal incision. The Hook knife is inserted into the submucosal layer, and the submucosal fibers are hooked and cut. The lesion then shrinks by the contraction of muscularis mucosa (Fig. 10.5). After that, mucosal incision

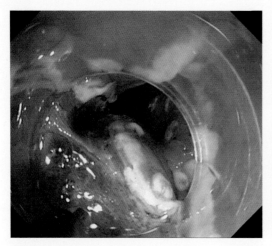

Fig. 10.5 The knife is inserted into the submucosal, and then the submucosal fibers are hooked and cut

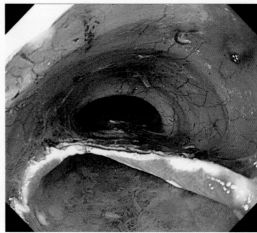

Fig. 10.7 After mucosal incision, a submucosal tunnel is made from the oral to anal side

Submucosal Dissection

The direction of gravity should be checked before submucosal dissection is started. Basically, submucosal dissection should be started from the lower side, because water and blood flow to the lower side causing the field of vision to become worse. Therefore, the operator should try to shift the lesion to the upper side. If submucosal dissection is begun from the upper side, the resected part will shift to the lower side, and submucosal dissection of the later half becomes difficult.

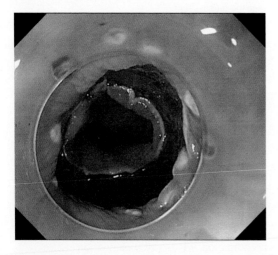

Fig. 10.6 Both oral and anal circumferential mucosal incisions were made

Tunneling Method

Tunnel-like dissection is necessary for circumferential ESD [12]. At first, a circumferential mucosal incision of the anal and oral parts is performed (Fig. 10.6). After that, a mucosal tunnel is made from oral to anal [12] (Figs. 10.7 and 10.8), and the second tunnel is made at the opposite side. Finally, the remaining submucosal fibers are dissected between the two tunnels (Fig. 10.9).

Clip-with-Line Method

If you can pull the target lesion, good countertraction can be made. The clip-with-line method was first reported in 2002 (Fig. 10.10) [13]. It is a simple and useful method for achieving countertraction during ESD. A long, 3-0, silk line is

of the distal side is performed and then circumferential incision is completed. When an IT-nano knife is used, the mucosal incision should be started from the anal side. The initial mucosal incision at the anal side is made by a needle knife after submucosal injection. After that, the mucosal incision is made with IT-nano knife by Endocut mode. The operator cannot see the next mark well, because the cutting direction is always from distal to proximal. Therefore, the operator should take care to avoid cutting inside of the marks.

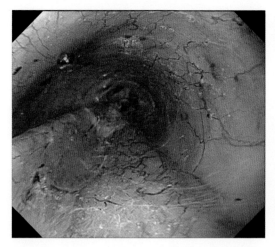

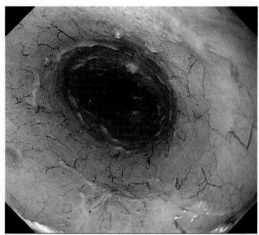

Fig. 10.8 At the opposite side, a second submucosal tunnel is made. The submucosal fibers remaining between the two tunnels are subsequently dissected

Fig. 10.9 En bloc ESD upon completion

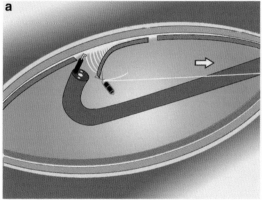

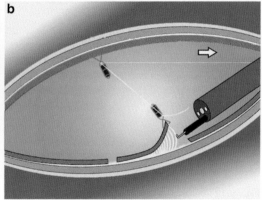

Fig. 10.10 Clip-with-line method. (**a**) A clip is placed at the distal edge of the target lesion once circumferential mucosal incision is complete. Countertraction and a clear field of view are obtained by pulling very gently on the line. (**b**) A second clip can be used to change the direction of the countertraction. (Originally from *Oyama T, Yuichi K, Shimaya S*, et al. *Endoscopic mucosal resection using a hooking knife—intra gastric lesion lifting method. Stomach and Intestine. 2002;37:1159. Japanese with English summary*)

tied to the arm part of the clip (HX-610-135; Olympus, Tokyo, Japan) (Fig. 10.11). Then the clip-with-line is reset in the cassette. The scope is withdrawn when the circumferential incision is finished. A clip applicator device (HX-110QR; Olympus) is inserted into the accessory channel of the endoscope, and the clip-with-line is mounted onto the tip of the applicator. The scope is inserted again, and the submucosal side of the target lesion is grasped (Fig. 10.12).

After that, the line is pulled very gently. Only a small amount of tension is required to create countertraction. This method also creates a clear field of vision (Figs. 10.13 and 10.14). During submucosal dissection, tension is maintained with a 10 g weight, such as a bite block mouthpiece, attached to the line. The 10 g weight creates sufficient countertraction and tension without threatening to tear the submucosal layer [14].

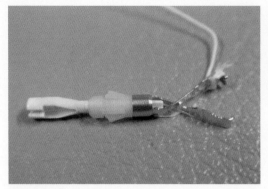

Fig. 10.11 A long silk line is attached to the arm part of a clip (HX-610-135, Olympus, Tokyo, Japan)

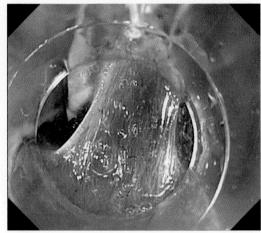

Fig. 10.13 Gentle pulling of the clip with traction line is used to provide countertraction

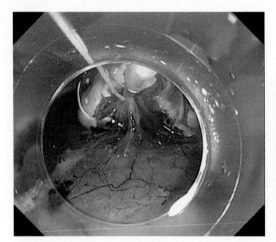

Fig. 10.12 The clip is used to grasp the submucosal side of the target lesion

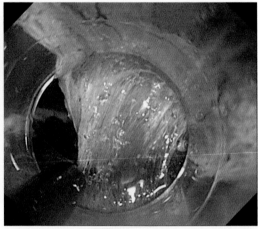

Fig. 10.14 Gentle pulling of the clip to provide counter-traction facilitates submucosal dissection

Hemostasis

Bleeding makes the visual field worse; therefore hemostasis should be performed as early as possible. When bleeding occurs during mucosal incision or dissection, the area should be flushed to find the origin of bleeding.

Hemostasis Using Knife

Hemostasis using an endoknife is useful for controlling oozing bleeds [15, 16]. The tip of the knife is brought close to the origin and electrical discharge is done with Spray mode to obtain hemostasis (Effect 2, 60 W) [16, 17]. Since prolonged electrical discharge may cause perforation, electrical discharge should be performed very briefly. Therefore, it is important to maintain optimal distance using a transparent hood. A scope equipped with a water jet should be selected for esophageal ESD as it is used to confirm the precise origin of the bleeding.

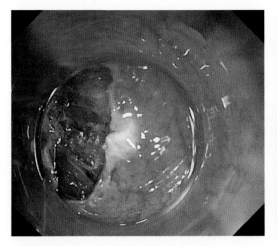

Fig. 10.15 If a vessel is large (≥1 mm), precut coagulation to prevent bleeding should be performed

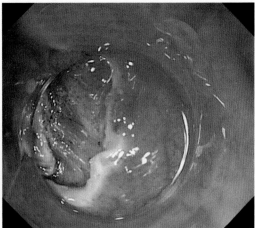

Fig. 10.17 The vessel can then be cut using the ESD knife and spray coagulation (Effect 2) without occurrence of any bleeding

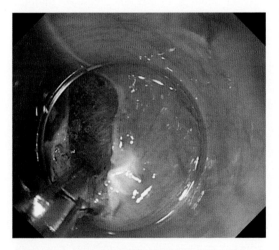

Fig. 10.16 Hemostatic forceps are used to grasp the large vessel, and it is coagulated with soft coagulation (Effect 5, 60 W)

Hemostatic Procedures Using Hemostatic Forceps

Hemostatic forceps, such as FD-410LR (Olympus, Tokyo, Japan), are useful in cases of more active or spurting bleeding. After flushing with a water jet to locate the origin of the bleed, the origin is grasped with the hemostatic forceps. After that, re-flushing with a water jet enables determination of whether the origin is grasped accurately. Then, the forceps are elevated a little to remove forceps from the proper muscular layer followed by electrical discharge with soft coagulation (Effect 5, 40 W), momentarily, to obtain hemostasis.

Prevention of Bleeding

Bleeding may worsen the visual field, leading to a higher risk of accidental complications. There are many vessels in the deep submucosal layer. A small vessel, 1 mm or less, could be cut using the Hook knife without bleeding when spray coagulation mode is used (Effect 2, 60 W). However, if the size of the vessel is 1 mm or larger, precut coagulation should be performed to prevent bleeding (Fig. 10.15). Larger vessels are grasped with the hemostatic forceps (Fig. 10.16) and coagulated by soft coagulation (Effect 5, 60 W). After that, the vessel can be cut using the Hook knife and spray coagulation (Effect 2, 60 W) without any bleeding occurring (Fig. 10.17).

Complications

Perforation

The major complication of EMR/ESD is perforation, as well as air embolization and aspiration pneumonia. Perforations may cause mediastinal emphysema, which increases the mediastinal pressure and crushes the esophageal lumen, leading to difficulty in securing the visual field. Severe mediastinal emphysema may be complicated by pneumothorax, which can lead to shock; therefore, electrocardiography, arterial oxygen saturation, and blood pressure (using an automated sphygmomanometer) monitoring should be conducted during ESD, as well as periodic observation for subcutaneous emphysema through palpation. CO_2 insufflation is useful for preventing such severe mediastinal emphysema.

Since the esophagus has no serous membrane and the intramediastinal pressure is lower than that of the esophageal lumen, mediastinal emphysema may occur in the absence of perforation. Dissection immediately above the proper muscular layer may damage the proper muscular layer during electrical discharge, which often causes mediastinal emphysema. Therefore, it is important to dissect the submucosal layer making sure to leave the lowest one-third without any exposure of the proper muscular layer. Under intubation general anesthesia, the mediastinal pressure is higher than the intraesophageal pressure, enabling prevention of mediastinal emphysema and/or subcutaneous emphysema. Therefore, intubation general anesthesia is preferable for large lesions that are expected to take two or more hours for complete resection.

The perforation rate caused by esophageal EMR has been reported as 0–2.4 %, and that of ESD as 0–6.4 % [7–10]. The shape and size of perforation caused by EMR is different from that caused by ESD. Muscle removed by EMR can be up to 1 cm or larger, and sometimes closure by clips is difficult. On the other hand, the shape of perforation caused by ESD is linear, without defect of proper muscle, and so closure by clips is usually easier than that of EMR. However, sometimes the clip may injure the remaining proper muscle and make the perforation larger. Therefore, the operator should be skilled at clipping. Usually such perforations can be treated by fast insertion of a nasoesophageal tube and intravenous antibiotic administration, without need for surgery.

Water jets are useful for the detection of the bleeding point. However, sometimes water reflux causes aspiration pneumonia. A flexible overtube (Sumitomo Bakelite, Akita, Japan) is a useful device for prevention of aspiration pneumonia. General anesthesia with tracheal intubation is necessary for the cervical esophageal ESD because the risk of aspiration pneumonia is high.

Stricture

Stricture is a major complication after ESD. Multivariate analysis has shown that a mucosal defect of more than three-quarters of the circumference is a reliable predictor of stricture [17–20]. Post-ESD stricture substantially decreases a patients' quality of life and requires multiple endoscopic balloon dilation (EBD) sessions. Preventive EBD has been the treatment of choice to prevent stricture; however, even after six sessions of preventive EBD, stricture is a frequent complication.

Recently, the efficacy of prophylactic oral prednisolone for prevention of post-ESD stricture was described [21]. Although this method reduced the stricture rate, the cumulative dose of prednisolone was approximately 1,000 mg, and exposure to such a high prednisolone dose raises concerns regarding adverse effects.

The efficacy of intralesional triamcinolone injection to prevent stricture after esophageal ESD has also been described [22, 23]. Especially worth noting is research by Hanaoka et al., where the effect of a single session of intralesional steroid injections immediately after ESD was studied. In this prospective study they compared the results with a historical control group of patients who underwent ESD without intralesional steroid injection. The treatment group had a significantly lower stricture rate (10 %, 3/30 patients vs. 66 %, 19/29 patients; $p < 0.0001$) and a lower number of EBD sessions (median 0, range 0–2 vs. median 2, range 0–15; $p < 0.0001$) [23].

A novel, unique method to prevent stricture after esophageal ESD has been published [24]. Specimens of oral mucosal tissue were collected from nine patients with superficial esophageal neoplasms. Epithelial cell sheets were fabricated ex vivo by culturing isolated cells for 16 days on temperature-responsive cell culture surfaces. After a reduction in temperature, these sheets were endoscopically transplanted directly to the ulcer surfaces of patients who had just undergone ESD. Complete re-epithelialization occurred within a median time of 3.5 weeks. No patients experienced dysphagia, stricture, or other complications following the procedure, except for one patient who had a full circumferential ulceration that expanded to the esophagogastric junction [24]. For additional discussion of stricture management, please Chaps. 14 and 15.

Conclusions

The advantage of ESD is the ability to achieve R0 resection, and a low local recurrence rate. However, esophageal ESD is technically more difficult than gastric ESD due to the narrower space of esophagus for endoscopic maneuvers. Also, the risk of perforation is higher because of the thinner muscle layer of the esophageal wall. The clip-with-line method is useful for maintaining a good endoscopic view with added countertraction. ESD for esophageal cancer is a procedure that requires high technical ability, and therefore, only operators who have adequate skills should perform esophageal ESD.

References

1. Makuuchi H. Endoscopic mucosal resection for early esophageal cancer: indication and techniques. Dig Endosc. 1996;8:175–9.
2. Makuuchi H, Yoshida T, EII C. Four-step endoscopic esophageal mucosal resection tube method of resection for early esophageal cancer. Endoscopy. 2004;36:1013–8.
3. Inoue H, Takeshita K, Hori H, et al. Endoscopic mucosal resection with a cap-fitted panendoscope for esophagus, stomach and colon mucosal lesions. Gastrointest Endosc. 1993;39:58–62.
4. Pech O, Gossner L, May A, et al. Endoscopic resection of superficial esophageal squamous-cell carcinomas: western experience. Am J Gastroenterol. 2004;99:1226–32.

5. Momma K. Endoscopic treatment of esophageal mucosal carcinomas: indications and outcomes. Esophagus. 2007;4:93–8.
6. Oyama T, Kikuchi Y. Aggressive endoscopic mucosal resection in the upper GI tract: hook knife EMR method. Min Invas Ther Alied Technol. 2002;11:291–5.
7. Oyama T, Tomori A, Hotta K, et al. Endoscopic submucosal dissection of early esophageal cancer. Clin Gastroenterol Hepatol. 2005;3:S67–70.
8. Fujishiro M, Yahagi N, Kakushima N, et al. Endoscopic submucosal dissection of esophageal squamous cell neoplasms. Clin Gastroenterol Hepatol. 2006;4:688–94.
9. Ishihara R, Iishi H, Uedo N, et al. Comparison of EMR and endoscopic submucosal dissection for en bloc resection of early esophageal cancers in Japan. Gastrointest Endosc. 2008;68:1066–72.
10. Takahashi H, Arimura Y, Hosokawa M, et al. Endoscopic submucosal dissection is superior to conventional endoscopic resection as a curative treatment for early squamous cell carcinoma, of the esophagus. Gastrointest Endosc. 2010;71:255–64.
11. Dunbar K, Spechler S. The risk of lymph-node metastases in patients with high-grade dysplasia or intramucosal carcinoma in Barrett' s esophagus: a systematic review. Am J Gastroenterol. 2012;107:850–62.
12. Oyama T, Tomori A, Hotta K, et al. ESD with a hook knife for early esophageal cancer. Stom Intest. 2006;41:491–7. Japanese with English summary.
13. Oyama T, Yuichi K, Shimaya S, et al. Endoscopic mucosal resection using a hooking knife – intra gastric lesion lifting method. Stom Intest. 2002;37:1155–61. Japanese with English summary.
14. Oyama T. Counter traction makes endoscopic submucosal dissection easier. Clin Endosc. 2012;45:375–8.
15. Oyama T. Endoscopic submucosal dissection using a hook knife. Tech Gastrointest Endosc. 2011;13:70–3.
16. Oyama T, Akihisa T, Hotta K, Miyata Y. Hemostasis with hook knife during Endoscopic submucosal dissection. Dig Endosc. 2006;18:S128–30.
17. Katada C, Muto M, Manabe T, et al. Esophageal stenosis after endoscopic mucosal resection of superficial esophageal lesions. Gastrointest Endosc. 2003;57:165–9.
18. Mizuta H, Nishimori I, Kuratani Y, et al. Predictive factors for esophageal stenosis after endoscopic submucosal dissection for superficial esophageal cancer. Dis Esophagus. 2009;22:626–31.
19. Ono S, Fujishiro M, Niimi K, et al. Predictors of postoperative stricture after esophageal endoscopic submucosal dissection for superficial esophageal squamous cell neoplasms. Endoscopy. 2009;41:661–5.
20. Takahasi H, Arimura Y, Okahara S, et al. Risk of perforation during dilation for esophageal strictures after endoscopic resection in patients with early squamous cell carcinoma. Endoscopy. 2011;43:184–9.
21. Yamaguchi N, Isomoto H, Nakayama T, et al. Usefulness of oral prednisolone in the treatment of

esophageal stricture after endoscopic submucosal dissection for superficial esophageal squamous cell carcinoma. Gastrointest Endosc. 2011;73:1115–21.

22. Hashimoto S, Kobayashi M, Takeuchi M, et al. The efficacy of endoscopic triamcinolone injection for the prevention of esophageal stricture after endoscopic submucosal dissection. Gastrointest Endosc. 2011;74: 1389–93.

23. Hanaoka N, Ishihara R, Takeuchi Y, et al. Intralesional steroid injection to prevent stricture after endoscopic submucosal dissection for esophageal cancer: a controlled prospective study. Endoscopy. 2012;44:1007–11.

24. Ohki T, Yamato M, Ota M, et al. Prevention of esophageal stricture after endoscopic submucosal dissection using tissue-engineered cell sheets. Gastroenterology. 2012;143:582–8.

ESD Technique: Stomach

Hiroyuki Ono

Introduction

Endoscopic therapy for early gastric cancer has been attempted since the 1960s, but it came to be widely performed after the development of endoscopic mucosal resection (EMR) in the 1980s. However, en bloc resection by EMR is difficult to perform for lesions larger than 1 cm and lesions arising with ulcer scars [1]. To overcome these issues, endoscopic submucosal dissection (ESD) was developed in Japan in the mid-1990s [2].

In the 2000s, ESD for early gastric cancer spread rapidly, first across Japan and then across other Asian countries that have a high incidence of gastric cancer, such as Korea, Taiwan, and China. At present, the technique is widely used for lesions in the esophagus, duodenum, and colon.

The first high-frequency knife developed for use with ESD was the IT knife [2]. An improved IT knife 2 for the treatment of early gastric cancer followed [3], and later the IT knife nano was introduced for the treatment of esophageal and colon cancer [4] (Fig. 11.1). Several other designs have subsequently been developed [5–7].

Preparation

Informed Consent

Informed consent should be obtained from patients only after they have received an explanation about the nature of their cancerous disease, the indications and need for treatment, surgical techniques, other treatment modalities, potential procedural complications and their frequency, and the option to voluntary withdraw their consent. Patients with expanded-indication lesions must be told that surgical resection is currently regarded as standard therapy, and a meeting with the surgeon is desirable.

Preoperative Endoscopic Examination

This examination is essential for determining the extent of the lesion, invasion depth, and histological type. Preoperative endoscopy should be done to ensure that ESD is performed to treat the indicated lesions appropriately and to avoid residual disease and recurrence. The basic idea is to perform normal, white-light endoscopy and chromoendoscopy to determine the extent of resection preoperatively. If the extent is

Electronic supplementary material is available in the online version of this chapter at 10.1007/978-1-4939-2041-9_11. Videos can also be accessed at http://www.springerimages.com/videos/978-1-4939-2040-2.

H. Ono, M.D., Ph.D. (✉)
Division of Endoscopy, Shizuoka Cancer Center,
1007 Shimonagakubo Nagaizumi-cho, Suntogun,
Shizuoka 411-8777, Japan
e-mail: h.ono@scchr.jp

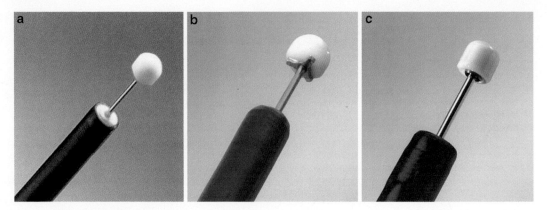

Fig. 11.1 (**a**) IT knife, (**b**) IT knife 2, and (**c**) IT knife nano

unclear, biopsies are taken from various points outside the cancer margin that are believed to be normal tissue. Defining the non-cancerous region and correctly determining the line of incision are important goals of the preoperative endoscopic examination. Magnifying endoscopy and narrow band imaging-magnifying endoscopy (NBI-ME) are also useful to define the lesion.

Preoperative Examination

Interview on Medical History and History of Present Illness

Patients must be interviewed in detail about their history of drug allergies, the presence of a cardiac pacemaker, cardiovascular disease, glaucoma, hypertensive disease, cerebrovascular disease, and prostatic hypertrophy. When asking about drugs that are taken on a daily basis, patients should be asked specifically about oral anticoagulants (e.g., warfarin) and various anti-platelet agents.

Blood Biochemistry and Physiological Examination

Blood type, presence of infectious diseases (e.g., HBV, HCV, HIV, and syphilis), general blood biochemistry, prothrombin time, and activated partial thromboplastin time should be checked. Cardiopulmonary screening must be conducted by performing electrocardiography (ECG), chest X-ray, and lung function tests.

Instruments

Electrosurgical Unit (ESU; Power Generator)

The high-frequency electric current in cauterization devices provides an incision wave, a coagulation wave, or a mixed wave, and, depending on the device, a mode to change the rate and timing of incision and coagulation.

The ICC-200, ICC-300, VIO300D (ERBE, Tubingen, Germany), and ESG100 (Olympus Medical Systems, Tokyo, Japan) are widely used. The Endocut mode has become standard following the emergence of these ESUs, and it is now possible to perform incisions and dissections with less frequent immediate hemorrhage. This has helped facilitate the widespread use of ESD.

Regardless of which ESU or mode is used, the optimal settings depend on the target lesion and the type of local injection solution used. It is important, therefore, for the endoscopist to choose the proper output mode. For reference, the authors use the following settings for the stomach. With the VIO300D, incision is made using Endocut, Effect 2, Cut duration 2, and Cut interval 2, and submucosal dissection is performed using Swift coagulation and Effect 4 or 5 at 100 W.

Endoscopes
Standard Endoscopes for ESD

Most ESD procedures can be performed under direct visualization using a normal single-channel scope. However, it may be preferable in some cases to use a 2-channel scope.

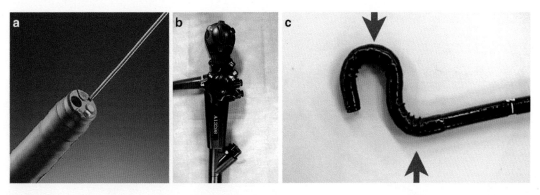

Fig. 11.2   (**a**) Endoscope with an auxiliary water jet function. (**b**) A multibending scope with two independently curving segments

Scopes Equipped with an Auxiliary Water Jet (Fig. 11.2a)

An auxiliary water jet helps to maintain a clear view during ESD by flushing water from a nozzle at the tip of the endoscope into the immediate operative field during hemorrhage. This feature can even be used with the device for incision or hemostasis still being within the accessary channel, and so helps to prevent perforation or mucosal incision by flushing a surgical field when obscured by blood. It is also extremely useful for pinpointing and confirming petechiae (a potential source of bleeding). Water-jet enabled scopes allow ESD to be performed safely and quickly.

Multi-Bending Scope (Fig. 11.2b)

To secure the position of a normal scope in difficult-to-operate sites, such as the lesser curvature in the lower gastric body and the anterior wall in the upper body, the multi-bending scope is provided with an additional flexure in front of the normal flexure. It is advisable to prepare the use of one of these multi-bending scopes when performing ESD if available.

Incision and Dissection Devices
IT Knife (Insulation-Tipped Diathermic Knife)

A ceramic ball is attached to the tip for insulation, and the knife is used for incision and dissection with the blade placed in a horizontal orientation.

These Other Knives Are Classified as So-Called Tip Knives

Examples include: Hook knife, Dual knife, Flush knife, and Hybrid knife.

Intraprocedural Monitoring

Intraprocedural monitoring is essential during ESD. At a minimum, blood pressure, degree of oxygen saturation, ECG, and pulse should be monitored.

ESD Procedure

The ESD procedure, as a rule, involves a circumferential incision being made around the lesion and submucosal dissection. The actual process may differ depending on the devices used and required experience.

When using IT knife, the basic movement is from distal to proximal direction (Fig. 11.3).

ESD Using an IT Knife (Fig. 11.4)

Examination of the Lesion

The endoscope is inserted into the stomach, and taking the biopsy sites of the preoperative endoscopic examination into consideration, the lesion is once again sufficiently examined to determine its extent (Fig. 11.4a).

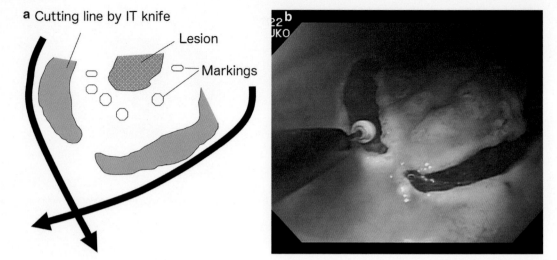

Fig. 11.3 (**a** and **b**) As a rule, the main movement of the IT knife is cutting by drawing the knife anteriorly from the interior

Marking

Marking of the entire circumference is conducted at intervals of a few millimeters, approximately 2–5 mm laterally from the lesion margin. When this is performed, some kind of landmark should be used to differentiate the oral and anal ends of the resection specimen. An additional marking should be placed as a landmark as it will be useful when arranging the specimen after the completion of ESD (Fig. 11.4b).

Local Injection

The local injection needle is placed somewhat laterally to the markings, and injections are performed so as to create sufficient mucosal protrusion. The injection solution used is normal saline or sodium hyaluronate, to which epinephrine or indigo carmine is added as desired for their effect (Fig. 11.4c).

Precutting and Circumferential Mucosal Incision

Using the incision wave, the needle knife is used to create small incisions of approximately 1–2 mm (precutting) approximately 5 mm lateral to the markings for insertion of the IT knife into the mucosa. As the incision wave is used for precutting, the tip of the needle knife is not insulated, so it is important to take care not to perforate into surrounding tissue (muscularis propria or serosa) but adequate enough to cut to reach submucosal layer. Precutting is conducted distal to the lesion (Fig. 11.4d).

The tip of the IT knife is inserted into the small incisions created during precutting, and the mucosa lateral to the lesion is cut circumferentially using the Endocut or Dry cut mode. In this example photo, because the mucosal incision is shallow, making an incision and dissecting the submucosal layer would be difficult, so the muscularis mucosae needs to be incised further (Fig. 11.4e, f).

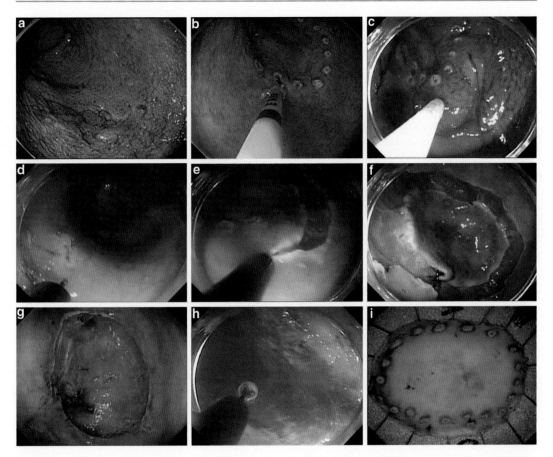

Fig. 11.4 (**a**) 0-IIc type early gastric cancer located at the greater curvature of the antrum. (**b**) Marking. (**c**) Submucosal injection of saline or hyaluronic acid solution. (**d**) Precutting for insertion of the IT knife. (**e**) Mucosal dissection. (**f**) Circumferential cutting. (**g**) Submucosal dissection. (**h**) Ulcer after resecting the lesion. (**i**) Resected specimen

Incision and Dissection of the Submucosa

When the circumferential incision has been completed, local injection of the entire lesion is repeated to make it further protrude to widen the submucosal layer. While confirming the submucosal layer, the submucosal tissue is cut and dissected using the Endocut mode or the Swift coagulation mode. Basic dissection is performed by sliding the IT knife parallel to the gastric wall while applying sufficient tension to the submucosal tissue (Fig. 11.4g).

After sufficient submucosal dissection has been performed, the IT knife is used to complete the dissection of the submucosa resulting in completion of the resection, or a snare may be used for final resection (Fig. 11.4h). The resected specimen is withdrawn using the grasping forceps.

Hemostasis

After withdrawal of the resected specimen, the scope is reinserted to confirm hemostasis. If hemorrhage is observed, hemostasis is accomplished using hemostatic forceps or by APC.

Dealing with Difficult Lesions with Submucosal Fibrosis (e.g., Ulcer Scar)

Tips for Procedure

Selection of Electrosugical Knives

First, this section deals with selection of an appropriate device for use in scarred regions. However, it is still possible to use the IT knife 2, which can be used without major concern even in cases of mild fibrosis, and it is also possible to achieve resection using the normal method of dissection. When there is a large degree of fibrosis, tip knives such as the needle knife or hook knife require higher skills for manipulation. Tip knives are used for dissection after visually confirming the layer structure under direct visualization, but the layer structure is disrupted when there is a high degree of fibrosis, which makes it difficult to determine the incision line. To avoid perforation or incision of the mucosal surface, it is necessary to cut carefully, in stages, which tends to take more time.

The IT knife 2 is composed of a needle knife with three short blades attached to the back of a ceramic tip, and these are able to grasp and incise the indurated fibrotic tissue. So, although they do not have the same incision capabilities as the tip knife, they function well in situations where there is a high degree of fibrosis. The advantage of incising fibrotic areas with the IT knife 2 is that instead of cutting after visually confirming the layer structure, the cutting is done parallel to the gastric wall and the muscularis layer is dissected. For this reason, even if the submucosal layer and muscle layer are adhered to the ulcer, the curvature of the gastric wall and the line of the muscularis layer can be estimated.

It is better to perform circumferential incisions in regions where there is no scarring, but difficulty increases when the ulcer is wider than the lesion and when the resection specimen is too large. In such cases, the only choice is to run the incision line through the ulcer. When the fibrosis is particularly extensive and it is not possible to perform incision with an IT knife, the IT knife should be used in conjunction with a needle knife (or tip knife).

Case Study

Figure 11.5 shows a difficult case. This variation is due to an ulcer scar on the angular incisure of the lesser curvature. A 0-IIc lesion, 10 mm in diameter, is apparent within the scar (Fig. 11.5a). After making a circumferential incision, dissection of the submucosa was initiated. The images

in Fig. 11.5b–d,f were taken while viewing the angular incisure from below. When making the incision, the IT knife 2 was moved from the posterior wall toward the anterior wall (right to left on the photo with retroflexed position of the endoscope). First, the knife was placed at the margin of the posterior wall and next, as shown in Fig. 11.5c, it was traced along the angular incisure to move in the direction to the anterior wall. Figure 11.5d shows incision of areas with marked scarring where the knife was further advanced along the anterior wall. The path of the IT knife 2 where it was advanced to cut the areas with marked fibrosis is clearly visible. Under such circumstances, it is important to move the scope closer to the area of incision and hold the knife firmly. When the knife is moved from a distance, it may be repelled by the indurated fibrotic area, which may result in perforation or incision of the mucosal surface. When it is difficult to position the scope close to the lesion, a multi-bending scope (Olympus Medical Systems) or an air-assisted balloon (Top, Tokyo, Japan) should be used. In the case shown in Fig. 11.5, the required proximity was achieved using an Olympus Q260J (standard single channel upper endoscope with water jet). The resection specimen was removed in one piece (Fig. 11.5g) and the procedure was completed uneventfully (specimen diameter 35×30 mm, en bloc resection, resection time of 41 min).

Conclusions

When considering ESD for gastric cancer, a procedure commonly performed in Japan and other Asian countries, physicians should practice and master the basic maneuvers needed to examine and perform resection in the stomach. If patient numbers are too small to gain sufficient experience, animal models should be used to learn and practice these basic maneuvers. Use of an IT knife is useful in gastric ESD, and specific maneuvers described in this chapter should help all endoscopists to complete gastric ESD.

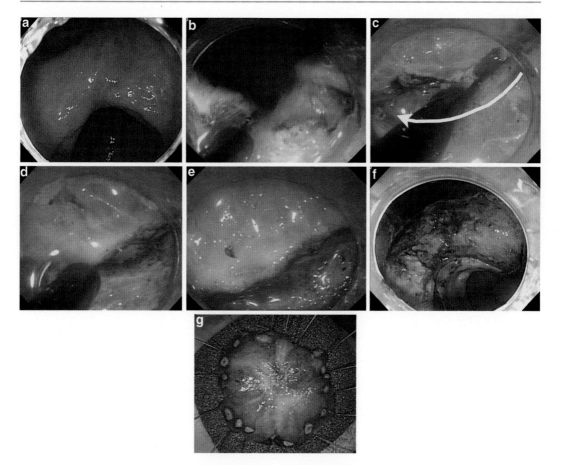

Fig. 11.5 (**a**) A IIc lesion on a gastric ulcer on the angular incisure of the lesser curvature. (**b**) Dissection of the submucosa after making a circumferential incision. (**c**) The IT knife is moved along the muscle layer, parallel to the line of the gastric wall from the posterior wall toward the anterior wall in the direction shown by the *yellow arrow*. (**d**) The dissection region is approached as closely as possible in the areas with marked scarring, and the knife is grasped firmly in order to cut through the fibrotic tissue. (**e**) Incision of the fibrotic area. (**f**) Ulcer after resection. (**g**) Resected specimen shows contraction of the scar on the mucosal surface after resection, but no incision of the mucosa and the lesion was resected en bloc

References

1. Ono H. Early gastric cancer: diagnosis, pathology, treatment techniques and treatment outcomes. Eur J Gastroenterol Hepatol. 2006;18(8):863–6.
2. Ono H, Kondo H, Gotoda T, Shirao K, Yamaguchi H, Saito D, et al. Endoscopic mucosal resection for treatment of early gastric cancer. Gut. 2001;48(2):225–9.
3. Ono H, Hasuike N, Inui T, Takizawa K, Ikehara H, Yamaguchi Y, et al. Usefulness of a novel electrosurgical knife, the insulation-tipped diathermic knife-2, for endoscopic submucosal dissection of early gastric cancer. Gastric Cancer. 2008;11(1):47–52.
4. Hotta K, Yamaguchi Y, Saito Y, Takao T, Ono H. Current opinions for endoscopic submucosal dissection for colorectal tumors from our experiences: indications, technical aspects and complications. Dig Endosc. 2012;24 Suppl 1:110–6.
5. Oyama T, Kikuchi Y. Aggressive endoscopic mucosal resection in the upper GI tract: hook knife EMR method. Min Invas Ther All Technol. 2002;11:291–5.
6. Yahagi N, Fujishiro M, Kakushima N, Kobayashi K, Hashimoto T, Oka M, et al. Endoscopic submucosal dissection for early gastric cancer using the tip of an electro-surgical snare (thin type). Dig Endosc. 2004;16:34–8.
7. Neuhaus H, Wirths K, Schenk M, Enderle MD, Schumacher B. Randomized controlled study of EMR versus endoscopic submucosal dissection with a water-jet hybrid-knife of esophageal lesions in a porcine model. Gastrointest Endosc. 2009; 70(1):112–20.

ESD for Colorectal Lesions

Naohisa Yahagi

Introduction

ESD for colorectal lesions is considered more technically demanding than ESD in the stomach for a variety of reasons. Basically, the colonic wall is thinner and softer than the gastric wall, and therefore, the risk of perforation is much higher than in the stomach. Control of the endoscope is sometimes more difficult as well, and it can even become unstable or move in a paradoxical manner due to the flexional structure of the colon. Colorectal lesions are often located on or behind a prominent fold, and there are limitations in the retroflex approach due to the narrow lumen of the colon. Because of the above-mentioned difficulties, the equipment and techniques used in gastric ESD are not always suitable for colorectal ESD. To perform ESD safely in the colon and rectum, it is important to use specific equipment and proper techniques.

Although there are some technical difficulties, ESD has great potential for achieving reliable en bloc resection, even for large and difficult colorectal lesions. Published data from high-volume Japanese centers have shown excellent short- and long-term clinical outcomes [1–5]. And clinical outcomes of European experts have suggested that ESD would become feasible even in the Western countries after appropriate training and experience with a certain number of ESD procedures [6, 7]. In this chapter, the necessary equipment and an outline of technical tips for colorectal ESD are described.

Indications for Colorectal ESD and Assessment of Its Curability

Almost all kinds of superficial neoplastic lesions with negligible risk for lymph node metastasis can be treated by endoscopic submucosal dissection (ESD); however, true targets of this technique are large and difficult lesions that are almost impossible to remove by conventional endoscopic mucosal resection (EMR). Consequently, large superficial lesions, especially laterally spreading tumors (LSTs), and lesions with some fibrosis due to previous attempts at endoscopic resection, are considered as candidates for ESD.

N. Yahagi, M.D., Ph.D. (✉)
Division of Research and Development for Minimally Invasive Treatment, Cancer Center, School of Medicine, Keio University, 35 Shinanomachi, Shinjuku-ku, Tokyo 160-8582, Japan
e-mail: yahagi-tky@umin.ac.jp

In order to determine whether the resection was curative, the risk of lymph node metastasis should be carefully assessed by a detailed histopathological examination of the resected specimen. Endoscopic complete resection of neoplastic lesions diagnosed as a benign adenoma or as a noninvasive or minimally invasive carcinoma without vessel infiltration is considered curative regardless of the size of the lesion [8]. According to the guidelines for the treatment of colorectal carcinomas published by the Japanese Society for Cancer of the Colon and Rectum [9], additional surgical colectomy and lymph node dissection is recommended for submucosal cancers that have one of five factors: a positive vertical resection margin; a depth of invasion >1,000 μm; vessel infiltration; poorly differentiated type; and tumor budding at the invasive front. Vessel infiltration, both lymphatic and venous, indicates a high risk of lymph node metastasis [10].

Necessary Equipment for Colorectal ESD

Endoscope

Maneuverability of the endoscope is the key factor for successful ESD. Retroflex manipulation is required when the oral edge of those lesions straddling a fold is to be incised. Therefore, a smaller diameter endoscope, such as a pediatric colonoscope or gastroscope, is much better than a regular colonoscope in order to allow smooth maneuverability in the retroflexed position. And a built-in water jet mechanism is extremely important for clear visualization of the operating field, especially in the occasion of bleeding. It is necessary to use normal saline for water irrigation to maintain good electrical conductivity.

Transparent Hood

It is strongly recommended to use a transparent hood throughout the procedure in order to perform ESD safely. The edge of the hood can be used like surgical forceps to open the incision in order to get a better view of the operating field, and to give appropriate traction to the target tissue. A soft distal attachment (Olympus Co. Ltd., Tokyo, Japan, Fig. 12.1a) is usually used for the majority of colorectal ESDs. In those cases where it is difficult to open the mucosal incision adequately, the short ST hood (Fujifilm, Tokyo, Japan, Fig. 12.2a) is very useful. It can open a narrow submucosal space very easily, although the visual field becomes a bit smaller.

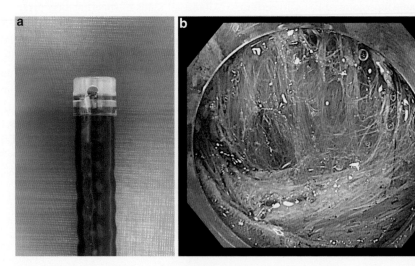

Fig. 12.1 A straight soft distal attachment (Olympus Medical Systems, Tokyo, Japan)

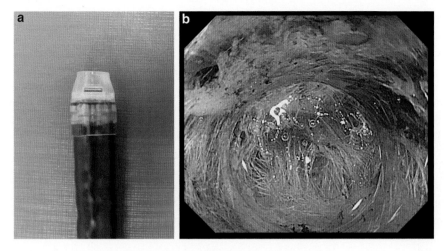

Fig. 12.2   A short ST hood (small-caliber tip hood) (Fujifilm, Tokyo, Japan)

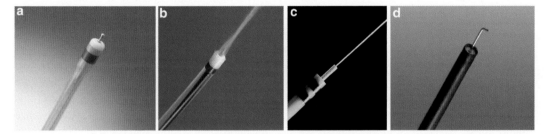

Fig. 12.3   Various ESD knifes suitable for colorectal ESD

Knives

Short needle type knives, such as the Dual Knife (Olympus Medical Systems, Tokyo, Japan, Fig. 12.3a) and the Flush Knife (Fujifilm, Tokyo, Japan, Fig. 12.3b), are the most popular devices for colorectal ESD. The Dual Knife is the most maneuverable device, owing to its soft and flexible nature, and it is ideal for colonic ESD [11]. The Flush Knife has water flushing function through its sheath, thus it is able to give additional submucosal fluid cushion during the procedure [12]. Both of the knives have a small disk or ball at the tip of the needle that can get hold of the target tissue.

The Hybrid Knife (ERBE, Tubingen, Germany, Fig. 12.3c) is also a length adjustable short needle knife. The particular specification of this knife is the pressure-controlled water jet function through its needle. It can inject some solution without using an injection needle, even through the mucosa, by setting appropriate water pressure [13]. It is a promising technology for ESD; however, precise control of the knife within a narrow space is rather difficult due to its rigidity and the relatively thick knife tip.

Many standard colorectal ESD procedures can be smoothly done with the above-mentioned short needle type knives, but in the case of a difficult situation, one had better to switch to the Hook knife (Olympus Medical Systems, Tokyo, Japan, Fig. 12.3d). It has a rotatable small hook part at the tip. One can hook and pull the target tissue with this hook before cutting it, which aids safety [14].

Hemostatic Forceps and Endoclips

Before starting ESD, it is necessary to have readily available hemostatic forceps (Pentax Co. Ltd. and Olympus Medical Systems, Tokyo, Japan) and rotatable clip fixing devices (Olympus Medical Systems, Tokyo, Japan, Boston Scientific, Boston, U.S.A.) to use anytime for bleeding and perforation. The hemostatic forceps must not be confused with a hot biopsy forceps, the latter being much larger and not pointed at the tip. The use of hot biopsy forceps is not recommended for colonic procedures, mainly for fear of a delayed perforation owing to focal over-coagulation.

Injection Solutions

Normal saline is the most popular injection fluid for conventional EMR. However, the mucosal protrusion created with the injection of normal saline does not last long enough to provide sufficient time for submucosal dissection [15]. In order to create a long-lasting submucosal fluid cushion, several other fluids have been used for ESD; among those, Glyceol solution (consisted of 10 % glycerin, 5 % fructose, and 0.9 % sodium chloride) is the most popular solution for the standard procedure. And a much more viscous agent, such as sodium hyaluronate [15–17], is preferable for larger and more difficult lesions. A sodium hyaluronate solution at a concentration of 0.4 % (MucoUp, Seikagaku Kougyo Co., Tokyo, Japan; derived from rooster comb) can create a prominent, long-lasting effect and is approved in Japan for use in the endoscopic resection of colorectal lesions [18]. A mixture with a small amount of added epinephrine is effective for the control of bleeding during the procedure. A further additive, indigocarmine dye, is useful for aiding clear visualization of the submucosal layer and visual differentiation from muscle.

Carbon Dioxide Insufflation

The safety and efficacy of carbon dioxide (CO_2) insufflation during ESD with the patient under conscious sedation and deep sedation have been reported [19–21]. Since the procedure time of ESD is much longer than other ordinary endoscopic procedures, it is mandatory to use CO_2 insufflation for ESD procedure. Moreover, even in the event of perforation, with CO_2 insufflation there is enough time to close the perforation with clip placement because leaked CO_2 into the abdominal cavity and/or retroperitoneal space is quickly absorbed.

Strategy for Colorectal ESD

The demarcation of colonic lesions is usually quite obvious and clear, so initial marking is not necessary for colorectal ESD (Fig. 12.4a). And it is very important to make a strategy for the procedure in order to perform colorectal ESD successfully.

One usually starts the procedure at the proximal side of the lesion, along the uppermost part (in terms of gravity) (Fig. 12.4b). If it is possible to keep the endoscope in a retroflexed view, it is better to start the procedure in this position since the endoscope is more stable and the target lesion is more easily approximated to the working channel (Fig. 12.4c). Circumferential mucosal incision is not recommended, since injected solution can easily leak out from the incised area. Submucosal dissection should be started immediately after partial mucosal incision, tracing along the inner edge of the incision line (Fig. 12.4d) until a submucosal pocket is created (Fig. 12.4e). It is quite important to get into the submucosal space with the transparent hood after initial submucosal dissection; this makes it easier to continue submucosal dissection with a stable condition under good visualization of the submucosa (Fig. 12.4f). When it is necessary, change the patient position in order to open the submucosal space widely by utilizing gravity (Fig. 12.4g). After progressing through submucosal dissection of more than half of the lesion from the upper side, reverse the position of the patient so that the remaining side becomes easier to dissect for the rest of the procedure. Keeping the submucosal fluid cushion sufficient by additional injection when necessary, any remaining incision and

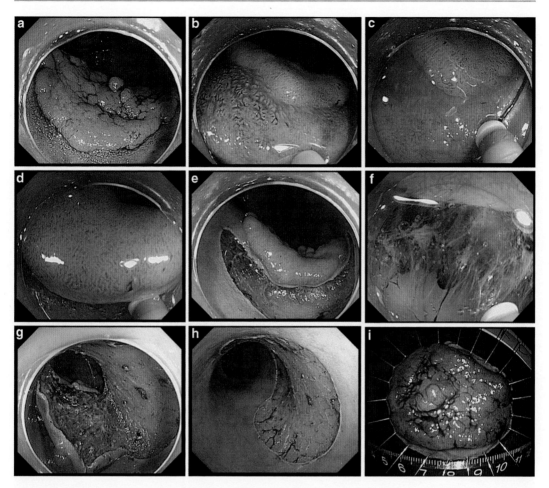

Fig. 12.4 Standard colonic ESD procedure for a mid-sized LST-G. The lesion was completely removed in an en bloc fashion. Resected specimen revealed a well-differen-tiated tubular adenocarcinoma with an adenomatous component; 46×38 mm, pSM (0.8 mm), INFa, ly0, v0, pHM0, pVM0

dissection can be safely done. Check the resected area and coagulate the exposed blood vessels carefully (Fig. 12.4h). Stretch the resected specimen on a cork board with pins before submitting it to the pathologist (Fig. 12.4i).

Difficult Situations for Colorectal ESD

Good maneuverability of the endoscope is the most important factor for a successful ESD procedure. There are some factors that can cause poor maneuverability of the endoscope. A long and strongly inflectional colon or severe adhesion of the colon due to previous surgery or some other diseases are major reasons for poor maneuverability of the endoscope. In these particular situation, ESD becomes almost impossible to do and even insertion of the endoscope becomes extremely tough. However, using a balloon assisted endoscope system, there is still some chance to perform ESD. Currently, a 152 cm universal double balloon endoscope (Fuji EI-530B, Fig. 12.5, Fujifilm Tokyo, Japan), which is a suitable length for standard ESD instruments, is commercially available. The majority of difficult situations caused by poor maneuverability of the endoscope can be under better control with this system. If one cannot get better control with the balloon-assisted endo-scope system, one had better not attempt ESD.

Other difficult situations usually arise due to the nature of the lesions themselves. Large lesions crossing the haustral hold (Fig. 12.6), large lesions invading the anal canal (Fig. 12.7) or those at the ileocecal valve (Fig. 12.8) are very

difficult situations for ESD. In order to dissect the submucosal tissue smoothly, one has to open the submucosal space by utilizing gravity and changing patient position. In the case of lesions with anal canal invasion, it is necessary to use some local anesthesia, such as 1 % lidocaine, when the operator cuts tissue within the anal canal. And in the case of lesions with ileocecal valve involvement, initial injection and incision should be started from the ileal side, otherwise it becomes almost impossible to cut the ileal side at later stages.

Severe fibrosis is the most difficult situation for ESD since it drastically increases technical difficulty and the risk of perforation, especially in the colon and rectum. One should approach the target lesion a little bit away from the scarred area and by first dissecting the surrounding submucosa. Subsequently, one can dissect the scarred, fibrotic area by connecting the dissection plane from both lateral sides (Fig. 12.9). This kind of treatment should be attempted only by well-experienced experts. One should check the situation carefully beforehand and work out a strategy for the treatment.

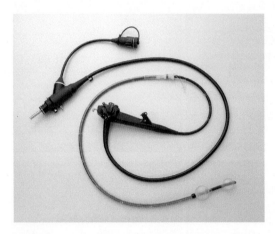

Fig. 12.5 Universal double balloon endoscope (Fujifilm, EI-530B, Tokyo, Japan)

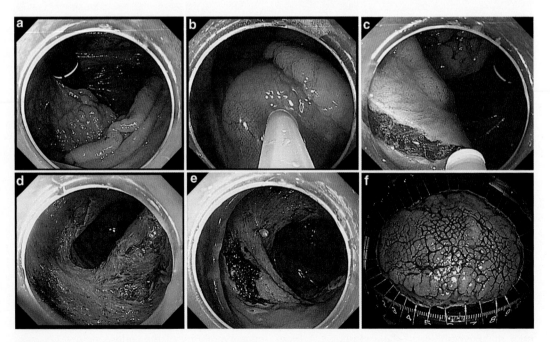

Fig. 12.6 A large LST-G located at ascending colon, straddling two folds. Resected specimen revealed a well-differentiated tubular adenocarcinoma, 78×56 mm, pM, ly0, v0, pHM0, pVM0

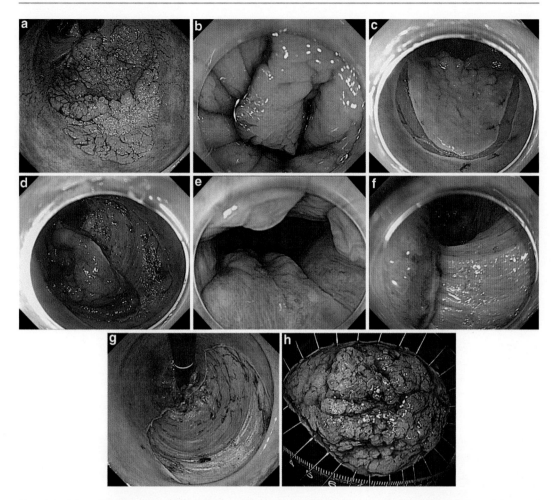

Fig. 12.7 A large LST-G invading to the anal canal. ESD was performed using 1 % lidocaine at the anal canal. Resected specimen revealed well-differentiated tubular adenocarcinoma, 65 × 48 mm, pM, ly0, v0, pHM0, pVM0

Training for Colorectal ESD

The basic technique for ESD is completely different from other ordinary therapeutic endoscopy procedures; therefore, specific training is necessary before attempting actual ESD procedures in humans. Step 1 is the observation of about ten ESD procedures at a high volume center to understand each step of the procedure; including how to delineate the border of lesions, how to create adequate submucosal fluid cushion, how to perform mucosal incision, how to perform submucosal dissection, how to manage complications, such as severe bleeding and perforation, and how to handle resected specimens.

Step 2 is participating in ESD procedures as an assistant to learn how to use the devices for ESD and to understand treatment strategy. Step 3 is the hands-on training of ESD using animal models in order to acquire the basic technical skills of ESD. Isolated porcine stomachs and bovine colon models are available for basic training (Fig. 12.10), and live pigs that can provide much more similar to live conditions, such as peristalsis, pulsation, and bleeding during the procedure, are available for advanced training. Hands-on training with animal models is highly recommended for beginners since it can facilitate a better learning curve when one begins to perform ESD in patients [22–24].

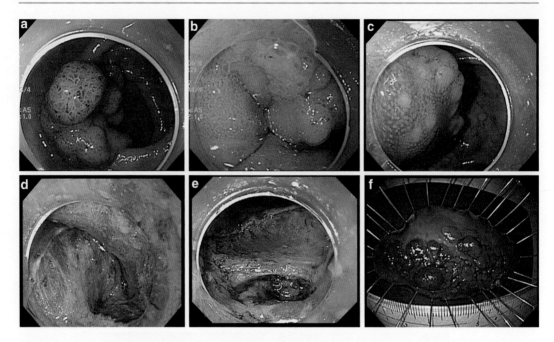

Fig. 12.8 A large LST-G involving the ileo-cecal valve. Complete resection was achieved and pathological diagnosis was a tubular adenoma with severe atypia, 60×30 mm, pHM0, pVM0

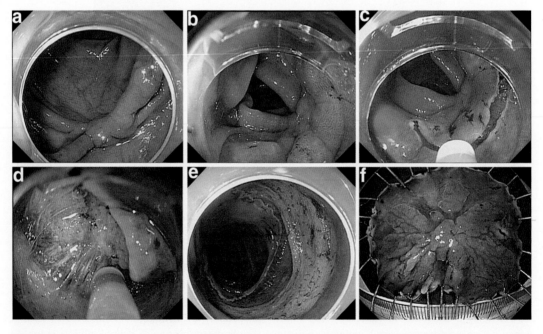

Fig. 12.9 Recurrent adenoma after piecemeal resection. Complete resection was achieved by dissecting the scarred tissue under direct vision. Pathological diagnosis was a tubular adenoma with severe atypia, 48×40 mm, pHM0, pVM0

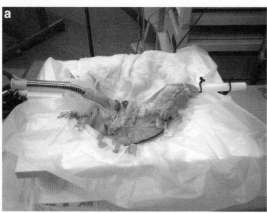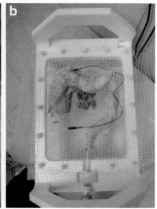

Fig. 12.10 (**a**) Isolated porcine stomach model, (**b**) Isolated bovine colon model

Step 4 is an actual human ESD procedure of a relatively easy case; however, for safety reasons and because there is a steeper learning curve in the early phases of clinical experience, appropriate guidance and supervision by an expert are essential. At least in Japan, experience with a minimum of 20 gastric ESD cases is recommended before initially performing colorectal ESD because of the technical difficulties and the higher risk of perforation in the colon. Based on extensive clinical experience at high volume centers in Japan, Kakushima et al. [25] and Yamamoto et al. [26] reported that someone with limited experience, such as a young trainee, can begin to handle gastric ESD cases independently after performing approximately 30 supervised ESD procedures. In addition, Niimi et al. [27] reported that colorectal ESD could be safely and efficiently taught to trainees competent in gastric ESD under the supervision of experts. Yet another study reported the safety of colorectal ESD independently performed by trainees after preparatory training and hands-on experience in 30 cases with the guidance by experts [28].

Although it is desirable to start actual ESD procedures with gastric case, under supervision of experts, it remains difficult to have enough volume of early gastric cancer cases and experts to supervise the procedure in most Western countries. Therefore, it might be unavoidable to start the procedure by oneself, without a supervisor. In such circumstances, it is highly recom-

mended to select a relatively small rectal case at the beginning since it is less risky and less difficult. And once an operator becomes confident at performing mucosal incision and submucosal dissection on an easy target, one may step ahead to larger lesions and different locations.

As for further incremental steps, we suggest performing ESD on lesions in the ascending, transverse, descending, and sigmoid colon, followed by flexures, in that order. The sigmoid colon and flexures are considered to be the most difficult locations because of the flexion and unstable scope position. Therefore, for those lesions located at flexional areas should be approached as a final step, only after having a certain amount of ESD experience. And, always, we have to think about the balance between risk and benefit of the procedure before attempting colorectal ESD.

Conclusions

Colorectal ESD is one of the most advanced and sophisticated therapeutic endoscopy procedures available for difficult lesions. Since it is technically demanding, it is necessary to have sufficient training. To avoid the potential risk of serious complications, one should understand the features of this procedure and conduct it very carefully using specific equipment and proper techniques.

Conflict of Interest Naohisa Yahagi has some patents for ESD devices together with Olympus Medical Systems and Pentax Corp.

References

1. Niimi K, Fujishiro M, Kodashima S, Goto O, Ono S, Hirano K, Minatsuki C, Yamamichi N, Koike K. Long-term outcomes of endoscopic submucosal dissection for colorectal epithelial neoplasms. Endoscopy. 2010;42:723–9.

2. Nishiyama H, Isomoto H, Yamaguchi N, Fukuda E, Ikeda K, Ohnita K, Mizuta Y, Nakamura T, Nakao K, Kohno S, Shikuwa S. Endoscopic submucosal dissection for colorectal epithelial neoplasms. Dis Colon Rectum. 2010;53:161–8.

3. Saito Y, Uraoka T, Yamaguchi Y, Hotta K, Sakamoto N, Ikematsu H, Fukuzawa M, Kobayashi N, Nasu J, Michida T, Yoshida S, Ikehara H, Otake Y, Nakajima T, Matsuda T, Saito D. A prospective, multicenter study of 1111 colorectal endoscopic submucosal dissections (with video). Gastrointest Endosc. 2010;72:1217–25.

4. Kuroki Y, Hoteya S, Mitani T, Yamashita S, Kikuchi D, Fujimoto A, Matsui A, Nakamura M, Nishida N, Iizuka T, Yahagi N. Endoscopic submucosal dissection for residual/locally recurrent lesions after endoscopic therapy for colorectal tumors. J Gastroenterol Hepatol. 2010;25:1747–53.

5. Yamamoto H. Endoscopic submucosal dissection–current success and future directions. Nat Rev Gastroenterol Hepatol. 2012;9:519–29.

6. Probst A, Golger D, Anthuber M, Markl B, Messmann H. Endoscopic submucosal dissection in large sessile lesions of the rectosigmoid: learning curve in a European center. Endoscopy. 2012;44:660–7.

7. Repici A, Hassan C, Pagano N, Rando G, Romeo F, Spaggiari P, Roncalli M, Ferrara E, Malesci A. High efficacy of endoscopic submucosal dissection for rectal laterally spreading tumors larger than 3 cm. Gastrointest Endosc. 2013;77:96–101.

8. Kitajima K, Fujimori T, Fujii S, et al. Correlations between lymph node metastasis and depth of submucosal invasion in submucosal invasive colorectal carcinoma: a Japanese collaborative study. J Gastroenterol. 2004;39:534–43.

9. Watanabe T, Itabashi M, Shimada Y, et al. Japanese Society for Cancer of the Colon and Rectum (JSCCR) guidelines 2010 for the treatment of colorectal cancer. Int J Clin Oncol. 2012;17:1–29.

10. Egashira Y, Yoshida T, Hirata I, et al. Analysis of pathological risk factors for lymph node metastasis of submucosal invasive colon cancer. Mod Pathol. 2004;17:503–11.

11. Yahagi N, Uraoka T, Ida Y, et al. Endoscopic submucosal dissection using the flex and the dual knives. Tech Gastrointest Endosc. 2011;13:74–8.

12. Toyonaga T, Man-I M, Fujita T, et al. The performance of a novel ball-tipped Flush knife for endoscopic submucosal dissection: a case–control study. Aliment Pharmacol Ther. 2010;32:908–15.

13. Yahagi N, Neuhaus H, Schumacher B, et al. Comparison of standard endoscopic submucosal dissection (ESD) versus an optimized ESD technique for the colon: an animal study. Endoscopy. 2009;41:340–5.

14. Oyama T, Tomori A, Hotta K, et al. Endoscopic submucosal dissection of early esophageal cancer. Clin Gastroenterol Hepatol. 2005;3(7 Suppl 1):S67–70.

15. Fujishiro M, Yahagi N, Kashimura K, et al. Comparison of various submucosal injection solutions for maintaining mucosal elevation during endoscopic mucosal resection. Endoscopy. 2004;36:579–83.

16. Yamamoto H, Yube T, Isoda N, et al. A novel method of endoscopic mucosal resection using sodium hyaluronate. Gastrointest Endosc. 1999;50:251–6.

17. Fujishiro M, Yahagi N, Kashimura K, et al. Different mixtures of sodium hyaluronate and their ability to create submucosal fluid cushions for endoscopic mucosal resection. Endoscopy. 2004;36:584–9.

18. Hirasaki S, Kozu T, Yamamoto H, et al. Usefulness and safety of 0.4% sodium hyaluronate solution as a submucosal fluid "cushion" for endoscopic resection of colorectal mucosal neoplasms: a prospective multicenter open-label trial. BMC Gastroenterol. 2009;9:1.

19. Kikuchi T, Fu KI, Saito Y, et al. Transcutaneous monitoring of partial pressure of carbon dioxide during endoscopic submucosal dissection of early colorectal neoplasia with carbon dioxide insufflation: a prospective study. Surg Endosc. 2010;24:2231–5.

20. Nonaka S, Saito Y, Takisawa H, et al. Safety of carbon dioxide insufflation for upper gastrointestinal tract endoscopic treatment of patients under deep sedation. Surg Endosc. 2010;24:1638–45.

21. Saito Y, Uraoka T, Matsuda T, et al. A pilot study to assess the safety and efficacy of carbon dioxide insufflation during colorectal endoscopic submucosal dissection with the patient under conscious sedation. Gastrointest Endosc. 2007;65:537–42.

22. Parra-Blanco A, Saito Y, Yahagi N, et al. Recommendations about training for colorectal endoscopic submucosal dissection in the western world. Results of a survey to experts. Gastrointest Endosc. 2011;73 Suppl 4:AB419–20.

23. Berr F, Ponchon T, Neureiter D, et al. Experimental endoscopic submucosal dissection training in a porcine model: learning experience of skilled western endoscopists. Dig Endosc. 2011;23:281–9.

24. Parra-Blanco A, Arnau MR, Nicolás-Pérez D, et al. Endoscopic submucosal dissection training with pig models in a Western country. World J Gastroenterol. 2010;16:2895–900.

25. Kakushima N, Fujishiro M, Kodashima S, et al. A learning curve for endoscopic submucosal dissection of gastric epithelial neoplasms. Endoscopy. 2006;38:991–5.

26. Yamamoto S, Uedo N, Ishihara R, et al. Endoscopic submucosal dissection for early gastric cancer performed by supervised residents: assessment of feasibility and learning curve. Endoscopy. 2009;41: 923–8.

27. Niimi K, Fujishiro M, Goto O, et al. Safety and efficacy of colorectal endoscopic submucosal dissection by the trainee endoscopists. Dig Endosc. 2012;24 Suppl 1:154–8.

28. Sakamoto T, Saito Y, Fukunaga S, Nakajima T, Matsuda T. Learning curve associated with colorectal endoscopic submucosal dissection for endoscopists experienced in gastric endoscopic submucosal dissection. Dis Colon Rectum. 2011;54:1307–12.

Hironori Yamamoto, Yoshikazu Hayashi, and Keijiro Sunada

Introduction

Endoscopic submucosal dissection (ESD) has been developed to overcome the limitations of endoscopic mucosal resection (EMR); namely, feasible en bloc resection specimen size and precise determination of resection margins. By performing ESD, reliable, complete en bloc resections for large superficial lesions in the GI tract have become feasible. With the advent of ESD, application criteria for endoscopic resection have expanded.

Although ESD is an ideal endoscopic resection technique, there are many factors that can contribute to potential difficulty. In such cases, ESD could have high rates of complications and could be extraordinarily time consuming.

In this chapter, the factors contributing to these difficulties are analyzed and some tips and techniques to conquer the difficulties are proposed.

Electronic supplementary material Supplementary material is available in the online version of this chapter at 10.1007/978-1-4939-2041-9_13. Videos can also be accessed at http://www.springerimages.com/videos/978-1-4939-2040-2.

H. Yamamoto, M.D., Ph.D., F.A.S.G.E. (✉)
Y. Hayashi, M.D., Ph.D. • K. Sunada, M.D.
Jichi Medical University, 3311-1, Shimotsuke, Tochigi 329-0498, Japan
e-mail: ireef@jichi.ac.jp

Factors that Contribute to Difficult ESD

1. Bleeding
2. Thin muscle layer
3. Difficulty in mucosal elevation (fibrosis, etc.)
4. Angle of approach
5. Direction of gravity
6. Endoscopic maneuverability and control

Differences Among Different Organs

The technical difficulties of ESD differ among each organ. In general, gastric ESD is considered easier than that of the esophagus and colon. However, each organ brings its own difficulties. In order to overcome these difficulties, the characteristics of each organ should be considered.

Gastric ESD

The gastric wall is thicker than the walls of the esophagus and colon. The thick muscle layer makes ESD easier, and the anatomical characteristics of the antrum of the stomach are especially suitable for ESD. In the antrum, the submucosal tissue is usually fine and clearly distinct from the muscle layer. Good mucosal elevation can be created by submucosal injection and the thickened submucosal layer can be easily maintained.

Besides, control of bleeding is also easy in the gastric antrum. However, ESD in the upper body of the stomach is much more difficult due to more abundant blood vessels and less clear distinction between the muscle fiber and the submucosal tissue. ESD in the greater curvature of the upper body and fundus can be very difficult.

Esophageal ESD

The angle of approach toward esophageal lesions is mostly tangential. Submucosal tissue in the esophagus is fine and, after submucosal injection, can be easily distinguished from the muscle layer. These factors make esophageal ESD technically easy.

However, the narrow lumen and both respiratory and cardiac movements make the procedure difficult. The esophageal wall is thin and lacks serosa. If an ESD knife is activated while it approaches the muscle layer, perforation can easily occur. Perforation of the esophagus can cause serious complications, such as pneumomediastinum, pneumothorax, hemothorax, and cardiac arrest. Therefore, it is particularly important in the esophagus to keep an adequate safety margin from the muscle layer by maintaining good mucosal elevation.

Colorectal ESD

Creation of good mucosal elevation is usually simple in the colon. The submucosal tissue is fine and is easily distinguished from the muscle layer after submucosal injection. Control of bleeding is usually easy in the colon as well. These factors make colorectal ESD rather easy.

However, endoscopic control is often difficult in the colon. Prominent folds and the location of lesions can make colorectal ESD very difficult. The colonic wall is much thinner and softer than in the stomach. These factors make the risk of perforation higher in the colon than in the stomach. But a short double-balloon endoscope is often useful for endoscopic control and stability, even in cases with unstable lesion location.

Duodenal ESD

Duodenal ESD is considered the most difficult and the most risky [1]. The difficulties of duodenal ESD will be discussed further.

The proper muscle layer of the duodenum is very thin and soft; even thinner than in the esophagus and colorectum. Therefore, the duodenal wall is prone to perforation. Just by exposing the muscle layer on the posterior wall, without obvious perforation, insufflation can cause an air leak to the retroperitoneal space through the thin muscle layer.

Risk of delayed perforation is also high in the duodenum, due to the thin muscle layer and the irritating effects of the duodenal content (mainly bile and pancreatic juice). Thermal injury to the thin muscle layer during submucosal dissection can easily cause necrosis of the muscle layer in the duodenum, which can lead to delayed perforation. Therefore, submucosal dissection should be performed with minimum thermal injury to the muscle layer, and a thin layer of submucosal tissue should be left on the muscular surface.

The submucosal tissue of the duodenum is coarse compared to that of the esophagus and colorectum. In the duodenal bulb, adequate mucosal elevation by submucosal injection is often difficult to obtain; most likely due to the presence of dense Brunner's glands in the submucosal layer. In the second and third portion of the duodenum, however, good mucosal protrusion is usually created by submucosal injection with relative ease, though it quickly disperses after mucosal incision. Therefore, it is difficult to maintain sufficient submucosal thickening during ESD in the duodenum.

Blood vessels are abundant in the duodenal submucosal layer, which often makes it difficult to control bleeding during dissection portion of duodenal ESD.

The mucosal layer of the duodenum has another unique feature from other parts of the GI tract. In the esophagus, stomach, and colorectum, the mucosa shrinks after incision, resulting in opening of the wound that exposes the submucosal layer. However, duodenal mucosa does not shrink after incision, making it difficult to expose the submucosa after mucosal incision.

In the second portion of the duodenum, there exists the major and minor papillae. Imprudent or accidental injuries to the papilla can cause pancreatitis. Therefore, the major and minor papillae should be identified to clarify involvement or proximity to the lesions before starting ESD in the second portion of the duodenum.

All of the above-mentioned anatomical features of the duodenum contribute to the technical challenge of duodenal ESD.

How to Overcome Difficulties in ESD

Bleeding and perforation are two major complications of ESD. Once such complications occur, ESD becomes even more difficult and sometimes impossible. Therefore, prevention of such complications is very important to make ESD not only safe but reliable.

Perforation occurs when recognition of muscle layer becomes difficult or endoscopic control becomes unstable. As long as good orientation of muscle layer in three-dimensional image and good control of the ESD device are maintained, perforation can be avoided. Bleeding is the factor that contributes most to increasing difficulty of muscle layer recognition. Therefore, control of bleeding is important for prevention of perforation.

Bleeding can be effectively controlled by coagulation of blood vessels before cutting. Recognition of blood vessels for effective coagulation is extremely important for safe and reliable ESD.

However, it is also important to acquire the skill required to handle such complications in case they occur. Hemostasis with hemostatic clips or forceps and wound closure with clips are mandatory skills to obtain before starting ESD.

Carbon dioxide (CO_2) insufflation is also important, not only for avoiding patient discomfort but also for endoscopic management of such complications. Especially in cases of perforation, CO_2 insufflation allows time to close the perforation with clips, because CO_2 leaked into the abdominal cavity and/or retroperitoneal space is quickly absorbed. Progression to catastrophic complications, such as tension pneumothorax, which causes respiratory and cardiac arrest, can be prevented (if air is used, insufflated air leaks into the abdominal cavity or mediastinum causing collapse of the lumen; continuous insufflation can cause accumulation of air in the abdominal cavity, the retroperitoneal space and/or the mediastinum). Endoscopic closure of the perforation and conservative management of the patient's course is usually possible when CO_2 insufflation is used.

The direction of gravity is another important factor contributing to the difficulty of ESD. Selection of patient position in terms of gravity is especially important in colonic ESD. Patient position should be selected in order to best locate the lesion at the top of the colonic lumen with regard to gravity. If the lesion is located at the top, the dissected part of the lesion is naturally pulled down by gravity, which allows sufficient opening of the incised wound with good visualization of the submucosal tissue during the procedure. In cases of unfavorable events such as bleeding and perforation, this positioning is beneficial to avoid or minimize further complications. In the case of bleeding, blood flows down from the bleeding point. If bleeding occurs at the bottom of the lumen, with regard to gravity, the bleeding point is immediately covered by a pool of blood that hampers appropriate hemostatic procedures. Conversely, if the bleeding point is at the top of the lumen, hemostasis can be performed reliably with accurate identification of the bleeding point because blood flows away. Even in cases of perforation, if the perforation occurs at the top of the lumen with regard to gravity, identification and closing of the perforation is easier as one can maintain a good view of the site of perforation. Only insufflated CO_2, not infected intestinal fluid, will flow out from the lumen to the abdominal cavity before closing the perforation, which is important to prevent diffuse peritonitis.

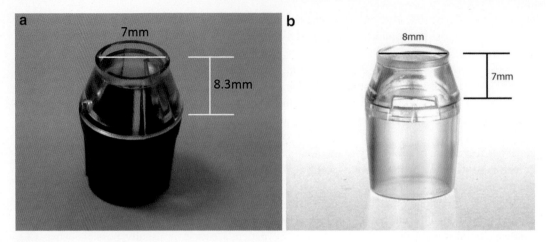

Fig. 13.1 Small-caliber-tip transparent hood (ST hood). (**a**) A conventional ST hood (DH-16GR; Fujifilm, Tokyo, Japan). (**b**) A short ST hood (DH-28GR; Fujifilm, Tokyo, Japan)

Traction Methods for ESD

Yet another difficulty of endoscopic therapeutic procedures, such as ESD, is the lack of assisting traction to aid exposure of the wound. In order to open and expose the incised wound, several assisting devices have been proposed. Those devices include an ESD traction device called the S-O clip [2], the clip with line method [3] and magnetic-anchor-guided ESD [4]. However, attachment of a transparent hood and the use of gravity are simple and useful methods for overcoming this hurdle to successful ESD.

Pocket-Creation Method for ESD

"Pocket-creation method" is a reliable ESD technique that makes recognition of blood vessels easy by maintaining good visualization of the submucosal tissue throughout the procedure. This unique ESD method makes the most of the assistance of a transparent hood. A regular cylindrical transparent hood, such as a soft, straight distal attachment (D-201-11804; Olympus, Tokyo, Japan), can be used in this technique. However, a small-caliber-tip transparent hood (ST hood: DH-16GR or DH-28GR; Fujifilm, Tokyo, Japan) (Fig. 13.1) [5, 6] is more suitable for this method. Needle-type ESD knives, such as

the Flush knife and Dual knife, are suitable for this method. This method is a modification of the tunneling method [6–8], and the sequence is as follows (Fig. 13.2).

Submucosal Injection to Create a Submucosal Fluid Cushion Under the Lesion

Creation and maintenance of an adequate submucosal cushion is key factor for successful ESD. In order to create a long-lasting submucosal cushion, a 0.4 % sodium hyaluronate solution (MucoUp; Johnson and Johnson, Tokyo, Japan) is often used in Japan [9]. Sodium hyaluronate is a viscous substance with a high molecular weight that creates long-lasting mucosal protrusion when injected into the submucosa. Despite its high viscosity, it is an isotonic solution that causes no damage to the injected tissue [10].

A thick submucosal cushion with enough injection should be created. This thickened submucosal tissue provides safety margins for both the proper muscle and mucosal layers. The vertical (deep) resection margin is important for histopathologic assessment of invasion of the cancer. The depth of invasion and involvement of vessels are strong indicators of lymph node metastasis.

Using the pocket-creation method, the thickened submucosal cushion can be maintained throughout the entire ESD procedure.

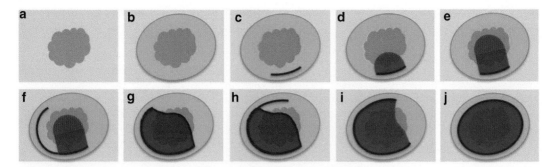

Fig. 13.2 Illustration showing the sequence of pocket-creation method. (**a**) A flat neoplastic lesion indicated by the orange area. (**b**) Mucosal elevation by enough submucosal injection (indicated by the *light blue area*). (**c**) Initial mucosal incision at the closer edge of the lesion (*blue line*). (**d**) Creation of a submucosal pocket (*blue area*). (**e**) Extension of the submucosal pocket under the lesion. (**f**) Mucosal incision at the down-side lateral edge of the lesion. (**g**) Opening of the pocket by submucosal dissection at the lateral edge. (**h**) Extension of the mucosal incision over the middle line of the lesion at the distant edge of the lesion. (**i**) Extension of the submucosal dissection to the distant edge. (**j**) Completion of ESD

Mucosal Incision at the Proximal Edge of the Lesion

After creation of a sufficient submucosal cushion, mucosal incision is made at the proximal edge of the lesion. The mucosal incision should be performed on the normal mucosa with enough distance (5–10 mm) from the edge of the lesion. The length of the initial mucosal incision should not be too long. Usually, about a 2 cm incision is enough for the initial mucosal incision for pocket creation (Fig. 13.3).

Submucosal Incision to Open the Incised Wound

After the mucosal incision, submucosal incision should be made to open the incised wound. At this initial stage, the incised wound cannot be opened with the tip of the hood yet, and so submucosal incision should be made by opening the wound with the tip of the sheath of the knife. Submucosal incision at the deep level close to the muscle layer is not necessary yet since it is still normal mucosa peripheral to the lesion. The submucosal layer right below the mucosa should be incised with the tip of the knife by moving the knife parallel to the muscle layer while slightly lifting the mucosa with its sheath (Fig. 13.4).

Creation of the Submucosal Pocket

After repeating submucosal incision with the tip of the knife a few times, the incised wound can easily be opened by the tip of the ST hood. By opening the incised wound with the tip of the hood, the submucosal tissue can be clearly visualized (Fig. 13.5). Further dissection of the submucosal tissue should be made all the way to the deeper tissue that is close to the muscle layer, very carefully, until the muscle layer can be seen through the submucosal tissue.

By continuing dissection of the submucosal layer, a submucosal pocket is created. Once the transparent hood on the tip of the endoscope is inserted into the submucosal pocket, mechanical stretching of the submucosal tissue occurs. By making a submucosal pocket, the endoscope tip is stabilized, which allows for precise control of the knife. With precise control of the knife and a good safety margin obtained by the stretching of the submucosal tissue, selection of a good level of dissection becomes feasible. Adjusting the approach angle of the knife to be tangential to the wall is also easier with this method, because an adjusting force with the endoscope tip can be applied in either direction by pushing the mucosa up or pushing the muscle wall down with the tip

Fig. 13.3 Initial mucosal incision at the closer edge of the lesion

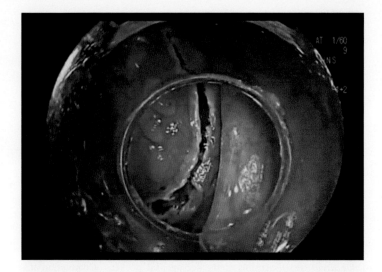

Fig. 13.4 Initial submucosal dissection with the tip of a Flush knife

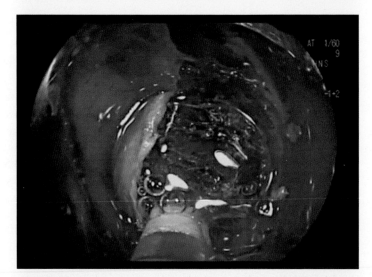

Fig. 13.5 Opening of the incised wound with the tip of the ST hood

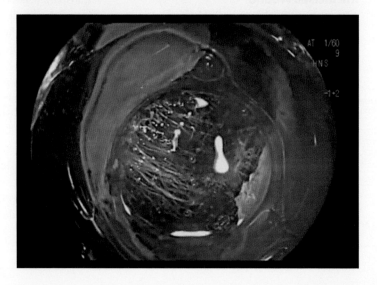

Fig. 13.6 Recognition of the muscle layer by pushing the tip of the hood down to the wall

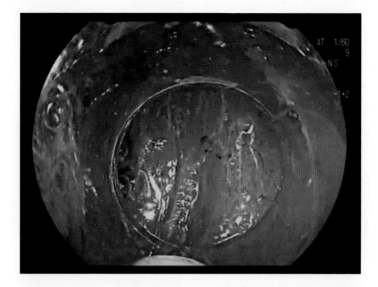

Fig. 13.7 Submucosal dissection after adjusting the approaching angle tangential to the muscle layer

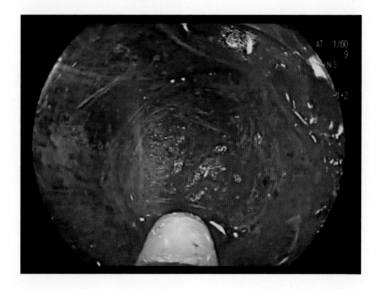

of the hood. For every bit of submucosal dissection, the tip of the hood should be pushed down against the wall to see through the muscle layer first (Fig. 13.6). Then, the tip of the hood should be moved to the direction of the mucosa to adjust the approaching angle to be tangential to the muscle layer (Fig. 13.7). The dissection level of the submucosa should be selected at the level close to the muscle layer leaving a small amount of submucosal tissue on top of the muscle layer.

With this pocket-creation method (Fig. 13.8), submucosal dissection can be happen under clear visualization of the submucosal tissue, and blood vessels can be carefully recognized for coagulation before cutting (Fig. 13.9). When a blood vessel is identified, it is better to dissect the submucosa around the vessel to isolate it (Fig. 13.10). By isolating the blood vessel, coagulation of the vessel becomes simple and effective. If bleeding occurs, the bleeding vessel should be pressed with the tip of the hood to temporarily stop the bleeding. Clear identification of the bleeding point makes hemostasis with hemostatic forceps easy. Good control of bleeding is a key factor for successful ESD.

Fig. 13.8 Submucosal pocket created by the submucosal dissection

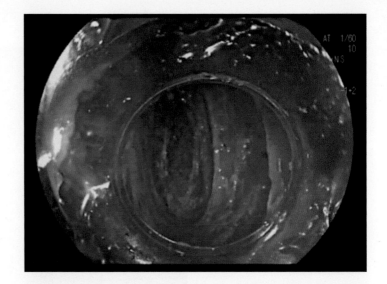

Fig. 13.9 Recognition of a blood vessel. A red blood vessel can be seen through the blue-stained submucosal tissue

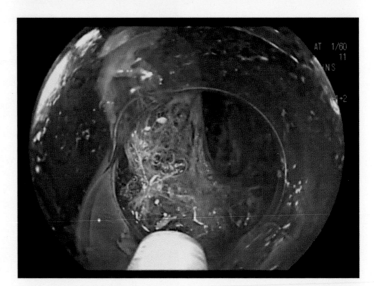

Fig. 13.10 The blood vessel is isolated by dissecting the submucosal tissue around the vessel

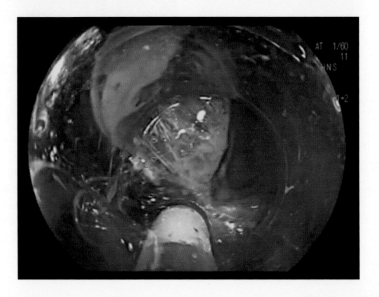

Fig. 13.11 Mucosal incision at the lateral edge of the lesion which is downside in terms of gravity. The mucosal opening at the right side of the view is the created submucosal pocket

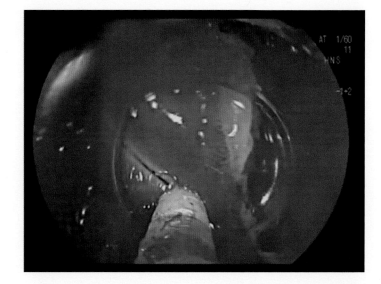

Fig. 13.12 Extension of the mucosal incision over the middle line of the lesion at the distant edge of the lesion

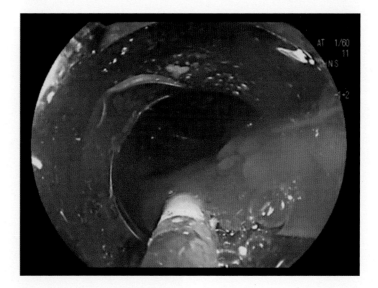

Incision and Dissection of the Lateral Edge of the Lesion

The difference between the pocket-creation method and the tunneling method is the presence or absence of tunneling completion by cutting through the opposite side of the mucosa. In the pocket-creation method, submucosal dissection is made under the tumor by creating the pocket. After completion of submucosal dissection under the tumor, incision and dissection of the lateral edge of the lesion should be made. At this stage, the lateral side that is on the bottom, in terms of gravity, should be cut first (Fig. 13.11).

Incision and Dissection of the Distal Edge of the Lesion

Mucosal incision and dissection should be extended over the central line of the lesion at the distal edge of the lesion, to reach the other lateral side (Fig. 13.12). If both lateral sides are cut, leaving the distant edge of the lesion, the incision and dissection of the distal edge becomes difficult.

Fig. 13.13 Mucosal incision and dissection of the other lateral side of the lesion

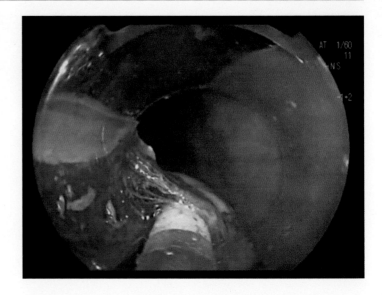

Fig. 13.14 Completion of the dissection of the lesion

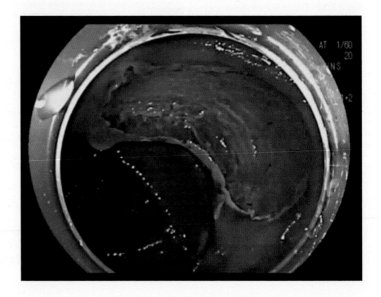

Completion of Dissection by Incision and Dissection of the Remaining Lateral Edge of the Lesion

After the pocket is opened by cutting the lower lateral side and the distal side, the lesion hangs down due to gravity, leaving the mucosa at the other lateral edge. Dissection of the lesion can easily be completed by simply cutting the mucosa from proximal to distal side (Figs. 13.13 and 13.14).

Pocket-Creation Method for a Lesion with Severe Fibrosis (Fig. 13.15)

The pocket-creation method is very useful for ESD of a lesion with severe fibrosis. If there is severe fibrosis at the center of the lesion, submucosal pockets should be created on both sides of the fibrosis. By making pockets on both sides of the fibrosis, the muscle layer can clearly be recognized, like the ridge of a mountain (Fig. 13.16).

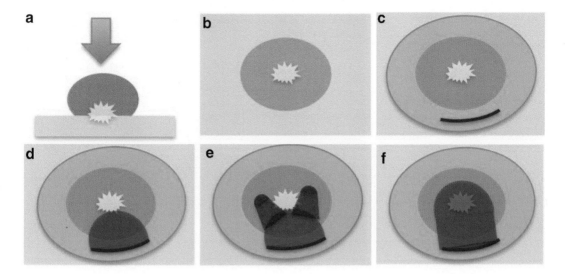

Fig. 13.15 Illustration showing the sequence of pocket-creation method for a lesion with a severe fibrosis. (**a**) A sessile lesion with a severe fibrosis at the center (lateral view). (**b**) A view of the same lesion from the top. (**c**) Initial mucosal incision at the closer edge after sufficient submucosal injection. (**d**) Creation of a submucosal pocket. (**e**) Extension of the submucosal pocket to the both sides of the fibrosis. (**f**) Dissection of the fibrosis

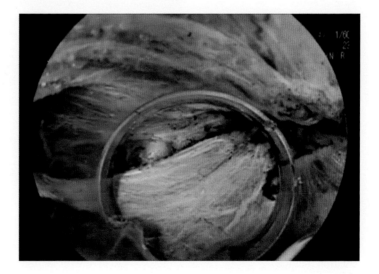

Fig. 13.16 The muscle layer recognized like a ridge of a mountain in the submucosal pocket. The fibrosis is on the right side of the view

The muscle layer is pulled up at the fibrosis, forming the shape of a mountain (Fig. 13.17). Dissection of the fibrosis can be made with the tip of the knife, little by little, along the imaginary line at the top of the "mountain," linking both sides of the ridge. Submucosal injection on the other side of the fibrosis should be made before dissecting the fibrotic area. Using an ST hood, and by creating the pockets, submucosal space can be opened even near the fibrosis. Just by cutting the fibrosis little by little, the fibrotic part gradually opens and the top of the "mountain" is pulled down to the base. When the fibrotic part is dissected through, the "mountain" becomes flat (Fig. 13.18). If dissection of the fibrotic area is successfully completed, the rest of

Fig. 13.17 The muscle layer forming a shape of a mountain due to the traction at the fibrosis. The fibrosis is on the left side of the view

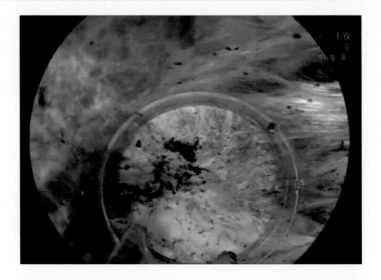

Fig. 13.18 The flattened fibrotic area after completion of the dissection

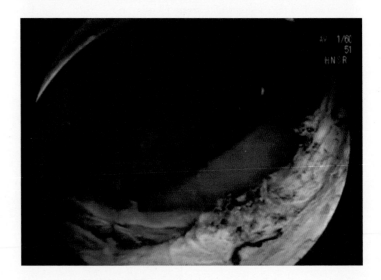

the procedure is the same as the regular pocket-creation method.

The summarized benefits of pocket creation for a lesion with severe fibrosis are: (1) Traction of the mucosa can be applied with the tip of the hood. (2) Pocket creation on both sides of the fibrosis makes recognition of the incision line feasible, even at the fibrosis. (3) By using a tangential approach, injection into the fibrosis is possible to create some elevation even at the fibrosis. (4) By stabilization of the target tissue with the tip of the hood, precise control of the

ESD knife becomes possible, enabling incision at the dissection line with a very narrow safety margin (Fig. 13.19).

Selection of Endoscopes in ESD

ESD requires precise control of the endoscope tip. Therefore, a thin endoscope is preferred over a robust therapeutic endoscope. For this reason, some operators select a single channel upper endoscope, even for colorectal ESD in the distal

Fig. 13.19 The dissection of the fibrosis with a needle knife

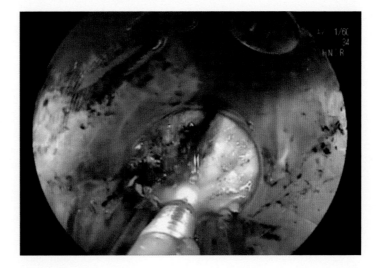

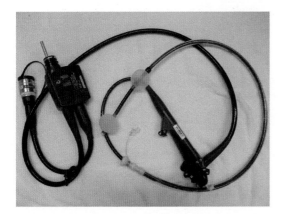

Fig. 13.20 A short-type DBE (EC-450BI5, Fujifilm, Tokyo)

colon or rectum. Even for the proximal colon, a thin single-channel colonoscope is preferred over a standard size colonoscope. Using a thin scope allows a retroflex approach in the colon and rectum. Yet, a relatively large accessory channel, at least 3.2 mm, and a waterjet function are preferred features for ESD.

ESD Using Double-Balloon Endoscopy

When lesions are located at a position of unstable control, the double-balloon endoscope (DBE) is useful for stabilizing control of the endoscope tip. A short-type DBE (EC-450BI5, Fujifilm,

Tokyo) (Fig. 13.20) is suitable for such situations as in colonic ESD [8]. ESD of lesions in the transverse colon near the hepatic flexure or the splenic flexure are often difficult due to unstable control. Stabilization by grip with an overtube balloon can make ESD possible even for these difficult cases.

Conclusions

There are a lot of factors that can cause ESD to be especially difficult, such as increased bleeding, thin muscle layers, difficulty in mucosal elevation, angle of approach, direction of gravity, and endoscopic control. There are many things to take into consideration, and they should be well understood and practiced under the supervision of an experienced endoscopist. Some possible ways to deal with especially difficult ESD are the pocket-creation technique and use of a double-balloon endoscope for stable control.

References

1. Yamamoto H, Miura Y. Duodenal ESD: conquering difficulties. Gastrointest Endosc Clin N Am. 2014;24:235–44.
2. Sakamoto N, Osada T, Shibuya T, Beppu K, Matsumoto K, Mori H, et al. Endoscopic submucosal dissection of large colorectal tumors by using a novel

spring-action S-O clip for traction (with video). Gastrointest Endosc. 2009;69(7):1370–4.

3. Oyama T. Endoscopic submucosal dissection using a hook knife Techniques. Gastrointest Endosc. 2011;13:70–3.

4. Gotoda T, Oda I, Tamakawa K, Ueda H, Kobayashi T, Kakizoe T. Prospective clinical trial of magnetic-anchor-guided endoscopic submucosal dissection for large early gastric cancer (with videos). Gastrointest Endosc. 2009;69(1):10–5.

5. Yamamoto H, Kawata H, Sunada K, Sasaki A, Nakazawa K, Miyata T, et al. Successful en-bloc resection of large superficial tumors in the stomach and colon using sodium hyaluronate and small-caliber-tip transparent hood. Endoscopy. 2003;35(8):690–4.

6. Yamamoto H, Osawa H. Endoscopic submucosal dissection using small-caliber-tip transparent hood and sodium hyaluronate. Tech Gastrointest Endosc. 2011;13(1):79–83.

7. Arantes V, Albuquerque W, Freitas Dias CA, Demas Alvares Cabral MM, Yamamoto H. Standardized endoscopic submucosal tunnel dissection for management of early esophageal tumors (with video). Gastrointest Endosc. 2013;78(6):946–52.

8. Yamamoto H. Endoscopic submucosal dissection for colorectal tumors. Interventional and therapeutic gastrointestinal endoscopy. Front Gastrointest Res. 2010;27:287–95.

9. Yamamoto H, Yahagi N, Oyama T, Gotoda T, Doi T, Hirasaki S, et al. Usefulness and safety of 0.4% sodium hyaluronate solution as a submucosal fluid "cushion" in endoscopic resection for gastric neoplasms: a prospective multicenter trial. Gastrointest Endosc. 2008;67(6):830–9.

10. Yamamoto H, Yube T, Isoda N, Sato Y, Sekine Y, Higashizawa T, et al. A novel method of endoscopic mucosal resection using sodium hyaluronate. Gastrointest Endosc. 1999;50(2):251–6.

Part V

Peri-procedural Considerations

Prevention of Stricture Formation After Esophageal Endoscopic Submucosal Dissection

14

Manabu Takeuchi

Introduction

Diagnosis of and ESD for Esophageal Cancer

With the dramatic advancement of esophageal endoscopy for the diagnosis and treatment of superficial carcinomas in recent years, there has been an increase in early detection of esophageal cancer as well as the percentage of cases where the disease can be cured with minimally invasive endoscopic resection. With the development of narrow band imaging (NBI) for endoscopic diagnosis within the esophageal region, lesions can be easily discovered without iodine staining; furthermore, it has been shown that NBI is significantly superior in detecting cancer compared to white light observation [1]. Moreover, by combining the use of NBI and magnifying endoscopy and through magnified observation of the esophageal mucosal surface microvasculature, represented by the intrapapillary capillary loop (IPCL) pattern classification of Inoue et al. [2] and the microvascular pattern classification of Arima et al. [3], detailed qualitative and depth of invasion diagnosis is now feasible. In addition, endoscopic submucosal dissection (ESD), a method that allows collective and accurate dissection of lesions [4], was developed as an endoscopic therapy method, and is currently widely used. Since the procedure is performed under direct visualization, lesions of any size can be resected, and so wide, superficially spreading lesions (including circumferential lesions) can be resected safely, collectively, and completely.

Indication of Esophageal ESD

However, according to the esophageal cancer diagnosis and treatment guidelines, the absolute indications for endoscopic therapy are a depth of invasion limited to the epithelium (EP) or lamina propria (LP) and $\leq$ two-thirds circumferential spread of the cancer, with lesions that exceed two-third circumferential spread considered relative indications [5]. The reason for circumferential spread being a relative indication for ESD stems from the technical perspective that postoperative strictures will undoubtedly occur in the lumen of the narrow esophagus, rather than an oncological perspective that risk of lymph node metastasis increases with greater width and area of the lesion; thus, even in lesions that exceed two-third circumferential spread, the disease can be cured with ESD, as long as the depth of invasion is EP or LP.

M. Takeuchi, M.D. (✉)
Department of Gastroenterology, Niigata University Medical and Dental Hospital, 1-754 Asahimachi-dori, Chuo-ku, Niigata 951-8520, Japan
e-mail: manabu@med.niigata-u.ac.jp

N. Fukami (ed.), *Endoscopic Submucosal Dissection: Principles and Practice*,
DOI 10.1007/978-1-4939-2041-9_14, © Springer Science+Business Media New York 2015

Problems with Other Therapies

Other treatments can also be chosen other than ESD, such as surgery or chemoradiation therapy (CRT). Minimally invasive surgical procedures, performed with thoracoscopy and/or laparoscopy, have been recently commonly performed as an alternative to conventional thoracotomy and laparotomy procedures. However, esophageal cancer patients are relatively older in age and tend to have increased rate of complications; a decrease in quality of life after the surgery and resulting organ loss is therefore unavoidable. Additionally, although CRT is advantageous due to its organ-preserving capability and is considered standard therapy because the treatment outcomes being comparable to that of surgery, CRT is associated with severe radiation-induced late effects, residual lesions, and recurrence in approximately 30–40 % of cases [6].

Management of Esophageal Stricture After ESD

Hence, at Niigata University Hospital, even in semi-circumferential lesions or those spreading over more than two-thirds of the circumference of the esophagus, if the depth of invasion is diagnosed as being restricted to the LP, we thoroughly explain to the patients that postoperative strictures always occur with endoscopic therapy and that long-term stricture-preventive measures are required after ESD. ESD is only performed after obtaining consent for the above prevention from the patients. As a preventive measure for postoperative strictures, endoscopic balloon dilatation (EBD) is performed [7] in the first half of ESD and local steroid injection therapy [8] in the second half of ESD. This chapter will discuss the specific methods, precautions, and outcomes of EBD and local steroid injection, as well as the future of preventive measures for postoperative esophageal strictures.

Endoscopic Balloon Dilatation (EBD)

EBD Protocol

We use GIF-Q240 or GIF-H260Z gastrointestinal endoscopes (Olympus Medical Systems, Japan), together with a 12–15 mm CRE Balloon Dilator for the esophagus (Boston Scientific, USA) for "through-the-scope" (TTS) balloon dilatation. Preventative dilatation is performed early after ESD (3–4 days post-operation). Previously, EBD was initiated when there was resistance to passage of the scope. However, since it has been shown that there is a greater risk of procedural complications, such as perforation, due to the high degree of fibrosis when stricture has already occurred, it is more effective to perform dilatation before fibrosis occurs [9]. Therefore, EBD is initiated soon after the procedure.

1. Since EBD is repeated several times, it is performed under intravenous anesthesia to relieve patients' pain. Both sedatives and analgesics, along with oxygen supplementation and appropriate monitoring, are used during all procedures.
2. The scope is inserted, and the state of the post-ESD resection plane is thoroughly examined. If the balloon is inserted from above the resection plane, the ulcer base can be damaged by the tip of the balloon catheter. Therefore, the tip of the scope is advanced to the point where it is beyond the resection plane, and subsequently the balloon is inserted from the working channel of scope. Once the entire balloon is inserted from the working channel, the scope is pulled back, and the balloon is finally aligned with the resection plane (Fig. 14.1).
3. The balloon is inflated using distilled water. At this time, the assistant's maneuver is more important than the endoscopist, since, during this step, it is essential to avoid maximal inflation too quickly. The slow careful dilation is done to prevent perforation and to prevent the balloon being drawn below the ulcer

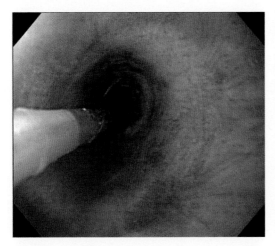

Fig. 14.1 The balloon is aligned with the resection plane

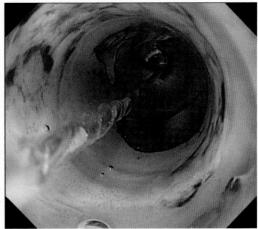

Fig. 14.3 The balloon is pulled slightly back to make close contact with the tip of the scope. It is then irrigated with water to visualize the adequacy of dilation

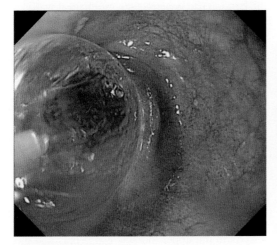

Fig. 14.2 The balloon is slowly pressurized

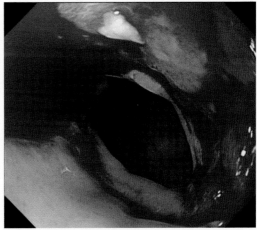

Fig. 14.4 The procedure is completed upon confirmation that there were no procedural complications, such as perforation of the resection plane

(Fig. 14.2). Dilatation to 15 mm requires a pressure of 8 atmospheres (atm). It takes about 30 s for the balloon to reach a pressure of 3–4 atm. Dilation is performed for approximately 1 min at this pressure, following which the pressure is increased in 1 atm increments over a similar amount of time, until a maximum diameter of 15 mm and pressure of 8 atm is reached. At this point, it is best to withdraw the balloon until it makes contact with the tip of the scope and irrigate the ulcer site with water to visualize the adequacy of dilatation (Fig. 14.3).

4. After dilatation, the ulcer site is inspected to ensure that there are no procedural complications, such as perforation. Bleeding essentially stops naturally and does not usually become a problem (Fig. 14.4).

EBD is initiated 3–4 days after ESD, and is repeated once a week for semi-circumferential resections and twice a week for circumferential resections. The interval between each EBD is gradually lengthened, and EBD is completed

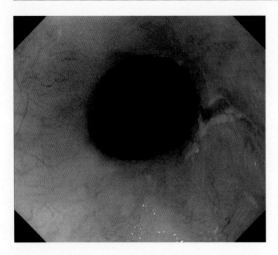

Fig. 14.5 EBD is discontinued upon confirming that there is complete epithelialization of the entire resection plane and easy passage of the scope with no dysphagia

upon confirming that there is complete epithelialization of the entire resection plane, easy scope passage, and absence of dysphagia (Fig. 14.5).

Procedural Complications Associated with EBD

The only case of perforation we experienced with EBD is shown below [10]. ESD was performed on a circumferential lesion (0-IIc, T1a-EP 60 mm) extending from the abdominal to the lower thoracic esophagus, thus requiring a circumferential resection (Fig. 14.6a, b). Four days after ESD, EBD was performed. The resection area had narrowed slightly, and there was resistance to passage of the scope. Thus, dilatation was performed by directly inserting the balloon up to the stricture site from the proximal side of the resection area. This resulted in the tip of the balloon penetrating the esophageal wall, and a large perforation was detected, through which the mediastinum was visible (blue arrow) (Fig. 14.6c). Since closure of the perforation was considered impossible, the patient's course was observed conservatively in collaboration with the surgical department. Although the patient

developed a fever for 2 days, the inflammation subsequently subsided, and no superior mediastinal abscess developed, as seen by computed tomography (CT). Further, since esophageal imaging 1 week later did not show any leakage, balloon dilatation was once again performed 10 days after the perforation, with a balloon diameter of 7 mm. The procedure was performed twice a week, and normal oral intake was possible 2 months later (Fig. 14.6d). In this case, the perforation was caused by not advancing the guidewire when the balloon was advanced from above the resection area. This indicates that it is very important to be extremely careful when performing EBDs, since resection planes that have not epithelialized are extremely soft and the tip of the balloon can penetrate the esophageal wall.

Outcome of EBD (Table 14.1)

There were 30 lesions in 29 patients that required postoperative balloon dilatation at our institution until December 2007. Of these 29 patients, 24 were men and 5 were women, with a mean age of 70 years (range: 49–90). Many of the lesions had $\geq$ two-thirds circumferential spread, and nearly all lesions exceeded semi-circumferential spread. Three of these were lesions that required full circumferential resection. There were two lesions in the upper thoracic esophagus that did not require semi-circumferential resection, although EBD was required since they were close to the physiological sphincter area. The overall mean number of EBDs performed was 7.1 times (1–20), although differences in the number of dilatations did not depend on the diameter or site of dissection. The mean number of EBDs performed in the 25 semi-circumferential resection lesions was 6.5 times (1–20), and 12.3 times (5–20) in the 3 circumferential resection lesions, demonstrating that dilatation tended to be required more frequently with full circumferential resection. The aforementioned case of perforation was the only complication associated with EBD.

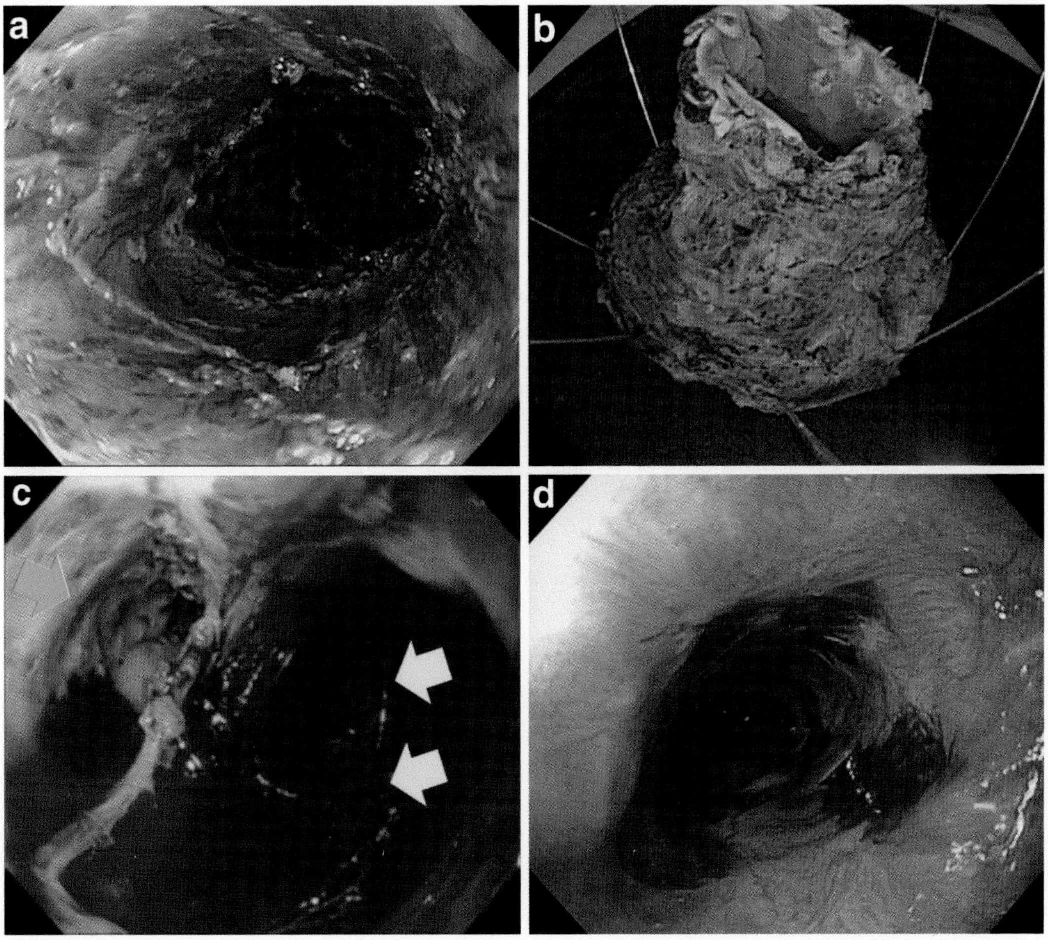

Fig. 14.6 (a) Image taken after circumferential resection of a 6 cm lesion extending from the abdominal esophagus to the lower esophagus. (b). Freshly resected specimen. (c). Giant perforation following balloon dilatation 4 days after ESD. The *blue arrow* indicates the original esopha- geal lumen. The *yellow arrows* indicate the mediastinum observed in the depths of the perforation site. (d) Post-balloon dilatation performed 2 months after ESD. Normal oral intake was possible despite the presence of mild lacerations

Table 14.1 Treatment outcome following EBD

	EBD group (30 lesions in 29 patients)	
Circumferential spread	Semi-circumferential dissection: 25	Circumferential dissection: 3
Mean number of dilatations	6.5 times (1–20)	12.3 times (5–20)

Endoscopic Triamcinolone Injection (ETI)

Local Steroid Injection Protocol

With EBD, normal oral intake became possible in all patients after ESD. However, frequent EBD, the requirement of dilatation over an extended period of time, and the risk of perforation during dilatation are some of the drawbacks of this treatment option. Thus, at our department, we introduced local steroid injection therapy, which had previously been used as post-dilatation treatment for esophageal inflammation or postoperative anastomotic strictures, to prevent strictures after ESD [8]. The protocol and precautions of the procedure are described below.

Steroid

Triamcinolone acetonide (Product name: Kenacort®-A), a synthetic corticosteroid, is used for the procedure (Fig. 14.7). One vial contains 5 ml of a white aqueous suspension (triamcinolone acetonide: 50 mg). Since esophageal inflammation (corrosive esophagitis after using an autoscope) and post-esophageal dilatation are listed as indications for the use of this drug, we selected triamcinolone acetonide for use at our institution.

Methods and Interval of Local Injection

Methods

A 25-guage local injection needle (TOP Corporation, Tokyo, Japan) is used. The solution of Kenacort®-A (need generic name, mg/cm³ vial) is used undiluted, and, using a 1 ml syringe, approximately 0.2 ml is injected at each site. At this step, it is important to inject the steroid with the needle inserted into the shallow layer of the ulcer base, nearly parallel to the esophageal wall, such that a bulge forms. This is done because the drug can be easily injected outside the wall if the needle is inserted deep into the ulcer base (Fig. 14.8a, b). The steroid is injected starting from the distal side of the lesion, following which the scope is withdrawn 1–1.5 cm at a time toward the proximal side, giving 2–3 injections at each level, to cover the whole lesion. The total amount of Kenacort®-A used for each local injection session is approximately 5–10 ml (1–2 V), and approximately 20–30 sites are injected.

Interval

Injection is initiated 2–3 days after ESD. The steroid is injected 2–4 times for ≥ three-quarter circumferential resection and 4 times for full circumferential resection, every 3–4 days.

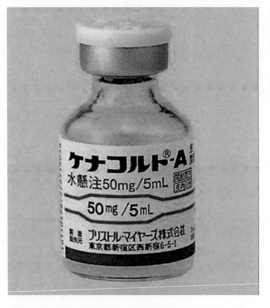

Fig. 14.7 Triamcinolone acetonide (Product name: Kenacort®-A)

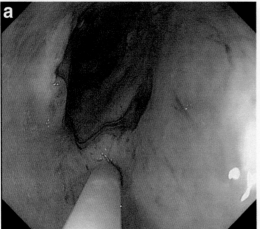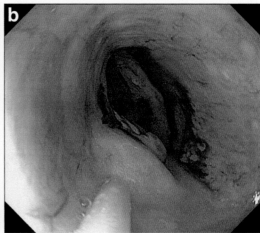

Fig. 14.8 (**a**) The steroid is injected with a needle that is inserted into the shallow layer of ulcer base, nearly parallel to the esophageal wall, (**b**) A bulge by injecting steroid appropriately is formed

Table 14.2 Interval between local steroid injections

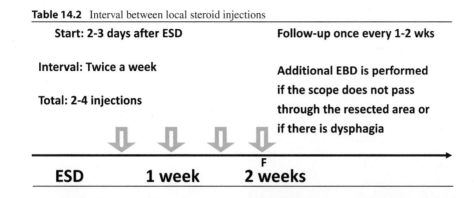

Start: 2-3 days after ESD	Follow-up once every 1-2 wks
Interval: Twice a week	Additional EBD is performed if the scope does not pass through the resected area or if there is dysphagia
Total: 2-4 injections	

ESD   1 week   2 weeks

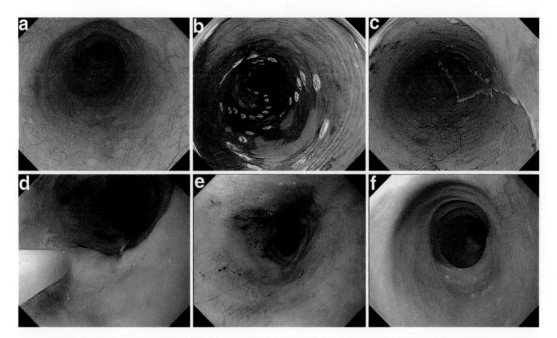

Fig. 14.9 Endoscopic images of the esophagus in which semi-circumferential resection was performed. (**a, b**). IIb lesions (30 and 15 mm) with slight redness and unstained areas on iodine staining were detected in the mid-thoracic esophagus under endoscopic observation. (**c**). After semi-circumferential resection. (**d**). Local steroid injection was initiated the second day after ESD. (**e**). The scope could be easily passed 10 days after ESD, although epithelialization had yet to occur. (**f**). One month after ESD, squamous epithelialization of the entire resection plane occurred, and no stricture was observed. EBD was never required

Subsequently, if there is a slight resistance to scope passage or if there is discomfort upon swallowing, EBD is performed at an interval of 1–2 weeks (Table 14.2).

Case Presentation 1 (Semi-Circumferential ESD)

A man in his 80s presented with IIb lesions (diameters 30 and 15 mm) in the mid-thoracic esophagus (29–34 cm from the incisor) (Fig. 14.9a, b). Slight redness was observed, and upon iodine staining chromoendoscopy, unstained (dysplastic) areas were seen. Since the lesions were near each other, they were resected together by ESD with a semi-circumferential resection area of 52×35 mm (Fig. 14.9c). Local injection of Kenacort®-A was started on the second day after ESD. The injection needle was inserted parallel to the esophageal wall into the shallow base of the

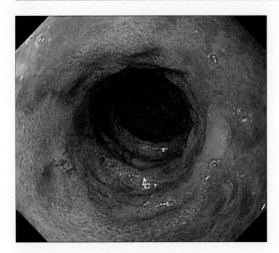

Fig. 14.10 A pseudodiverticulum-like recessed ulcer base can be observed after local injection

ulcer, at a dose of approximately 0.2 ml per injection, such that a bulge was created (Fig. 14.9d). The steroid was locally injected on a total of three occurrences. Endoscopic imaging 10 days after ESD demonstrated that the scope could be easily passed through the site of ESD, although epithelialization had not yet occurred (Fig. 14.9e). One month after ESD, squamous epithelialization had occurred in all the resection planes, there was no stricture, the scope easily passed through the site of ESD, and the patient did not have dysphagic symptoms (Fig. 14.9f). No dilatation was required in this patient after ESD.

Precautions

Extreme caution is required during the EBD procedure performed after local steroid injection. After the injection, the esophageal wall is weakened, leading to the risk of perforation if dilatation is not carefully performed. It is essential that the dilatation be performed slowly, with more time than usual allocated. In addition, due to reports of delayed perforation potentially caused by local injection into the muscularis propria, the steroid must be injected into the shallow layer of the ulcer base; a slight leak is preferable to a deep injection. Local injection of the steroid into a deeper layer can be recognized by formation of a pseudodiverticulum-like recessed ulcer base (Fig. 14.10).

Case Presentation 2 (Full Circumferential ESD)

A man in his 70s presented with circumferential IIb lesions approximately 55 and 45 mm in size in the mid to lower thoracic esophagus (Fig. 14.11a). Circumferential resection with ESD was performed on both these lesions together, with a resection area of 115×53 mm (Fig. 14.11b, c). Local injection of Kenacort®-A was administered a total of four times, starting the day after ESD (Fig. 14.11d). Endoscopic images 2 months after ESD showed that the scope passed smoothly through the resection site and that most of the resection plane had epithelialized, although some white plaques remained (Fig. 14.11e). Three months after ESD, the entire resection plane had epithelialized, and no stricture was observed (Fig. 14.11f). Post-ESD dilatation was not required in this patient as well.

Outcome of ETI (Table 14.3)

Between January 2008 and September 2010, we performed local steroid injection for 45 lesions in 44 patients, as stricture prophylaxis. These patients included 39 men and 5 women, with a mean age of 72 years (range, 52–89). With the exception of 8 lesions in the upper thoracic esophagus adjacent to the cervical esophagus and in the abdominal esophagus, all lesions (37 lesions) had ≥ two-third circumferential spread, and 16 of these lesions required full circumferential resection. Local steroid injection was performed soon after performing ESD in all cases, and the mean number of injections for all cases was 2.9 (2–5). Comparing the 21 semi-circumferential resection lesions and the 16 full circumferential resection lesions, the mean numbers of local injections were 2.8 and 3.5, respectively, indicating a slightly greater tendency in the number of injections for circumferential resection. In addition, for semi-circumferential resection, the mean number of additional EBD was 2.1 times, showing that the need for EBD was reduced significantly ($p < 0.001$) by local steroid injection, compared to performing EBD alone. Further, 17 of the 21 lesions (81.0 %) did not require EBD at all.

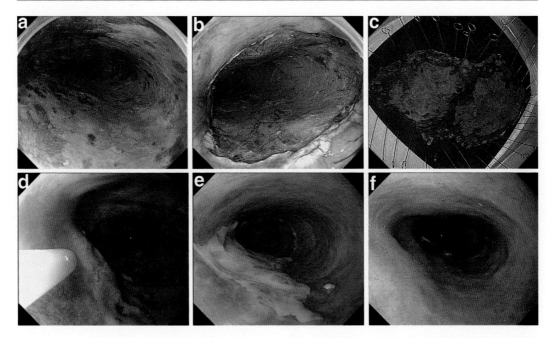

Fig. 14.11 (**a**) Circumferential IIb lesions (approximately 55 and 45 mm) were observed from the mid to lower thoracic esophagus. (**b, c**) Circumferential resection was performed with a resection area of 115×53 mm. (**d**) Steroid was injected a total of four times, commencing the day after ESD. (**e**). Two months after ESD, most of the resection plane had epithelialized, although some *white* plaque remained. (**f**). Three months after ESD, the entire resection plane had epithelialized and no stricture was observed. EBD was unnecessary in this case as well

Table 14.3 Treatment outcome following local steroid injection (in 37 lesions with ≥ 2/3 circumferential spread)

	Local injection group (37 lesions in 36 patients)	
Circumferential spread	Semi-circumferential dissection: 21	Circumferential dissection: 16
Mean number of local injections	2.8 times (2–4)	3.5 times (2–5)
Mean number of dilatations	2.1 times (0–25)	7.5 times (0–28)
Cases that did not require additional EBD	17 cases (81.0 %)	6 cases (37.5 %)

During follow-up examination after local steroid injection, the mean number of additional EBDs required was 7.5 times for 15 full circumferential resection lesions, excluding the lesion where perforation occurred. This demonstrates that additional EBD tends to be required less frequently following local steroid injection as compared to EBD alone. In addition, six of the circumferential lesions did not require EBD at all. While we consider local steroid injection to be effective stricture prophylaxis following circumferential resection, since we also experienced cases where additional EBD was required over a long period of time, further investigation is necessary to confirm the efficacy of this treatment modality.

Future Techniques

As methods of stricture prophylaxis following endoscopic resection for esophageal cancer, regenerative medicine techniques using transplantation of cultured autologous oral mucosal epithelial cell sheets [11, 12] and biodegradable stents [13] have been developed. In addition, stricture prevention measures using various drugs that aim to suppress fibrosis have also been employed. However, at present, these technologies are not available at every facility, and, therefore, further development is required for more widespread dissemination.

Conclusions

For semi-circumferential and circumferential superficial esophageal carcinoma, the ESD procedure that can safely and reliably allow resection of lesions is currently accepted as standard treatment. However, the procedure imposes a long-term burden on patients who have to receive multiple treatment sessions for postoperative strictures, in spite of undergoing a curative resection. If conventional EBD is repeated for an extended period of time, oral intake without dysphagia eventually becomes possible. However, local steroid injection therapy possibly eliminates the need for EBD in many patients who undergo semi-circumferential resection of lesions, and reduces the number of EBDs required in full circumferential resected lesions, indicating that it is a beneficial way to prevent post-procedural stricture in ESD patients.

References

1. Muto M, et al. Multicenter prospective randomized controlled study on the detection and diagnosis of superficial squamous cell carcinoma by back-to-back endoscopic examination of narrowband imaging and white light observation. Gastrointest Endosc. 2007;65:AB110.
2. Inoue H, Honda T, Nagai K, et al. Ultra-high magnification endoscopic observation of carcinoma in situ of the esophagus. Dig Endosc. 1997;9:16–8.
3. Arima M, Tada M, Arima H. Evaluation of microvascular patterns of superficial esophageal cancers by magnifying endoscopy. Esophagus. 2005;4:191–7.
4. Oyama T, Kikuchi Y. Aggressive endoscopic mucosal resection in the upper GI tract – hook knife EMR method. Min Invas Ther All Technol. 2002;11:291–5.
5. Japan Esophageal Association. Guidelines of diagnosis and treatment for esophageal cancer. 10th ed. Tokyo: Kanehara; 2008 (Revised version) (Japanese).
6. Hironaka S, Ohtsu A, Boku N, et al. Nonrandomized comparison between definitive chemoradiotherapy and radical surgery in patients with $T_{2-3}N_{any}M_0$ squamous cell carcinoma of the esophagus. Int J Radiat Oncol Biol Phys. 2003;57:425–33.
7. Katada C, Muto M, Manabe T, et al. Esophageal stenosis after endoscopic mucosal resection of superficial esophageal lesions. Gastrointest Endosc. 2003;57:165–9.
8. Hashimoto S, Kobayashi M, Takeuchi M, et al. The efficacy of endoscopic triamcinolone injection for the prevention of esophageal stricture after endoscopic submucosal dissection. Gastrointest Endosc. 2011;74: 1389–93.
9. Inoue H, Minami H, Sato Y, et al. Technical feasibility of circumferential ESD and preventive balloon dilation. Stom Intest. 2009;44:394–7.
10. Takeuchi M, Kobayashi M, Oyama T, et al. Complications in ESD for early esophageal carcinoma. Stom Intest. 2009;44:384–93.
11. Ohki T, Yamamoto M, Murakami D, et al. Treatment of oesophageal ulcerations using endoscopic transplantation of tissue-engineered autologous oral mucosal epithelial cell sheets in a canine model. Gut. 2007; 56(3):313–4.
12. Takagi R, Murakami D, Kondo M, et al. Fabrication of human oral mucosal epithelial cell sheets for treatment of esophageal ulceration by endoscopic submucosal dissection. Gastrointest Endosc. 2010;72:1253–9.
13. Saito Y, Tanaka T, Andoh A, et al. Novel biodegradable stents for benign esophageal strictures following endoscopic submucosal dissection. Dig Dis Sci. 2008; 53(2):330–3.

Regenerative Medicine for Stricture Management: What does the Future Hold?

15

Takeshi Ohki

Introduction

Following esophageal tumor excision procedures such as ESD, stricture can result in harmful outcomes for patients, especially if the induced area of ulceration is large. These strictures can be refractory to treatment [1, 2]. Steroids have been used to help control stricture, but they have many side effects [3]. Regenerative medicine techniques have recently been used together with endoscopy, and have been shown to be effective at controlling formation of stricture and inducing re-epithelialization following tumor excision [4–7]. One of the most important components of this procedure is *cell sheet technology* [8, 9]. Sheets of cells for auto-transplantation can be cultivated by using a culture dish coated with a temperature-responsive polymer and the patient's own oral mucosal epithelial cells. These cell sheets have proven to be effective at preventing post-esophageal ESD strictures. The prevention of post-esophageal ESD strictures using cell sheet technology will be summarized in this chapter.

Cell Sheet Technology

Temperature-responsive surfaces have been successfully developed by Okano et al. [10, 11] through covalent binding of a hydrophobic polymer of poly(N-isopropylacrylamide) to culture dishes. Cells are then seeded onto these dishes at 37 °C and allowed to attach to the surface (Fig. 15.1a). When the temperature is reduced to 20 °C, the surface of the dish becomes hydrophilic, and the cells become detached (Fig. 15.1b). To extract cells from culture dishes, conventional protocols utilize protease enzymes. However, these enzymes can destroy the adhesion proteins that hold cells together. In contrast, with temperature-responsive culture dishes, all of the cells can be harvested as a contiguous sheet of cells with the extracellular matrix deposited at the bottom of the cultured cell sheet (Fig. 15.1b) [12]. Adhesion proteins are retained on the surface of these cells, and then the sheet can be transplanted onto various tissues without sutures [13, 14].

Electronic supplementary material Supplementary material is available in the online version of this chapter at 10.1007/978-1-4939-2041-9_15. Videos can also be accessed at http://www.springerimages.com/videos/978-1-4939-2040-2.

T. Ohki, M.D., Ph.D. (✉)
Department of Surgery, Institute of Gastroenterology, Tokyo Women's Medical University, 8-1 Kawada-cho, Shinjuku-ku, Tokyo 162-8666, Japan

Institute of Advanced Biomedical Engineering and Science, Tokyo Women's Medical University (TWIns), 8-1 Kawada-cho, Shinjuku-ku, Tokyo 162-8666, Japan
e-mail: ohki@ige.twmu.ac.jp; ohki.takeshi@twmu.ac.jp

N. Fukami (ed.), *Endoscopic Submucosal Dissection: Principles and Practice*,
DOI 10.1007/978-1-4939-2041-9_15, © Springer Science+Business Media New York 2015

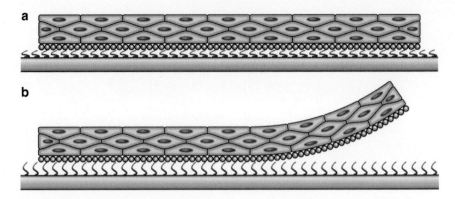

Fig. 15.1 (**a**) Confluent epithelial cells were strongly connected to each other and attached to the temperature-responsive surfaces of the culture dishes at 36 °C. (**b**) Cell sheets were harvested by decreasing the temperature to 20 °C, without use of any enzymes

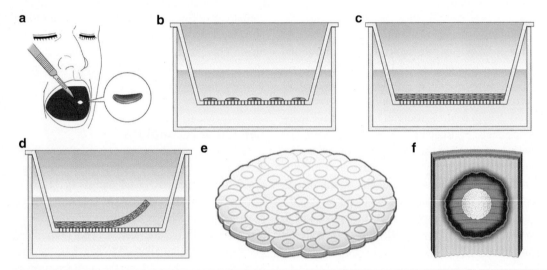

Fig. 15.2 (**a**) The patients' own oral mucosal tissues were used to obtain cells for culture. (**b**) Isolated cells were seeded onto temperature-responsive culture inserts. (**c**) Epithelial cells on temperature-responsive culture inserts were cultured by confluent growth for 16 days. (**d**) Epithelial cell sheets were harvested by reducing the temperature to 20 °C. (**e**) Harvested autologous oral mucosal epithelial cell sheet. (**f**) Cell sheets were endoscopically transplanted to the affected area immediately after esophageal ESD

Treatment for the Prevention of Esophageal Strictures: Autologous Oral Mucosal Epithelial Cell Sheets

We developed a treatment adapting regenerative medicine using tissue-engineered epithelial cell sheets [15–17]. Epithelial cells isolated from the patient's own oral mucosa (Fig. 15.2a) were seeded onto temperature-responsive culture inserts (Fig. 15.2b) and cultured for 16 days at 36 °C (Fig. 15.2c, d). The autologous cell sheets (Figs. 15.2e and 15.3) were then transplanted with endoscopic forceps onto the bed of the esophageal ulcer after ESD (Figs. 15.2f and 15.4). Nine cases involving oral mucosal epithelial cell sheet transplantation have been reported [17]. The results indicate that cell sheet transplantation effectively prevents post-esophageal ESD strictures (Fig. 15.5).

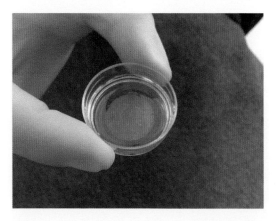

Fig. 15.3 Autologous oral mucosal epithelial cell sheet

Culture of Autologous Oral Mucosal Epithelial Cell Sheets

After each patient's oral cavity was sterilized, specimens of oral mucosal tissue were surgically taken from the buccal mucosa (Fig. 15.2a). Two types of specimens were used for the cell culture: multiple 6 mm diameter circular tissue samples and spindle-shaped tissue samples [18]. Oral mucosal epithelial cells were collected by removing all epithelial layers with dispase I (1,000 PU per milliliter, Godo Shusei, Tokyo, Japan) at 37 °C for 2 h. Next, the cells were placed in trypsin and ethylenediaminetetraacetic

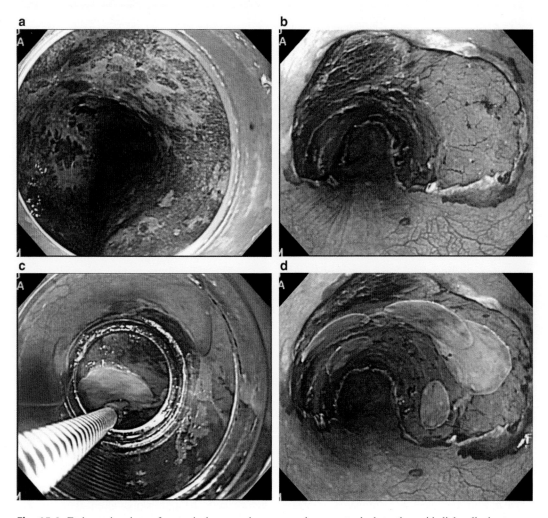

Fig. 15.4 Endoscopic view of a typical case where esophageal strictures were prevented using cell sheets. (**a**) Three quarters of the circumferential tumor is shown as an unstaining area with iodine dye chromoendoscopy. (**b**) An artificial ulceration immediately after ESD. (**c**) Support membranes attached to the epithelial cell sheet were grasped with endoscopic forceps and transplanted to the affected area by endoscopy. (**d**) The affected area immediately after endoscopic transplantation of cell sheets

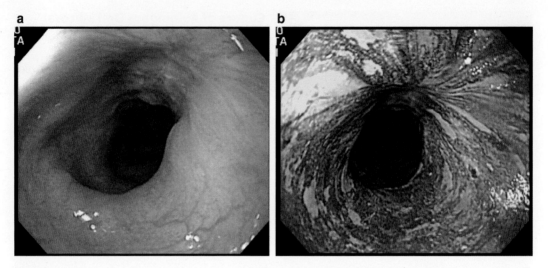

Fig. 15.5 (**a**) Three weeks after cell sheet transplantation; visualized under white light. (**b**) Three weeks after transplantation; visualized as well stained area with iodine dye chromoendoscopy

Table 15.1 Keratinocyte culture medium (KCM) for harvest of oral mucosal epithelial cell sheets

Culture medium	Dulbecco's modified Eagle's medium (DMEM); Sigma, St. Louis, MO	(3:1 DMEM:Ham's F-12)
	Ham's F-12; Sigma, St. Louis, MO	
Media supplements	2 nmol/L triiodothyronine; Wako Pure Chemicals, Osaka, Japan	
	5 µg/mL insulin; Eli Lilly, Indianapolis, IN	
	10 ng/mL epidermal growth factor (EGF); Higeta Shoyu, Chiba, Japan	
	0.4 µg/mL hydrocortisone; Kowa Pharmaceutical, Tokyo, Japan	
	1 nM cholera toxin; List Biological Laboratories, Campbell, CA	
	0.25 µg/mL amphotericin B; Bristol-Myers Squibb, New York, NY	
	40 µg/mL gentamicin; Schering-Plough, Kenilworth, NJ	
	5 % autologous human serum	

acid (EDTA) for 20 min to form single-cell suspensions. Temperature-responsive cell culture inserts (UpCell Insert, CellSeed, Tokyo, Japan) (23.4 mm in diameter) were prepared as previously described [19, 20]. Isolated cells were seeded onto these temperature-responsive culture inserts (Fig. 15.2a) and cultured with keratinocyte culture medium (KCM) (Table 15.1) by confluent growth for 16 days (Fig. 15.2c, d).

Preparation for Transplantation

Two incubators (36 and 20 °C) were used in an endoscopic procedure room to harvest the cell sheets. The patients' cell sheets were transferred from the cell processing center to the 36 °C incubator. The cell culture team staff carried those sheets to another incubator (20 °C) and harvested the cell sheets (Figs. 15.2e and 15.3) as instructed by the ESD operator. A sheet of polyvinylidene difluoride (PVDF) (Immobilon-P, Durapore; Millipore, Billerica, MA) was used as a support membrane.

Transplantation Technique (with Video 15.1)

An esophageal EMR tube (Create Medic, Yokohama, Japan) was inserted in the esophagus before cell sheet transplantation. The support membrane with the attached autologous oral mucosal epithelial cell sheet was grasped with endoscopic forceps and carefully carried at endoscopic tip and maneuvered to the ulcer site through the EMR tube (Fig. 15.4c). An endoscopic cap was used to protect the cell sheet. Cell sheets were then placed directly onto the ulcer site. The cell sheets stably adhered to the ulcer wound beds after 10 or more minutes (Fig. 15.4d). The support membrane was not removed, and this procedure was repeated with several transplanted cell sheets to cover portions of the ulcer.

Post-transplantation Patient Care

Patients received oral proton pump inhibitor (PPI) treatment before the procedure. After the procedure, they received a continuous intravenous drip of PPI through postoperative day 4, and oral PPI thereafter. Patients were allowed a liquid diet starting on day 5 and were allowed to consume rice porridge after day 6. Patients stayed in the hospital for approximately 8 days.

Limitations

Skilled technicians monitored each procedure during the course of the study. The cell-processing center had sterilized rooms, constantly followed the good manufacturing practice guidelines, and adhered to the standard operating procedures for regenerative medicine [21]. As these technologies are currently extremely expensive, for commercial use there is a need for industrialization and mass production before it can be scaled up for more widespread adoption [1, 22].

References

1. Sato H, Inoue H, Kobayashi Y, Maselli R, Santi EG, Hayee B, Igarashi K, Yoshida A, Ikeda H, Onimaru M, Aoyagi Y, Kudo SE, et al. Control of severe strictures after circumferential endoscopic submucosal dissection for esophageal carcinoma: oral steroid therapy with balloon dilation or balloon dilation alone. Gastrointest Endosc. 2013;78:250–7.

2. Takahashi H, Arimura Y, Okahara S, Uchida S, Ishigaki S, Tsukagoshi H, Shinomura Y, Hosokawa M. Risk of perforation during dilation for esophageal strictures after endoscopic resection in patients with early squamous cell carcinoma. Endoscopy. 2010;43:184–9.

3. Yamaguchi N, Isomoto H, Nakayama T, Hayashi T, Nishiyama H, Ohnita K, Takeshima F, Shikuwa S, Kohno S, Nakao K, et al. Usefulness of oral prednisolone in the treatment of esophageal stricture after endoscopic submucosal dissection for superficial esophageal squamous cell carcinoma. Gastrointest Endosc. 2011;73:1115–21.

4. Sakurai T, Miyazaki S, Miyata G, Satomi S, Hori Y. Autologous buccal keratinocyte implantation for the prevention of stenosis after EMR of the esophagus. Gastrointest Endosc. 2007;66:167–73.

5. Honda M, Hori Y, Nakada A, Uji M, Nishizawa Y, Yamamoto K, Kobayashi T, Shimada H, Kida N, Sato T, Nakamura T, et al. Use of adipose tissue-derived stromal cells for prevention of esophageal stricture after circumferential EMR in a canine model. Gastrointest Endosc. 2011;73:777.

6. Nieponice A, McGrath K, Qureshi I, Beckman EJ, Luketich JD, Gilbert TW, Badylak SF. An extracellular matrix scaffold for esophageal stricture prevention after circumferential EMR. Gastrointest Endosc. 2009;69:289–96.

7. Badylak SF, Hoppo T, Nieponice A, Gilbert TW, Davison JM, Jobe BA. Esophageal preservation in five male patients after endoscopic inner-layer circumferential resection in the setting of superficial cancer: a regenerative medicine approach with a biologic scaffold. Tissue Eng Part A. 2011;17:1643–50.

8. Yang J, Yamato M, Nishida K, Ohki T, Kanzaki M, Sekine H, Shimizu T, Okano T, et al. Cell delivery in regenerative medicine: the cell sheet engineering approach. J Control Release. 2006;116:193–203.

9. Yang J, Yamato M, Shimizu T, Sekine H, Ohashi K, Kanzaki M, Ohki T, Nishida K, Okano T, et al. Reconstruction of functional tissues with cell sheet engineering. Biomaterials. 2007;28:5033–43.

10. Okano T, Yamada N, Sakai H, Sakurai Y. A novel recovery system for cultured cells using plasma-treated polystyrene dishes grafted with poly(N-isopropylacrylamide). J Biomed Mater Res. 1993;27:1243–51.

11. Yamato M, Utsumi M, Kushida A, Konno C, Kikuchi A, Okano T. Thermo-responsive culture dishes allow the intact harvest of multilayered keratinocyte sheets without dispase by reducing temperature. Tissue Eng. 2001;7:473–80.

12. Kushida A, Yamato M, Konno C, Kikuchi A, Sakurai Y, Okano T. Decrease in culture temperature releases monolayer endothelial cell sheets together with deposited fibronectin matrix from temperature-responsive culture surfaces. J Biomed Mater Res. 1999;45:355–62.

13. Nishida K, Yamato M, Hayashida Y, Watanabe K, Yamamoto K, Adachi E, Nagai S, Kikuchi A, Maeda

N, Watanabe H, Okano T, Tano Y, et al. Corneal reconstruction with tissue-engineered cell sheets composed
of autologous oral mucosal epithelium. N Engl J Med.
2004;351:1187–96.

14. Sawa Y, Miyagawa S, Sakaguchi T, Fujita T,
Matsuyama A, Saito A, Shimizu T, Okano T, et al.
Tissue engineered myoblast sheets improved cardiac
function sufficiently to discontinue LVAS in a patient
with DCM: report of a case. Surg Today. 2011;42:
181–4.

15. Ohki T, Yamato M, Murakami D, Takagi R, Yang J,
Namiki H, Okano T, Takasaki K, et al. Treatment of
oesophageal ulcerations using endoscopic transplantation of tissue-engineered autologous oral mucosal
epithelial cell sheets in a canine model. Gut. 2006;55:
1704–10.

16. Ohki T, Yamato M, Ota M, Okano T, Yamamoto
M. Application of cell sheet technology for esopha-
geal endoscopic submucosal dissection. Tech
Gastrointest Endosc. 2011;13:105–9.

17. Ohki T, Yamato M, Ota M, Takagi R, Murakami D,
Kondo M, Sasaki R, Namiki H, Okano T, Yamamoto
M, et al. Prevention of esophageal stricture after endoscopic submucosal dissection using tissue-engineered
cell sheets. Gastroenterology. 2012;143:582–8.e1–2.

18. Sasaki R, Yamato M, Takagi R, Ohki T, Matsumine H,
Okano T, Ando T. Punch and spindle-shaped biopsies
for collecting oral mucosal tissue for the fabrication
of transplantable autologous epithelial cell sheets.
J Biomed Mater Res A. 2012;100:2849–54.

19. Takagi R, Yamato M, Murakami D, Kondo M, Yang J,
Ohki T, Nishida K, Kohno C, Okano T, et al.
Preparation of keratinocyte culture medium for the
clinical applications of regenerative medicine. J Tissue
Eng Regen Med. 2010;5:e63–73.

20. Takagi R, Yamato M, Murakami D, Kondo M, Ohki T,
Sasaki R, Nishida K, Namiki H, Yamamoto M, Okano
T, et al. Fabrication and validation of autologous
human oral mucosal epithelial cell sheets to prevent
stenosis after esophageal endoscopic submucosal dissection. Pathobiology. 2011;78:311–9.

21. Yamato M, Takagi R, Kondo M, Murakami D, Ohki T,
Sekine H, Shimizu T, Kobayashi J, Akiyama Y,
Namiki H, Yamamoto M, Okano T, et al. Grand
espoir: robotics in regenerative medicine. J Robot
Mechatron. 2007;19:500–5.

22. Yang F, Ma D, Cai QC, Li ZS. Esophageal strictures
after extensive endoscopic submucosal dissection:
steroid gel application, the ideal choice? J Gastroenterol Hepatol. 2013;28:1795–7.

Prevention, Identification, and Treatment of Hemorrhage

16

Kohei Takizawa

Introduction

Endoscopic submucosal dissection (ESD) has been a significant advancement in therapeutic endoscopy, with its major advantages being the ability to achieve a higher en bloc resection rate, accurate histological evaluation, and lower cancer recurrence rates compared to conventional endoscopic mucosal resection (EMR) [1–3]. ESD has become a standard therapy not only for early gastric cancer (EGC), but also for early esophageal cancer and early colorectal cancer in Japan [4, 5]. Compared to EMR, ESD requires a longer procedure time and a higher level of technical expertise, in addition to having a slightly greater risk of complications, especially at the beginning of the learning curve [6].

The most frequent complications are bleeding and perforation. Bleeding is more frequent in the stomach cases than esophageal and colorectal cases [4, 5, 7–57] (Tables 16.1 and 16.2). Cases of bleeding complications can be subdivided into immediate, intraprocedural bleeding and delayed bleeding taking place after the procedure, with respect to the time of onset. Immediate bleeding is difficult to define. In a previous study, it was defined as the diminution of 2 g/dL in hemoglobin (Hb) between pre-procedure and next-day levels. Delayed bleeding is usually defined as hematemesis or melena at 0–30 days after the procedure.

How to successfully manage bleeding both during and after ESD will be discussed in this chapter.

Preparation

Before starting training of ESD, pre-procedural, theoretic preparation is necessary. An endoscopist who intends to learn ESD must learn not only about the technique of ESD, but also the basic knowledge of bleeding (e.g. risk factors, incidence, management, etc.), as well as apparatuses such as electrosurgical units, endoscopic knives, and various other devices. The physician should also check all information of ESD patient, such as the past medical history and daily medications, especially anticoagulant agents.

The next steps for trainees are to observe expert endoscopists in action as they perform ESD procedures and assist experts performing the procedure, before beginning themselves. By assisting experienced endoscopists, trainees acquire the skills needed to troubleshoot various situations. Moreover, obtaining expertise in hemostasis before starting ESD is highly recommended since most of the difficulties surrounding the procedure are related to uncontrollable hemorrhage [58].

K. Takizawa, M.D. (✉)
Endoscopy Division, Shizuoka Cancer Center,
1007 Shimonagakubo Nagaizumi-cho, Sunto-gun,
Shizuoka 411-8777, Japan
e-mail: k.takizawa@scchr.jp

N. Fukami (ed.), *Endoscopic Submucosal Dissection: Principles and Practice*,
DOI 10.1007/978-1-4939-2041-9_16, © Springer Science+Business Media New York 2015

Table 16.1 The rate of delayed bleeding after ESD for stomach

Site	Author	Year	n	Delayed bleeding (%)	Reference
Stomach	Oda	2005	1,033	6.0	[8]
	Kakushima	2006	383	3.4	[9]
	Imagawa	2006	159	0	[10]
	Onozato	2006	171	7.6	[11]
	Oda	2006	303	0	[12]
	Hirasaki	2007	112	4.0	[13]
	Jung	2007	552	7.6	[14]
	Takizawa	2008	1,083	5.8	[15]
	Ono	2008	314	8.3	[16]
	Takenaka	2008	306	0.7	[17]
	Hoteya	2009	572	4.9	[18]
	Isomoto	2009	589	1.7	[19]
	Chung	2009	1,000	15.6	[20]
	Takizawa	2009	1,382	9.7	[21]
	Hotta	2010	703	0.3	[22]
	Mannen	2010	478	8.9	[23]
	Goto	2010	454	5.7	[24]
	Tsuji	2010	398	5.8	[25]
	Ahn	2011	833	5.3	[26]
	Akasaka	2011	1,188	3.1	[27]
	Lee	2011	806	4.2	[28]
	Higashiyama	2011	924	3.0	[29]
	Okada	2011	647	4.3	[30]
	Sugimoto	2012	485	3.7	[31]
	Goto	2012	1,814	5.5	[32]
	Toyokawa	2012	1,123	5.0	[33]

Instruments

An endoscope with a water jet function (GIF-Q260J, Olympus, Tokyo, Japan) mounted with a soft transparent hood (TOP Co. Ltd., Tokyo, Japan) is mainly used. This helps facilitate placement of the endoscope, especially during tumor dissection. Normal saline has been used as the injection solution for EMR; however, to achieve better lifting of the lesion in order to lessen the risk of perforation and to lessen tissue damage of the resected specimen, a solution containing sodium hyaluronate has been developed [59]. Many groups now use a commercially available solution of 0.4 % sodium hyaluronate (MucoUp, Johnson & Johnson, Tokyo, Japan). These solutions are usually combined with diluted epinephrine, which is used for the prevention of active bleeding.

Various knives can be used in ESD. At our institution, we developed IT knife-2 (KD-611L; Olympus, Tokyo, Japan). The difference between the IT knife (KD-610L; Olympus, Tokyo, Japan) and the IT knife-2 is the attachment of a short, three-prong blade between the needle and the ceramic tip (Fig. 16.1a, b). Drawbacks in cutting performance of the IT knife have been remarkably improved with the IT knife-2, such as cutting difficulty while the endoscope is looking downward and the relatively poor performance of cutting in a lateral direction. Consequently, the operating time using the IT knife-2 is reported to be much shorter than that using the original IT knife [16, 36, 60].

Since the development of IT knife-2 was mainly for application in the stomach, the insulated tip was too large to be used in the esophagus and colon where the submucosal layer is thinner

Table 16.2 The rate of delayed bleeding after ESD for esophagus and colorectum

Site	Author	Year	n	Delayed bleeding (%)	Reference
Esophagus	Fujishiro	2006	58	0	[34]
	Kakushima	2006	30	0	[35]
	Takizawa	2007	87	0	[36]
	Yoshinaga	2008	25	0	[37]
	Ishihara	2008	110	0	[38]
	Ono	2009	107	0	[39]
	Hirasawa	2010	58	5.2	[40]
	Ishii	2010	37	0	[41]
	Repici	2010	20	0	[42]
	Tanaka	2012	246	1.2	[43]
	Isomoto	2013	291	0.7	[5]
	Kanzaki	2013	48	2.1	[44]
Colorectum	Fujishiro	2007	200	1.0	[45]
	Saito	2007	200	2.0	[46]
	Tanaka	2007	70	1.4	[47]
	Hurlstone	2007	42	2.3	[48]
	Onozato	2007	35	0	[49]
	Tamegai	2007	71	0	[50]
	Toyonaga	2009	468	1.5	[51]
	Zhou	2009	74	1.3	[52]
	Isomoto	2009	292	0.7	[53]
	Yoshida	2010	119	1.6	[54]
	Saito	2010	1,111	1.5	[4]
	Hotta	2012	219	2.7	[55]
	Hotta	2012	146	1.4	[56]
	Yoshida	2013	530	2.3	[57]

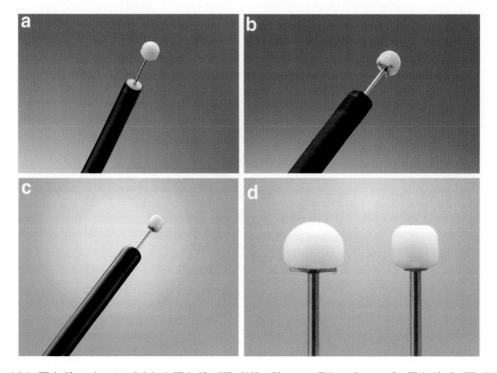

Fig. 16.1 IT knife series. (**a**) Original IT knife (KD-610L; Olympus, Tokyo, Japan). (**b**) IT knife 2 (KD-611L; Olympus, Tokyo, Japan). (**c**) IT knife nano (KD-612L; Olympus, Tokyo, Japan). (**d**) IT knife 2 and IT knife nano

Table 16.3 Instruments and conditions for ESD

	Stomach		Esophagus		Colorectum	
	Device	VIO300D	Device	VIO300D	Device	VIO300D
Marking	APC	Forced APC, 40 W, 1.8 L/min	APC	Precise APC, E3, 1.8 L/min	–	–
Precut	Needle knife	Dry cut, E 4, 50 W	Needle knife	Dry cut, E3, 30 W	Dual knife	Endocut Q, E3-D2-I2
Mucosal incision	IT-2	Endocut Q, E3-D1-I2	IT-nano	Endocut Q, E3-D1-I1	Dual knife	Endocut Q, E3-D2-I2
Submucosal dissection	IT-2	Swift coag, E5, 100 W	IT-nano	Swift coag, E5, 45 W	IT-nano/Dual knife	Swift coag, E3, 40 W
Minor oozing	IT-2	Swift coag, E5, 100 W	IT-nano	Swift coag, E5, 45 W	IT-nano/Dual knife	Swift coag, E3, 40 W
Major bleeding	Hot biopsy	Soft coag, E6, 100 W	Coagrasper	Soft coag, E6, 80 W	Coagrasper	Soft coag, E5, 80 W

IT-2 IT knife 2, *IT-nano* IT knife nano
E effect, *D* duration, *I* interval

a **b**

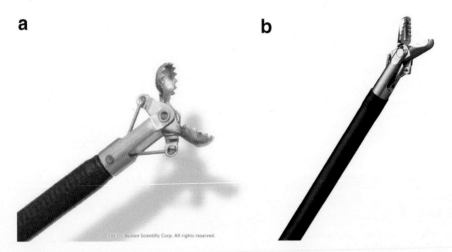

Fig. 16.2 Hemostatic forceps. (**a**) Hot biopsy forceps (Radial Jaw 4, Boston Scientific, Tokyo, Japan). (**b**) Coagrasper (FD-410LR, Olympus, Tokyo, Japan)

and the lumen is narrower. To solve these issues, the new IT knife nano (KD-612L; Olympus, Tokyo, Japan) was recently developed, which has a smaller insulated tip (Fig. 16.1c, d). Now, the IT knife-2 is mainly used for gastric ESD, and IT knife nano for esophageal and colonic ESD.

At our institution, the VIO300D (Erbe, Germany) is mainly used as the electrosurgical unit. The instruments and settings are shown in Table 16.3. For hematemesis, we use hot biopsy forceps (Radial jaw, Boston Scientific, Tokyo, Japan) for stomach, and Coagrasper (FD-410LR, Olympus, Tokyo, Japan) (Fig. 16.2) for esophagus and colon. In cases of severe bleeding that

could not be stopped by coagulation, endoclips were deployed. Because endoclips interfere with the subsequent resection procedure or dissection, one should dissect more submucosal tissue around the bleeding site in order to better expose the bleeding site before clipping.

Bleeding During ESD (Immediate Bleeding)

Bleeding during the procedure is infrequent with EMR techniques, but is quite common and almost unavoidable with ESD. It sometimes requires the

Table 16.4 Relation between immediate/delayed bleeding and lesion location, size (from Oda et al. [8])

		Immediate bleeding		Delayed bleeding	
Location	U	8 %	(14/176)	1 %	(1/176)
	M	8 %	(35/431)	6 %	(27/431)
	L	3 %	(14/426)	6 %	(31/426)
Size (mm)	−20	4 %	(32/719)	5 %	(35/719)
	21–30	8 %	(14/176)	7 %	(13/176)
	31–	12 %	(17/138)	8 %	(11/138)

procedure to be withheld or aborted; however, with the development of new endoscopic techniques and technology, it now only rarely becomes significant to the extent that requires the procedure to be aborted [8]. Management of immediate bleeding plays a critical role in the successful completion of ESD.

Immediate bleeding was found in 63 of 945 patients (7 %) in a previous report, in which immediate bleeding was defined as the diminution of 2 g/dL in hemoglobin (Hb) between pre-procedure and next-day levels [8]. The rates of significant immediate bleeding in the upper and middle thirds of the stomach are higher than in the lower third (Table 16.4) because of the larger diameter of the submucosal arteries in the upper and middle thirds of the stomach [61].

Immediate bleeding is not counted as a complication because this does not compromise the vital signs and the general condition of the patient [62]. However, the control of immediate bleeding (hemostasis) is vital to maintain a good visual field and for implementation of a safe procedure [8, 61].

Prevention of Bleeding During ESD (Immediate Bleeding)

As mentioned above, keeping a good visual field is very important for a safe and smooth procedure. Accidental injury to a large artery may occur during the procedure, immediately impairing endoscopic views with blood and making the procedure difficult. Such an accident can only be prevented by simultaneous visual observation and careful dissection of the submucosal layer and identification of the vessels prior to cutting through the tissue. Therefore, the most effective way of managing immediate bleeding is not how to stop bleeding (coping with bleeding), but how to manage vessels before bleeding (preventing bleeding), otherwise known as "precoagulation."

When a tiny vessel (<2 mm in diameter) is detected in the submucosa during ESD, it is cut using a cutting device such as the IT knife 2, Hook knife, Dual knife (KD-611L, KD-620LR, KD-650L; Olympus, Tokyo, Japan) in the swift coagulation mode (Effect 5, 100 W in VIO300D) to prevent hemorrhage (Fig. 16.3). When a large vessel (>2 mm in diameter) is detected, hemostatic forceps such as the Coagrasper (FD-410LR; Olympus, Tokyo, Japan) or hot biopsy forceps are used in the soft coagulation mode (Effect 6, 100 W in VIO300D) prior to cutting through the vessel to prevent hemorrhage (Fig. 16.4). Once the vessels are pretreated, dissection can be safely performed without bleeding.

Hemostasis for Bleeding During ESD (Immediate Bleeding)

Endoscopists must be aware of not only the risk factors for, and incidence of, complications, but also how to effectively treat such complications. During ESD, immediate minor bleeding is not uncommon, but it can be successfully treated by electrocautery on the bleeding vessels. Endoclips are only deployed for severe bleeding that cannot be controlled by coagulation, because endoclips interfere with the subsequent resection procedure [6, 61, 63].

Electrocautery is usually carried out using different devices, depending on the degree of bleeding. Minor oozing can be controlled by electrocautery using a cutting device such as the IT knife 2. For arterial bleeding, application of electrocautery using hemostatic forceps such as the Coagrasper or hot biopsy forceps is more suitable.

The most important key to achieving good hemostasis is an identification of the exact bleeding point by using water flushing and clearance of blood in the field. Endoscopes equipped with water jet systems (GIF-Q260J; Olympus, Tokyo,

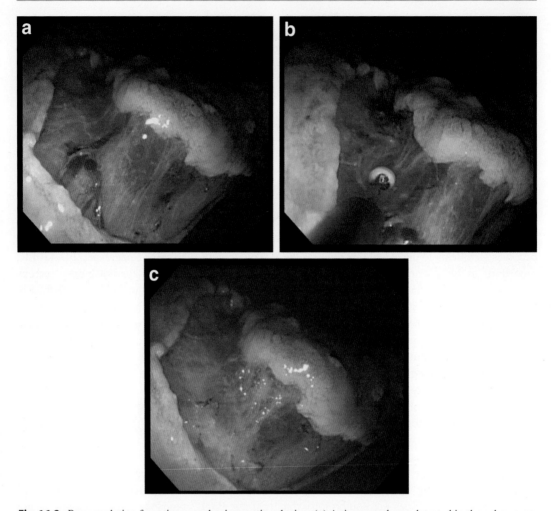

Fig. 16.3 Precoagulation for a tiny vessel using cutting device. (**a**) A tiny vessel was detected in the submucosa. (**b**, **c**) Slowly cut down using IT knife 2 in the swift coagulation mode to prevent hemorrhage

Japan) have recently become available for use in precisely determining the bleeding point. Once the bleeding point is securely clamped, hemostasis is always achievable. If the bleeding point cannot be identified due to constant blood flow, hemostasis could be possible by grasping the roughly estimated bleeding site with larger forceps (hot biopsy forceps, Boston Inc.). However, the operators should keep in mind that inappropriate hemostasis, such as accumulated coagulation energy, will increase the risk of delayed perforation.

Bleeding makes the scope view extremely limited and leads to significant complications such as perforation. Even slight bleeding should therefore be completely stopped as soon as it occurs.

Bleeding After ESD (Delayed Bleeding)

As reported previously [8], both perforation and immediate bleeding are easily recognized at the time of the procedure and can be successfully treated endoscopically [64]. On the other hand, delayed bleeding manifested as hematemesis or melena may occur days after the procedure, even

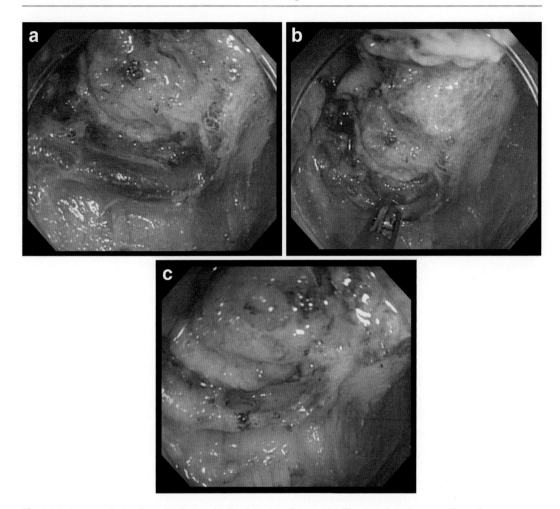

Fig. 16.4 Precoagulation for a thick vessel using hemostatic forceps. (**a**) Thick vessels were detected in the submucosa. (**b**) The vessels were grasped by the hot biopsy forceps. (**c**) The vessels and surrounding submucosa were coagulated and became whitish. Dissection could be safely performed without bleeding

many days after discharge from the hospital. As any delay in recognition of such an event may result in cardiovascular compromise, prevention of delayed bleeding is very important [15].

Delayed bleeding, which is usually defined as hematemesis or melena at 0–30 days after the procedure, should be confirmed and treated with urgent endoscopy. Delayed bleeding after ESD has been reported to range from 0 to 15.6 % [8–33] (Table 16.1). This wide variation is partly due to differences in the definition of delayed bleeding as used in the reported studies. The incidence of delayed bleeding after ESD is as common as in conventional EMR, and usually the

bleeding occurs within 12 h after the procedure. The frequency of delayed bleeding differs with location and size of lesions, patient age, and procedure time [8, 15, 30, 33].

Oda et al. reported that delayed bleeding occurred more frequently after ESD for lesions in the lower and middle thirds of the stomach compared to the upper third of the stomach [8, 15] (Table 16.4). The reasons for this remain unclear, but antral peristaltic activity and the alkaline effect of bile juice reflux may contribute to some extent. It is also speculated that this increase in the risk of delayed bleeding for lesions in the lower third of the stomach could be due to the fact that immediate bleeding in such cases is less common; therefore, the need for intraoperative hemostatic treatment is less than for lesions located in the upper third of the stomach [8, 15].

Okada et al. reported that resected specimen size of 40 mm was the only significant factor associated with delayed bleeding after ESD [30]. Toyokawa et al. reported that patient age ≥ 80 years and lengthier procedure time were associated with a significantly higher risk of delayed bleeding after ESD [33]. With regards to antiplatelet drugs, the possible influence on delayed bleeding of such drugs is controversial [65, 66].

Delayed bleeding mainly occurs during hospitalization; however, it sometimes occurs after the patient has been discharged from the hospital, and in such cases any delay in recognition may result in patient's serious condition. At our institution, clinicopathological data of 1,432 lesions in 1,250 consecutive patients with gastric neoplasms undergoing ESD from September 2002 to May 2008 were reviewed [21]. Median admission period was 5 days. Delayed bleeding occurred in 143 of 1,432 lesions, of which 22 % (32/143) occurred after the patient was discharged from the hospital. Univariate analysis showed that only gender (male, 3.1 % vs. female, 0.7 %) was a significant factor. Of 32 cases that occurred in patients discharged from the hospital, 28 cases underwent planned endoscopy on the next day of ESD and nine cases (32 %) required endoscopic hemostasis. The signs of delayed bleeding were hematemesis (56 %), melena/tarry stool (28 %), stomachache (10 %), and unconsciousness (6 %). The median period from ESD to bleeding was 10 days (range 5–19). All cases were controlled by endoscopic treatments (hemoclipping and/or electrocoagulation), and none required any surgical intervention. Blood transfusion was required in only three patients [21].

Prevention of Bleeding After ESD (Delayed Bleeding)

To prevent delayed bleeding, hemostasis of any vessels that appear on the artificial ulcer after removing the specimen is essential [15]. All visible, exposed vessels on the artificial ulcer should be coagulated using hemostatic forceps with soft coagulation mode, even if there was no evidence of bleeding at the end of ESD (Fig. 16.5). However, excess coagulation should be avoided because perforation may occur. After removing the specimen, if bleeding cannot be stopped easily, one should not persist with electrocautery, and endoclips should be considered.

It is important to recognize delayed bleeding as soon as possible. For such purposes, at our institution, a nasal tube is routinely inserted into the stomach until the following day.

The effectiveness of second-look endoscopy (SLE) after hemostasis of peptic ulcer bleeding has previously been shown [67, 68]. SLE is routinely performed the day after gastric ESD to detect and prevent bleeding after ESD. However, use of routine SLE in patients without any signs of bleeding has not yet been validated with regard to clinical outcomes. In a retrospective study in Japan, Goto et al. reported that SLE after gastric ESD may contribute little to the prevention of delayed bleeding [24]. And from Korea, Ryu et al. also suggested that SLE is not routinely necessary, because it does not affect clinical outcomes, including bleeding and morbidity after ESD, based on a prospective, randomized study [69].

Hemostasis for Bleeding After ESD (Delayed Bleeding)

Different modalities are applied according to the period of delayed bleeding. In the early days of delayed bleeding, the artificial ulcer floor is still soft with less granulation tissue so endoscopic clips or electrocautery using hemostatic forceps can be applied to control this complication. In the later days of delayed bleeding, the artificial ulcer floor hardens with granulation tissue so the injection method is preferable [6].

Medical Management After ESD

Hospitalization and Diet

In Japan, ESD is performed on hospitalized patients. Patients without complication start

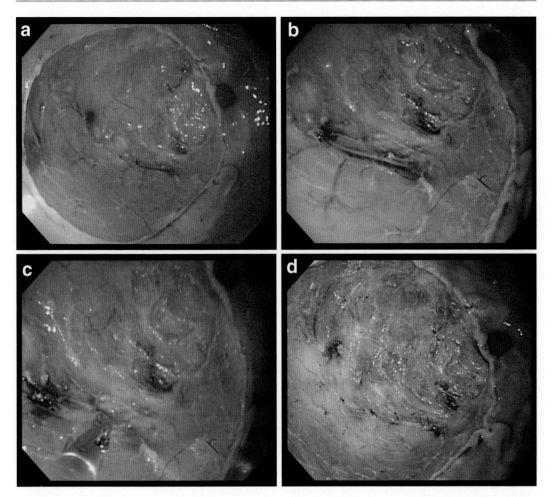

Fig. 16.5 Post-ESD coagulation (PEC) therapy [15]. Endoscopic appearance of endoscopic submucosal dissection (ESD) defect. (**a**, **b**) Before post-ESD coagulation (PEC). (**c**) All visible exposed vessels on the artificial ulcer was coagulated using hemostatic forceps with the soft coagulation mode, even if there was no evidence of bleeding. (**d**) ESD defect after PEC

drinking water on the day after ESD and start eating a soft diet 2 days after ESD, and were discharged within 4 ± 7 days.

Acid-Suppressing Medications

Acid-suppressing medications are generally used after gastric ESD; however, the choice of medication and the duration of treatment remain controversial. Kakushima et al. reported that healing occurred within 8 weeks with proton pump inhibitor (PPI) administration for 8 weeks, irrespective of ulcer size or location [70]. It has also been reported that administration of PPI for 2 weeks for artificial ulcers after ESD may be sufficient in helping them to heal [71]. Uedo et al. reported that PPI therapy was more effective at preventing delayed bleeding of ulcers created by ESD than H2-receptor antagonist (H2RA) treatment [72]. In contrast, Yamaguchi et al. reported that there were no differences in the incidence of delayed bleeding or ulcer size 30 and 60 days after gastric EMR between PPI and H2RA treatment [73].

It remains controversial about which type of acid-suppressing medication should be given after gastric ESD. At our institution, PPIs are prescribed for up to 2 months (double dose for 1 month and regular dose for 1 month) after gastric ESD. PPIs are not usually used for esophageal ESD, except for those lesions near the esophagogastric junction.

Antiplatelet and Anticoagulation Drugs

Recently published guidelines recommend discontinuation of all antiplatelet agents, including aspirin, before EMR or ESD, in case of the low risk of a thrombotic event [74]. However, this is a low-grade recommendation without results of large-scale trials, and there is no specific guideline for patients with high thrombotic risks.

Cho et al. reported that continuous aspirin use increases the risk of bleeding after gastric ESD, and they concluded that aspirin use should be stopped in patients with a low risk for thromboembolic disease to minimize bleeding complications [66]. In contrast, Lim et al. reported that in ESD for antiplatelet users, continuous administration was not found to have an independent significant association with bleeding [65]. There is still room for further research on this issue.

Conclusions

Management of (preferably prevention of) immediate bleeding is the most important key to successful completion of ESD. But prevention of delayed bleeding is also very important, because any delay in recognition of such an event may result in severe cardiovascular compromise. The endoscopist who intends to learn ESD must first obtain expertise in hemostasis and learn the basic knowledge of bleeding, including risk factors, incidence, and management, as well as the variety and features of devices used for hemostasis. A regimented training program is an important part of learning and performing successful ESD.

References

1. Ono H, Kondo H, Gotoda T, Shirao K, Yamaguchi H, Saito D, Hosokawa K, Shimoda T, Yoshida S. Endoscopic mucosal resection for treatment of early gastric cancer. Gut. 2001;48:225–9. PMID: 11156645.
2. Tanaka M, Ono H, Hasuike N, Takizawa K. Endoscopic submucosal dissection of early gastric cancer. Digestion. 2008;77 Suppl 1:23–8.
3. Gotoda T, Yamamoto H, Soetikno MR. Endoscopic submucosal dissection of early gastric cancer. J Gastroenterol. 2006;41:929–42.
4. Saito Y, Uraoka T, Yamaguchi Y, Hotta K, Sakamoto N, Ikematsu H, Fukuzawa M, Kobayashi N, Nasu J, Michida T, Yoshida S, Ikehara H, Otake Y, Nakajima T, Matsuda T, Saito D. A prospective, multicenter study of 1111 colorectal endoscopic submucosal dissections (with video). Gastrointest Endosc. 2010;72:1217–25.
5. Isomoto H, Yamaguchi N, Minami H, et al. Management of complications associated with endoscopic submucosal dissection/endoscopic mucosal resection for esophageal cancer. Dig Endosc. 2013;25 Suppl 1:29–38.
6. Oda I, Suzuki H, Nonaka S, Yoshinaga S. Complications of gastric endoscopic submucosal dissection. Dig Endosc. 2013;25 Suppl 1:71–8.
7. Kakushima N, Fujishiro M. Endoscopic submucosal dissection for gastrointestinal neoplasms. World J Gastroenterol. 2008;14(19):2962–7.
8. Oda I, Gotoda T, Hamanaka H, Eguchi T, Saito Y, Matsuda T, Bhandari P, Emura F, Saito D, Ono H. Endoscopic submucosal dissection for early gastric cancer: technical feasibility, operation time and complications from a large consecutive series. Dig Endosc. 2005;17:54–8.
9. Kakushima N, Fujishiro M, Kodashima S, Muraki Y, Tateishi A, Omata M. A learning curve for endoscopic submucosal dissection of gastric epithelial neoplasms. Endoscopy. 2006;38:991–5.
10. Imagawa A, Okada H, Kawahara Y, Takenaka R, Kato J, Kawamoto H, Fujiki S, Takata R, Yoshino T, Shiratori Y. Endoscopic submucosal dissection for early gastric cancer: results and degrees of technical difficulty as well as success. Endoscopy. 2006;38:987–90.
11. Onozato Y, Ishihara H, Iizuka H, Sohara N, Kakizaki S, Okamura S, Mori M. Endoscopic submucosal dissection for early gastric cancers and large flat adenomas. Endoscopy. 2006;38:980–6.
12. Oda I, Saito D, Tada M, et al. A multicenter retrospective study of endoscopic resection for early gastric cancer. Gastric Cancer. 2006;9:262–70.
13. Hirasaki S, Kanzaki H, Matsubara M, Fujita K, Ikeda F, Taniguchi H, Yumoto E, Suzuki S. Treatment of over 20 mm gastric cancer by endoscopic submucosal dissection using an insulation-tipped diathermic knife. World J Gastroenterol. 2007;13:3981–4.
14. Jung HY, Choi KD, Song HJ, Lee GH, Kim JH. Risk management in endoscopic submucosal dissection using needle knife in Korea. Dig Endosc. 2007;19 Suppl 1:S5–8.

15. Takizawa K, Oda I, Gotoda T, et al. Routine coagulation of visible vessels may prevent delayed bleeding after endoscopic submucosal dissection – an analysis of risk factors. Endoscopy. 2008;40:179–83.

16. Ono H, Hasuike N, Inui T, Takizawa K, et al. Usefulness of a novel electrosurgical knife, the insulation-tipped diathermic knife-2, for endoscopic submucosal dissection of early gastric cancer. Gastric Cancer. 2008;11:47–52.

17. Takenaka R, Kawahara Y, Okada H, et al. Risk factors associated with local recurrence of early gastric cancers after endoscopic submucosal dissection. Gastrointest Endosc. 2008;68:887–94.

18. Hoteya S, Iizuka T, Kikuchi D, Yahagi N. Benefits of endoscopic submucosal dissection according to size and location of gastric neoplasm, compared with conventional mucosal resection. J Gastroenterol Hepatol. 2009;24:1102–6.

19. Isomoto H, Shikuwa S, Yamaguchi N, et al. Endoscopic submucosal dissection for early gastric cancer: a large-scale feasibility study. Gut. 2009;58:331–6.

20. Chung IK, Lee JH, Lee SH, et al. Therapeutic outcomes in 1000 cases of endoscopic submucosal dissection for early gastric neoplasms: Korean ESD Study Group multicenter study. Gastrointest Endosc. 2009;69:1228–35.

21. Takizawa K, Tanaka M, Kakushima N, Yamaguchi Y, Matsubayashi H, Ono H. Delayed bleeding of gastric Endoscopic submucosal dissection in patients discharged from the hospital. Gastroenterol Endosc. 2009;51 Suppl 2:2190 (Abstract in Japanese).

22. Hotta K, Oyama T, Akamatsu T, et al. A comparison of outcomes of endoscopic submucosal dissection (ESD) for early gastric neoplasms between high-volume and low-volume centers: multi-center retrospective questionnaire study conducted by the Nagano ESD Study Group. Intern Med. 2010;49:253–9.

23. Mannen K, Tsunada S, Hara M, et al. Risk factors for complications of endoscopic submucosal dissection in gastric tumors: analysis of 478 lesions. J Gastroenterol. 2010;45:30–6.

24. Goto O, Fujishiro M, Kodashima S, et al. A second-look endoscopy after endoscopic submucosal dissection for gastric epithelial neoplasm may be unnecessary: a retrospective analysis of postendoscopic submucosal dissection bleeding. Gastrointest Endosc. 2010;71:241–8.

25. Tsuji Y, Ohata K, Ito T, et al. Risk factors for bleeding after endoscopic submucosal dissection for gastric lesions. World J Gastroenterol. 2010;16:2913–7.

26. Ahn JY, Jung HY, Choi KD, et al. Endoscopic and oncologic outcomes after endoscopic resection for early gastric cancer: 1370 cases of absolute and extended indications. Gastrointest Endosc. 2011;74: 485–93.

27. Akasaka T, Nishida T, Tsutsui S, et al. Short-term outcomes of endoscopic submucosal dissection (ESD) for early gastric neoplasm: multicenter survey by Osaka University ESD study group. Dig Endosc. 2011;23:73–7.

28. Lee H, Yun WK, Min BH, et al. A feasibility study on the expanded indication for endoscopic submucosal dissection of early gastric cancer. Surg Endosc. 2011;25:1985–93.

29. Higashiyama M, Oka S, Tanaka S, et al. Risk factors for bleeding after endoscopic submucosal dissection of gastric epithelial neoplasm. Dig Endosc. 2011;23: 290–5.

30. Okada K, Yamamoto Y, Kasuga A, et al. Risk factors for delayed bleeding after endoscopic submucosal dissection for gastric neoplasm. Surg Endosc. 2011; 25:98–107.

31. Sugimoto T, Okamoto M, Mitsuno Y, et al. Endoscopic submucosal dissection is an effective and safe therapy for early gastric neoplasms: a multicenter feasible study. J Clin Gastroenterol. 2012;46:124–9.

32. Goto O, Fujishiro M, Oda I, et al. A multicenter survey of the management after gastric endoscopic submucosal dissection related to postoperative bleeding. Dig Dis Sci. 2012;57:435–9.

33. Toyokawa T, Inaba T, Omote S, et al. Risk factors for perforation and delayed bleeding associated with endoscopic submucosal dissection for early gastric neoplasms; analysis of 1123 lesions. J Gastroenterol Hepatol. 2012;27:907–12.

34. Fujishiro M, Yahagi N, Kakushima N, Kodashima S, Muraki Y, Ono S, Yamamichi N, Tateishi A, Shimizu Y, Oka M, Ogura K, Kawabe T, Ichinose M, Omata M. Endoscopic submucosal dissection of esophageal squamous cell neoplasms. Clin Gastroenterol Hepatol. 2006;4:688–94.

35. Kakushima N, Yahagi N, Fujishiro M, Kodashima S, Nakamura M, Omata M. Efficacy and safety of endoscopic submucosal dissection for tumors of the esophagogastric junction. Endoscopy. 2006;38:170–4.

36. Takizawa K, Hasuike N, Ono H, Ikehara H, Otake Y, Matsubayashi H, Yamaguchi Y. Endoscopic submucosal dissection of oesophageal neoplasms using Improved IT knife (IT knife2). Endoscopy. 2007;39: A29.

37. Yoshinaga S, Gotoda T, Kusano C, Oda I, Nakamura K, Takayanagi R. Clinical impact of endoscopic submucosal dissection for superficial adenocarcinoma located at the esophagogastric junction. Gastrointest Endosc. 2008;67:202–9.

38. Ishihara R, Iishi H, Uedo N, et al. Comparison of EMR and endoscopic submucosal dissection for en bloc resection of early esophageal cancers in Japan. Gastrointest Endosc. 2008;68:1066–72.

39. Ono S, Fujishiro M, Niimi K, et al. Long-term outcomes of endoscopic submucosal dissection for superficial esophageal squamous cell neoplasms. Gastrointest Endosc. 2009;70:860–6.

40. Hirasawa K, Kokawa A, Oka H, et al. Superficial adenocarcinoma of the esophagogastric junction: long-term results of endoscopic submucosal dissection. Gastrointest Endosc. 2010;72:960–6.

41. Ishii N, Horiki N, Itoh T, et al. Endoscopic submucosal dissection with a combination of small-caliber-tip transparent hood and flex knife is a safe and effective

treatment for superficial esophageal neoplasias. Surg Endosc. 2010;24:335–42.

42. Repici A, Hassan C, Carlino A, et al. Endoscopic submucosal dissection in patients with early esophageal squamous cell carcinoma: results from a prospective Western series. Gastrointest Endosc. 2010;71: 715–21.

43. Tanaka M, Ono H, Kakushima N, Takizawa K, et al. Endoscopic submucosal dissection for widespread superficial esophageal neoplasm doesn't increase the incidence of perioperative complication except for esophageal stricture. Gastrointest Endosc. 2012;75: AB450–1.

44. Kanzaki H, Ishihara R, Ohta T, et al. Randomized study of two endo-knives for endoscopic submucosal dissection of esophageal cancer. Am J Gastroenterol. 2013;108:1293–8.

45. Fujishiro M, Yahagi N, Kakushima N, Kodashima S, Muraki Y, Ono S, Yamamichi N, Tateishi A, Oka M, Ogura K, Kawabe T, Ichinose M, Omata M. Outcomes of endoscopic submucosal dissection for colorectal epithelial neoplasms in 200 consecutive cases. Clin Gastroenterol Hepatol. 2007;5:678–83. quiz 645.

46. Saito Y, Uraoka T, Matsuda T, Emura F, Ikehara H, Mashimo Y, Kikuchi T, Fu KI, Sano Y, Saito D. Endoscopic treatment of large superficial colorectal tumors: a case series of 200 endoscopic submucosal dissections (with video). Gastrointest Endosc. 2007;66:966–73.

47. Tanaka S, Oka S, Kaneko I, Hirata M, Mouri R, Kanao H, Yoshida S, Chayama K. Endoscopic submucosal dissection for colorectal neoplasia: possibility of standardization. Gastrointest Endosc. 2007;66: 100–7.

48. Hurlstone DP, Atkinson R, Sanders DS, Thomson M, Cross SS, Brown S. Achieving R0 resection in the colorectum using endoscopic submucosal dissection. Br J Surg. 2007;94:1536–42.

49. Onozato Y, Kakizaki S, Ishihara H, Iizuka H, Sohara N, Okamura S, Mori M, Itoh H. Endoscopic submucosal dissection for rectal tumors. Endoscopy. 2007; 39:423–7.

50. Tamegai Y, Saito Y, Masaki N, Hinohara C, Oshima T, Kogure E, Liu Y, Uemura N, Saito K. Endoscopic submucosal dissection: a safe technique for colorectal tumors. Endoscopy. 2007;39:418–22.

51. Toyonaga T, Man-I M, Morita Y, Sanuki T, Yoshida M, Kutsumi H, Inokuchi H, Azuma T. The new resources of treatment for early stage colorectal tumors: EMR with small incision and simplified endoscopic submucosal dissection. Dig Endosc. 2009;21 Suppl 1:S31–7.

52. Zhou PH, Yao LQ, Qin XY. Endoscopic submucosal dissection for colorectal epithelial neoplasm. Surg Endosc. 2009;23:1546–51.

53. Isomoto H, Nishiyama H, Yamaguchi N, Fukuda E, Ishii H, Ikeda K, Ohnita K, Nakao K, Kohno S, Shikuwa S. Clinicopathological factors associated with clinical outcomes of endoscopic submucosal

dissection for colorectal epithelial neoplasms. Endoscopy. 2009;41:679–83.

54. Yoshida N, Naito Y, Sakai K, Sumida Y, Kanemasa K, Inoue K, Morimoto Y, Konishi H, Wakabayashi N, Kokura S, Yagi N, Yanagisawa A, Yoshikawa T. Outcome of endoscopic submucosal dissection for colorectal tumors in elderly people. Int J Colorectal Dis. 2010;25:455–61.

55. Hotta K, Shinohara T, Oyama T, et al. Criteria for non-surgical treatment of perforation during colorectal endoscopic submucosal dissection. Digestion. 2012;85:116–20.

56. Hotta K, Yamaguchi Y, Saito Y, et al. Current opinions for endoscopic submucosal dissection for colorectal tumors from our experience: indications, technical aspects and complications. Dig Endosc. 2012;24: 110–6.

57. Yoshida N, Yagi N, Inada Y, et al. Prevention and management of complications of and training for colorectal endoscopic submucosal dissection. Gastroenterol Res Pract. 2013;2013:287173.

58. Yamamoto S, Uedo N, Ishihara R, Kajimoto N, Ogiyama H, Fukushima Y, Yamamoto S, Takeuchi Y, Higashino K, Iishi H, Tatsuta M. Endoscopic submucosal dissection for early gastric cancer performed by supervised residents: assessment of feasibility and learning curve. Endoscopy. 2009;41:923–8.

59. Fujishiro M, Yahagi N, Nakamura M, et al. Successful outcomes of a novel endoscopic treatment for GI tumors: endoscopic submucosal dissection with a mixture of high-molecular-weight hyaluronic acid, glycerin, and sugar. Gastrointest Endosc. 2006;63: 243–9.

60. Kakushima N, Ono H, Tanaka M, Takizawa K, et al. Endoscopic dissection using the insulated-tip knife. Tech Gastrointest Endosc. 2011;13:63–9.

61. Toyonaga T, Nishino E, Hirooka T, Ueda C, Noda K. Intraoperative bleeding in endoscopic submucosal dissection in the stomach and strategy for prevention and treatment. Dig Endosc. 2006;18:S123–7.

62. Tajiri H, Kitano S. Complications associated with endoscopic mucosal resection: definition of bleeding that can be viewed as accidental. Dig Endosc. 2004;16:S134–6.

63. Muraki Y, Enomoto S, Iguchi M, Fujishiro M, Yahagi N, Ichinose M. Management of bleeding and artificial gastric ulcers associated with endoscopic submucosal dissection. World J Gastrointest Endosc. 2012;16:1–8.

64. Minami S, Gotoda T, Ono H, Oda I, Hamanaka H. Complete endoscopic closure of gastric perforation induced by endoscopic resection of early gastric cancer using endoclips can prevent surgery. Gastrointest Endosc. 2006;63:596–601.

65. Lim JH, Kim SG, Kim JW, et al. Do antiplatelets increase the risk of bleeding after endoscopic submucosal dissection of gastric neoplasms? Gastrointest Endosc. 2012;75:719–27.

66. Cho SJ, Choi IJ, Kim CG, et al. Aspirin use and bleeding risk after endoscopic submucosal dissection in

patients with gastric neoplasms. Endoscopy. 2012;44: 114–21.

67. Villanueva C, Balanzó J, Torras X, Soriano G, Sáinz S, Vilardell F. Value of second-look endoscopy after injection therapy for bleeding peptic ulcer: a prospective and randomized trial. Gastrointest Endosc. 1994;40:34–9.

68. Chiu PW, Lam CY, Lee SW, et al. Effect of scheduled second therapeutic endoscopy on peptic ulcer rebleeding: a prospective randomised trial. Gut. 2003;52:1403–7.

69. Ryu YH, Kim WJ, Kim SH, et al. Second-look endoscopy is not associated with better clinical outcomes after gastric endoscopic submucosal dissection: a prospective, randomized, clinical trial analyzed on an as-treated basis. Gastrointest Endosc. 2013;78:285–94.

70. Kakushima N, Yahagi N, Fujishiro M, et al. The healing process of gastric artificial ulcers after endoscopic submucosal dissection. Dig Endosc. 2004;16:327–31.

71. Niimi K, Fujishiro M, Goto O, et al. Prospective single-arm trial of two week rabeprazole treatment for ulcer healing after gastric endoscopic submucosal dissection. Dig Endosc. 2012;24:110–6.

72. Uedo N, Takeuchi Y, Yamada T, et al. Effect of a proton pump inhibitor or an H2-receptor antagonist on prevention of bleeding from ulcer after endoscopic submucosal dissection of early gastric cancer: a prospective randomized controlled trial. Am J Gastroenterol. 2007;102:1610–6.

73. Yamaguchi Y, Katsumi N, Tauchi M, et al. A prospective randomized trial of either famotidine or omeprazole for the prevention of bleeding after endoscopic mucosal resection and the healing of endoscopic mucosal resection-induced ulceration. Aliment Pharmacol Ther. 2005;21 Suppl 2:111–5.

74. Boustière C, Veitch A, Vanbiervliet G, et al. ESGE guideline: endoscopy and antiplatelet agents. Endoscopy. 2011;43:445–58.

Selvi Thirumurthi and Gottumukkala S. Raju

Introduction

At the beginning of the twenty-first century, endoscopists started exploring curative resection of early stage gastrointestinal neoplasms (defined as localized disease without lymph node or distant metastases) as an alternative to surgery. Although polypoid neoplasms can be removed with a biopsy or snare resection, these techniques are unsuitable for complete and safe resection of large non-polypoid lesions [1]. Endoscopic submucosal dissection (ESD) and endoscopic mucosal resection (EMR) allow complete resection of such flat lesions, as they utilize submucosal fluid injection to lift the lesion and make it accessible for complete resection. However, perforation is a serious risk as these procedures involve cutting the mucosa and submucosa while sparing the deep submucosa and muscularis propria of the rather thin gut wall. Advances in clinical practice as well as investigative work in the animal laboratory have helped us to develop techniques for successful

endoluminal closure of perforations. A detailed review of the literature will be presented to help the reader who is interested in EMR and ESD to gain further insight on this topic.

ESD Versus EMR: An Overview

Credit goes to the Japanese endoscopists for their enthusiasm to develop endoluminal resection techniques to avoid gastrectomy in patients with early gastric cancer. En bloc resection of larger lesions can be accomplished with ESD, while the same lesion could only be removed in a piecemeal fashion, instead of en bloc, with EMR. However, piecemeal resection poses a risk of recurrence as shown in a Japanese study, where gastric cancer recurred in 2.8 % of patients after piecemeal resection of >15 mm early gastric cancer lesions compared to no recurrences in patients treated with en bloc resection [2]. Other studies have described even higher rates of cancer recurrence of lesions treated with EMR; for instance, Saito et al. reported higher local cancer recurrence rate of after colorectal EMR compared to ESD (14 % vs 2 %; $p < 0.0001$) [3]. Still others have quoted a range of 2 % up to 35 %, from a variety of studies on endoscopic resection of gastric cancer [4]. In a meta-analysis of 15 published studies, ESD was associated with a higher rate of en bloc resection (OR 13.87, 95 % CI 10.12–18.99) and curative resection (OR 3.52, 95 % CI 2.57–4.84) compared to EMR [5].

S. Thirumurthi, M.D., M.S. • G.S. Raju, M.D., F.A.S.G.E. (✉)
Department of Gastroenterology, Hepatology, and Nutrition, The University of Texas MD Anderson Cancer Center, 1400 Pressler Street—Unit 1466, Houston, TX 77030, USA
e-mail: graju@mdanderson.org

N. Fukami (ed.), *Endoscopic Submucosal Dissection: Principles and Practice*,
DOI 10.1007/978-1-4939-2041-9_17, © Springer Science+Business Media New York 2015

Although EMR and ESD offer the advantage of complete resection of early neoplasms and a less invasive alternative to surgery, both are associated with risk of complications such as bleeding, perforation, and stricture. The ESD perforation rate is significantly higher than that of EMR (4–10 % vs. 0.3–0.5 %) [6]. A single-center, single-operator Japanese study of 1635 early gastrointestinal neoplasms of the esophagus, stomach, and colon reported ESD perforation rates of 0 %, 1.8 %, and 1.9 % respectively [7].

Identification of Perforation and Tension Pneumoperitoneum

Perforation is a serious complication of ESD. Perforations can be classified by size: microperforations and macroperforations, and by time of onset: immediate and delayed [8].

Microperforations are detected after the procedure as free air on routine post ESD imaging due to the escape of air through invisible perforations in a wall thinned by cautery and dissection.

Macroperforations are obvious to the endoscopist during the procedure and result from inadvertent deep cautery during the incision or dissection phase of ESD or entrapment of muscularis propria during snare resection of EMR. These perforations can be closed with clips, and the resection completed during the same session.

In a retrospective study of 1,711 patients undergoing ESD for early gastric cancers, Jeon et al. described an overall perforation rate of 2.1–3.2 % [9]. A total of 26 macroperforations and 13 microperforations occurred over 5 years. All patients with microperforations recovered with conservative management, but one patient with a macroperforation required emergent surgery. Though ESD was successfully completed in all patients after clip closure of macroperforations, the rate of incomplete resection and recurrence of tumor was greater among this group of patients, though not statistically significant. Perforation is an inherent risk in performing ESD,

and the identification and rapid management of perforation is of utmost importance while maintaining a high quality resection.

Tension Pneumoperitoneum results from the rapid escape of air through a perforation. Although tension pneumoperitoneum from escaped luminal gases can occur, it has become infrequent since the use of CO_2 for insufflation during EMR and ESD has become routine. Immediate abdominal decompression using an 18-gauge needle puncture is required to relieve tension pneumoperitoneum. Subsequently, patients should be kept nil by mouth, adequately hydrated with intravenous fluids, and started on broad-spectrum intravenous antibiotics. Patients who do not improve with these clinical interventions may require emergency surgery for repair [8, 9].

Risk Factors for ESD Perforation

Risk factors for ESD perforation include some related to the operator and others related to the lesion itself.

Operator-related factors include utilization of a precise endoscopic technique, adequate experience with ESD, and the volume of ESD performed at a particular center.

Lesion-related factors include the size and the luminal distribution of the lesion and its location, whether esophagus, stomach, duodenum, or colon. Large lesions and lesions that are difficult to access are at a higher risk for complications.

Endoscopic Closure Options

Binmoeller and colleagues were the first to describe the use of endoclips to close a gastric perforation after EMR of a leiomyoma in the early 1990s [10]. The ability to immediately close perforations endoscopically often spares the patient a surgical intervention and all the intrinsic risks and costs associated with it. Several models of through-the-scope clips, over-the-scope clips, and endoscopic suturing device prototypes are available on the market for endoscopic closure of perforations.

Through-The-Scope Clips

Through-the-scope clips (TTSC) were initially introduced in Japan in the 1970s to mark lesions and achieve hemostasis [10]. Currently available TTSC products include: Quick Clip (Olympus America Inc., Center Valley PA), which is free 360° bidirectionally rotatable; Resolution Clip (Boston Scientific Inc., Natick MA), which allows reopening prior to final clip deployment; and Instinct Clip (Cook Medical Inc., Bloomington IN), which has 360° bidirectional rotation as well as reopening capability.

TTSCs have been used in a variety of clinical situations, including closure of gastrointestinal fistulae and leaks as well as spontaneous and iatrogenic perforations. TTSCs can be used to successfully manage both fresh perforations and chronic fistulae and, with appropriate technical expertise, even close defects up to 25 mm in size [11]. Limitations of these TTS endoclips include their limited wing-span when open and their lower closure force that can lead to sub-optimal tissue apposition and often necessitate the placement of multiple endoclips [12]. The larger endoclips offer greater tissue grasp and a better leak proof seal, but may interfere with continuation of the ESD procedure.

Over-The-Scope Clips

The introduction of over-the-scope clips (OTSC) in 2007 helped to overcome some of the limitations of through-the-scope endoclips. OTSC are composed of nitinol (nickel titanium alloy) and are housed within a metal applicator cap that is fitted over the distal tip of the scope (Ovesco Endoscopy AG, Tubingen Germany). These clips are deployed by the release of a wire attached to a hand wheel mounted on the scope at the biopsy valve, in a mechanism similar to esophageal variceal rubber band ligation. Caps and clips are available in three sizes to accommodate different endoscope diameters. OTSC are offered in two depths (3 mm and 6 mm), to vary the amount of tissue that can be grasped

within the clip [13]. The clips have different shapes of teeth, rounded, pointed, and longer pointed, and the clinical indication for using OTSC will determine which clip configuration is used. The rounded teeth OTSC are used for hemostasis and are especially helpful in the esophagus and colon where the organ wall is thinner. The pointed teeth clip has the ability to grasp tissue with minimal slippage and can be useful for closing perforations and fistulae. The longer pointed teeth clip is effective in the thicker-walled stomach [13]. Since OTSC are able to grasp more tissue, they produce a more durable closure than TTSCs and can apply eight to nine Newtons of permanent closing force [14]. The U.S. Food and Drug Administration approved the use of OTSCs in 2010.

The initial clinical experience with OTSC was described by Kirschniak et al. when they used OTSC to achieve hemostasis in seven patients and successfully closed iatrogenic perforations in four patients [14]. Investigators have subsequently used OTSC to treat post-surgical leaks and chronic fistulae, and have diversified the clinical experience in closing iatrogenic perforation and bleeding with varying degrees of success [12, 15, 16]. Baron et al. described the clinical experience using OTSC in the first multi-center study in the United States [17]. OTSC were successful in closing 65 % of fistulae and post-surgical leaks and 75 % of iatrogenic perforations and achieved hemostasis in all seven patients. One clinical failure in this study was due to shifting of the OTSC and tissue away from the gastro-cutaneous fistula site. The clip was sectioned using argon plasma coagulation on the highest setting to remove it from the tissue [17]. In a recent systematic review, Weiland et al. reviewed 17 published clinical studies that involved closure of gastrointestinal perforations and leaks by OTSC [18]. The intervention was technically successful between 80 and 100 % of the time, and clinically successful (when no further intervention was necessary) 60–100 % of the time. The failure of OTSC was associated with necrotic tissue around the wound edges that prevented adequate clip deployment [18].

Endoscopic Suturing

The U.S. Food and Drug Administration approved an endoscopic suturing device in 2000 for gastro-esophageal reflux disease [19]. Much of the experience with endoscopic suturing devices comes from experimental models that were developed for natural orifice translumenal endoscopic surgery (NOTES). In NOTES, the reliable closure of controlled perforations made in the wall of the gastrointestinal tract is essential.

Organ-Specific Endoscopic Closure

Esophagus

The application of the aforementioned techniques for managing esophageal, gastro-duodenal, and colonic perforation after EMR and ESD will now be discussed, as well as the animal work that laid foundation for development of endoscopic closure techniques in clinical practice.

Experimental Studies

Endoscopic suturing has been evaluated in experimental studies. Fritscher-Ravens et al. have investigated the role of endoscopic suturing to close iatrogenic defects created in the esophagus [20]. One such study was performed to compare different techniques of iatrogenic esophageal perforation closure. The investigators created a small esophageal full-thickness perforation in 18 pigs and randomized them to closure with TTSC, endoscopic suturing with a custom-made suturing system, or standard thoracoscopic closure. Each of the study animals had a technically successful closure. One animal in the suturing group had a mediastinal abscess and another animal in this group and in the surgical group expired prematurely. Closure with TTSC was statistically significantly faster than either of the other groups (9 min vs. 21 min in suturing group and 42 min for surgery, $p=0.006$). On necropsy, peri-esophageal adhesions were most pronounced in the suturing group. In this small study, although TTSC, suturing and surgery were all comparable, the animals treated with endoclips had a better outcome.

Another NOTES study involving trans-esophageal mediastinoscopy by these investigators revealed no adhesions and on histological examination on necropsy; sutured closure had normal wall healing while there was disruption of the muscle layer but healing of the mucosal and submucosal layers after TTSC closure [21].

In another study, where a 2 cm full-thickness resection of the esophagus followed by closure with a prototype endoscopic suturing device, necropsy after 3 months revealed no complications related to incision, resection, or closure; there was no evidence of mediastinitis and all but one animal had well-healed scars [22]. This study demonstrates the feasibility of successful suture closure of full-thickness resection of a segment of the esophagus in an animal model.

Clinical Studies

Esophageal perforations can occur in a variety of other clinical settings, including spontaneous rupture, Boerhaave's syndrome, iatrogenic rupture (after endoscopic dilation, EMR, or surgical intervention), or secondary to foreign body ingestion [23, 24]. The treatment modality of choice is usually TTSC as these clips are readily available in the endoscopy suite and most gastroenterologists have experience using them. In a multicenter European cohort study, Voermans et al. described five cases where iatrogenic esophageal perforations were treated with OTSC. All five lesions were successfully closed. Three patients required a combination of OTSC and TTSC placement, while the other patients each had two OTSC deployed to close the defect [25]. Nishiyama et al. described one elderly patient who experienced an iatrogenic perforation of the distal esophagus after stomach feeding tube placement that was successfully treated with a 9 mm OTSC [26].

ESD has traditionally been used to treat superficial squamous cell carcinoma in the esophagus. ESD esophageal perforation rates vary among the published clinical studies but are generally below 10 % [27, 28]. Fujishiro et al. published some of the earliest esophageal ESD experience with their study of 58 squamous cell carcinoma lesions in 43 patients performed between 2002 and 2005.

An R0 resection was achieved in 78 % of lesions, which ranged between 2 and 66 mm in size. The majority of the lesions were in the thoracic esophagus and occupied less than half of the luminal circumference. In this particular study, perforation occurred in 7 % of cases (4/57) and was detected during the course of ESD and immediately closed with endoscopic clips. All patients demonstrated pneumomediastinum on chest X-ray and were treated conservatively with good clinical improvement and resolution of pneumomediastinum within 1 week. Pneumomediastinum was not seen in any patients without perforation noted during endoscopy [27]. Others have reported pneumomediastinum on post-procedure X-ray, without detection of perforation during ESD [29, 30]. In another study, a perforation was detected and presumably treated (likely with TTSC, though this is not certain) with good result [31].

Yamashina et al. described their ESD experience on esophageal lesions greater than 50 mm in diameter [32]. In 39 patients, the en bloc resection rate was 100 %, with tumor-free margins achieved in 92 %. The procedure was curative in 70 % with a complication rate of 2.5 %. One patient experienced mediastinal emphysema without perforation (microperforation), and stricture developed in 11 of 39 patients, as would be expected after large ESDs in the esophagus [32].

Sato et al. summarized the clinical presentation and management of esophageal perforations that occurred during or after EMR/ESD [33]. They treated 472 esophageal neoplasms (171 EMR, 306 ESD), and seven patients (1.9 %) experienced esophageal perforation. Three perforations occurred intra-operatively, three during balloon dilation for stricture prevention, and one due to food impaction. All were treated endoscopically and did not require surgery.

Although a great deal of ESD work has been done to treat early squamous cell carcinoma of the esophagus, recently there is growing interest in defining its role in esophageal adenocarcinoma. This condition occurs more commonly in the West where ESD experience is often limited to fewer skilled gastroenterologists. Nonetheless, a few Japanese investigators have described their experience in the literature [34–36]. En bloc resection rates were high (97–100 %) and R0 resection rates ranged between 79 % and 100 %. In these three studies where 112 patients were treated, only one perforation occurred during ESD, and it was successfully treated with TTSC placement [34–36]. Further study is required in the treatment of esophageal adenocarcinoma with ESD.

Stomach

Experimental Studies

Many investigators have described the role of different devices to close gastric perforations in experimental studies. OTSC have the ability to grasp a larger volume of tissue than TTSC and lead to full-thickness, more durable closure due to the greater force of closure. The superiority of OTSC over TTSC in repairing gastrotomies was demonstrated by von Renteln et al. with their in vivo study of 20 female swine [37]. Swine were randomized to gastrostomy repair with either TTSC or OTSC. Four TTSC pigs had a positive leak test after closure, compared to none in the OTSC group. Peri-gastric abscesses were present in two of the OTSC pigs and three of the TTSC pigs, but peritonitis and adhesions were only present in the TTSC group. These differences were not statistically significant, given the small number of animals in the study. It is interesting to note that not all closures with OTSC were full-thickness. 70 % of the closures involved mucosa and submucosa, 20 % also included the muscularis mucosa, and only 10 % involved the serosa; in contrast, 20 % of the closures with TTSC incorporated the mucosa and submucosa while the remainder were mucosal closures alone [37].

In another study, Voermans et al. compared OTSC closure with hand surgical suturing of gastrostomies [38]. Gastrotomies were created with a needle knife puncture followed by dilation with an 18 mm balloon in 26 ex vivo porcine stomachs. Eleven specimens were closed with OTSC and 15 specimens had surgical suturing. All defects were successfully closed; specimens repaired with OTSC showed air leakage at pressures

(233 mm Hg, SD 47) that were non-inferior to the gold standard of hand suturing (206 mm Hg, SD 59), thereby confirming the potential role for OTSC gastric perforation closures.

Matthes et al. conducted an ex vivo study to determine maximal closure capacity and pressure threshold for a single OTSC placed over gastrotomies [39]. Full-thickness gastric defects were created measuring 5, 10, 15, 20, and 25 mm and closed with a single OTSC. There was a linear inverse relationship between the size of the defect and the pressure associated with rupture of the closure. Optimal results were seen with the use of a single OTSC for defects up to 15 mm in diameter, and though adequate closure was achieved in 20 mm gastrotomies, the burst pressures were significantly lower, indicating the need for more than one OTSC for larger gastrotomies or supplemental endoclip placement [39].

Zhang et al. studied the feasibility of using OTSC to close perforations created in the gastric fundus of an in vivo canine model [40]. Seven canines underwent needle knife gastrostomy followed by placement of OTSC, which was technically difficult in two canines because of the retroflexed nature of the endoscope. Leak testing was performed with air insufflation and methylene blue solution instilled into the stomach and detected by laparoscopy. A minor leak, defined as a slight detection of methylene blue solution in the peritoneal cavity, was observed in one of the two canines in which OTSC placement was technically difficult. No OTSC-related complications were noted at necropsy. The feasibility and successful placement of OTSC over gastric fundal defects was demonstrated in this small study [40].

Suturing devices have also been used to successfully close gastric defects. Rajan et al. performed endoscopic suturing (Overstitch, Apollo Endosurgery Inc.) to close the mucosal defect after obtaining a full-thickness gastric biopsy using submucosal endoscopy with mucosal flap technique [41]. Defects were successfully closed in all 12 pigs with an uneventful clinical course. Endoscopy at 2 weeks showed stellate scarring without mucosal ulceration, and necropsy showed complete serosal healing in all study animals [41].

Park et al. conducted a study comparing closure of gastrotomies with a tissue apposition system comprised of tissue anchors against surgical repair in an in vivo porcine model [42]. After gastrotomy and peritoneoscopy, 32 pigs were randomized to endoscopic or surgical closure. All repairs were technically successful, recovery times were similar in both groups, and all closures remained secure at necropsy. Two pigs in the endoscopic group died, one from gastric distention and another was euthanized for rectal prolapse, while one pig was euthanized in the surgical group for wound dehiscence. One animal in the surgical group had a leak detected at necropsy and animals in both groups had signs of peritonitis, adhesions, and abdominal abscesses, though adhesions were significantly higher in the surgical group [42]. Since endoscopic treatment was comparable to surgery, this shows the potential use of endoscopic closure in NOTES and ESD.

Other endoscopic closure techniques include threaded tags (T tags) or tissue anchors. Dray et al. conducted an in vivo study comparing histologic healing after closure of gastrotomy using TTSC versus T tags in 12 pigs [43]. Closure was technically successful in all 12 animals followed by an uneventful 2-week follow up. Transmural healing was seen in 75 % (n = 3) of pigs treated with Resolution clips (Boston Scientific Corporation) and in 12 % (n = 1) of the T tag group. The authors concluded that although TTSC only perform mucosal closure, it consistently resulted in layer-to-layer closure and transmural healing. T tags form a tight plication and cause inversion of the gastric edges, which impairs layer-to-layer healing [43]. Sumiyama et al. performed a short-term animal survival study to evaluate the performance of tissue anchors in closure of gastric perforations [44]. These investigators created 12 large gastric perforations (median 3 cm) in 6 pigs and closed them using a flexible needle-catheter tissue-anchoring device. All closures were technically successful and all animals survived for 1 week without complications. At follow up endoscopy and necropsy, all perforations were secure and there were no findings of peritonitis; however, 12.5 % of the tissue anchors had penetrated surrounding organs [44].

Stapling devices have been studied to close gastrotomies in animal models with the goal of using this technology in closing access points in NOTES procedures. Magno et al. did an initial evaluation of the feasibility and effectiveness of a novel stapling device, which delivered a 6 cm long staple line (NOLC60, Power Medical Interventions, Langhorne, PA, USA) [45]. Leak-resistant gastric closure was achieved in all four pigs with an unremarkable clinical course. Necropsy demonstrated full-thickness healing confirmed by histologic examination. However, intra-mural micro abscesses were also seen in the two pigs that underwent the procedure using non-sterile technique [45]. Meireles et al. performed a follow-up study using this automated flexible stapling device (SurgASSIST, Power Medical Interventions, Langhorne, PA, USA), which delivered four rows of staples with each firing of the device and successfully created full-thickness closure of gastric defects in four pigs [46].

Surgical glues have been used with success in the treatment of variceal bleeding, embolization, and fistulae. Ersoy et al. conducted a study comparing suture, endoclip and combination of endoclip and topical cyanoacrylate glue to close gastric perforation in 60 rats [47]. Burst pressure levels were higher in the cyanoacrylate group along with improved histological healing indices (tissue granulation, chronic inflammation, and collagen deposition), however this was counterbalanced by significantly increased adhesion formation in this group [47]. The use of cyanoacrylate glue is a promising technique for closure of gastric perforations in ESD and NOTES.

Experiments using other bioprosthetics to close gastric perforations have been conducted. Agents that are successful in closing gastrointestinal perforations must form an effective seal, allow tissue ingrowth, and tolerate the local environment (for example, low gastric pH) [48]. The Gore Bioabsorbable Hernia Plug, which is made from the biodegradable polymer polyglycolide, trimethylene carbonate (PGA:TMC, W.L. Gore & Associates Inc, Flagstaff, AZ USA), was used to plug a surgically created 1 cm perforation on the anterior wall of the stomach in 12 canines. The bioprosthesis closed the perforation without leak in all animals when ex vivo testing was performed. Animals were sacrificed at different intervals to further examine the closure. At week one, the perforation was closed but there was no tissue ingrowth. However, at weeks four through twelve, the injury site was healed and the luminal portion of the plug had been absorbed. Bioprosthesis seem to offer a durable closure of gastric perforation with physiologic healing of the injury site [48].

Standard surgical treatment of gastro-duodenal perforations involves the placement of an omental patch over the defect. Hashiba et al. conducted one of the first published studies of experimental endoscopic repair with an omental patch in 2001 in ten pigs [49]. These investigators created a gastric perforation in two steps, first using a variceal band ligation cap fitted over the tip of the endoscope and a polypectomy snare to complete a mucosal resection. In the next step, they completed the perforation by repeating the first step with a smaller cap. To seal the perforation, omentum was aspirated into the defect and affixed to the muscularis propria layer with endoclips. Nine pigs had an uneventful clinical course, with an ulcer seen at the repair site on follow-up endoscopy. The omentum was completely adhered to the external gastric wall at necropsy without evidence of peritonitis. Histologic examination revealed complete healing without microabscess. One animal, in which the muscularis propria could not be clearly seen during omental patch placement, died prematurely, and postmortem examination revealed a persistent leak indicative of an unsuccessful repair with subsequent peritonitis [49].

More recently, Dray et al. have conducted experiments with omentoplasty [50]. Nine pigs were assigned to one of three groups: endoscopic full-thickness gastric resection using an EMR kit without closure, similar resection with omental closure (attaching the omentum to the intact gastric mucosa, away from the perforation site) or full-thickness resection using needle knife and balloon dilation followed by similar omental closure. All animals that did not have gastrotomy closure developed peritonitis. Complete healing was seen on endoscopy in all of the remaining animals except for a small ulceration seen in one animal from each of the omental closure groups. No complication was seen at necropsy or on histologic examination in these animals except for one animal in the group resected with the EMR kit that developed an abscess of the omental patch. As omentoplasty is the standard surgical repair for gastro-duodenal perforations and the greater omentum has known antibacterial, hemostatic, angiogenic, and adhesive properties, further studies for endoscopic placement of an omental patch are indicated [50]. As we have described, several novel techniques have been used to close gastric perforation in experimental models. Many of these have translated to clinical application in patients to address gastro-duodenal perforation and closure.

Clinical Studies

ESD has a several-fold increased risk of perforation over EMR of the stomach and duodenum. Gastroenterologists who perform ESD should be aware of the risk factors associated with perforation in the gastro-duodenum. Several investigators have retrospectively evaluated the experience at their centers to determine predictive risk factors for perforation during ESD for these upper gastrointestinal lesions.

Toyokawa et al. performed 1,123 gastric ESD between 2003 and 2010 and described an overall perforation rate of 2.4 % [51]. Lesions located in the upper or proximal stomach had a significantly higher risk of perforation (OR 4.9, 95 % CI 2.2–10.7) than in other parts of the stomach. They also described a lower rate of en bloc resection and a lower curative resection rate among patients who experienced a perforation (74 % versus 94 %, and 48 % versus 85 %, respectively).

Ohta et al., in a different center in Japan, performed 1795 gastric ESDs over an 8 year period [52]. Their overall perforation rate was 2.8 %, and risk factors for perforation again included proximal location of the gastric lesion (OR 2.4, 95 % CI 1.3–4.6). Another significant risk factor was tumor diameter greater than 2 cm (OR 1.9, 95 % CI 1.0–3.5). These investigators noted an improvement in perforation rate over their study period as there were significantly fewer perforations that occurred over the second half of the study period than had happened earlier in the study (OR 4.5, 95 % CI 2.1–9.4) [52].

Kim et al. described their experience with 1289 gastric ESDs between 2003 and 2010 [53]. Their overall perforation rate was 2.7 % and they also found that location of the lesion within the stomach impacted the risk for perforation: lesions in the gastric body had a higher risk for perforation than antral lesions (OR 2.6, 95 % CI 1.3–5.2). Also, lesions that required piecemeal resection had a significantly higher risk of perforation (OR 2.6, 95 % CI 1.0–6.6). The antrum appears to be a safer location to perform ESD as the en face position allows greater access to the lesion. The antral wall is also thicker and has fewer and smaller caliber blood vessels compared to the gastric body. The authors attribute the increased risk of perforation with piecemeal resection to intrinsic features of such lesions, including anatomic location, difficult scope maneuvering, or deeper invasion of the tumor [53].

Watari et al. reported a perforation rate of 8.2 % in 98 consecutive gastric neoplasms that underwent ESD; all patients were managed conservatively. Procedure time greater than 115 min was associated with an increased risk of perforation (OR 9.15, 95 % CI 1.08–77.54, $p = 0.04$). Subgroup analysis revealed similar post-ESD clinical course regardless of whether perforation was detected endoscopically versus those diagnosed on post-ESD imaging [54].

Investigators have reported not only their rates of perforation, but have further subdivided this into rates of microperforation and macroperforation. The clinical outcomes for patients experiencing micro- or macroperforation are favorable and comparable [9]. Kim et al. report a rate of 2.1 % microperforation and 0.6 % macroperforation [53]. Yoo et al., another group from Korea, performed 823 gastric ESD from 2005 to 2010 [55]. Their rate of microperforation was 2.1 % and was associated with patient age over 81 years (OR 20), tumor depth of invasion into the muscularis mucosa (OR 5.4) and procedure time greater than 2 h (OR 5.9). Macroperforation rate was 7.5 % and was associated with proximal gastric location of lesion (OR 7.9), fibrosis seen during submucosal dissection (OR 3.0) and prolonged procedure time of over 2 h (OR 3.3) [55].

The gastric fundus is a difficult area for resection, with a correspondingly higher risk of perforation. Li et al. reported ESD of gastric fundus subepithelial tumors (<3 cm) in 10 patients, followed by clip closure of the post-ESD defect [56]. Perforation occurred in 30 %, all of which were successfully closed with clips.

Minami et al. have described nearly two decades of experience at their center in Japan [57]. In 2,460 patients who underwent endoscopic resection of early gastric cancer, perforation occurred in 5 % of patients ($n = 121$). One quarter of the patients had EMR and the remaining patients were treated with ESD. The initial four patients who experienced gastric perforation were treated with emergent surgery. The remaining 117 patients were treated with either TTSC for small lesions or an omental patch for larger lesions, of which two such patients were referred for surgery due to failure of endoscopic closure. In the last 6 years of the study, patients treated with endoscopic closure of gastric perforation had a recovery rate similar to that of non-perforation patients. Over time, with this particular group, perforation rates have remained steady, despite performing seven times as many procedures (1987–1993: 155 procedures, 2003–2004: 833 procedures). The post-procedure fasting period for patients and their length of hospital stay have also declined over the years, however. Prior to 1998, patients fasted for a mean of 6 days with a 10-day hospital course. After 1999, patients fasted an average of 2 days and spent 7 days in the hospital. Patients who did not experience a perforation fasted for 1–2 days and were admitted for 4–7 days post-procedure. There was no statistically significant difference in the rates of perforation between EMR and ESD. Although rates of perforation were higher for lesions located in the upper third of the stomach, in this study it was not statistically significant.

Experience with EMR/ESD of gastric lesions over the years, along with successful closure of perforations and post-procedure management of these patients has been encouraging.

Duodenum

Clinical Studies

Both TTSC and OTSC are utilized for closure of gastro-duodenal perforations. Unlike other sites, the duodenum is prone to high risk of perforation.

Matsumoto et al. were among the first to describe their experience using ESD exclusively in the duodenum [58]. They reported 85.7 % en bloc ESD on 14 early cancers, adenomas, and neuroendocrine tumors (3–60 mm; mean 12.7 mm) arising from the duodenal bulb or the non-ampullary descending duodenum; and one piecemeal resection of a large elevated adenoma. Three perforations (21 %) occurred; perforation during the resection of an invasive neuroendocrine tumor required surgical repair and excision, while the remaining two perforations during resection of duodenal bulb submucosal tumor and descending duodenum depressed type adenocarcinoma were repaired endoscopically [58].

Fifteen duodenal lesions (duodenal bulb, $n = 3$; descending duodenum, $n = 12$) 12–39 mm in size were resected by either EMR or ESD by Honda et al. over a 3 year period [59]. Ampullary tumors were again excluded from this study. Perforations occurred in 13 %; one perforation during the procedure was closed with endoclips and delayed perforation in another patient required surgery [59].

Min et al. reported their results for endoscopic treatment of 36 non-ampullary sporadic duodenal adenomas in 35 consecutive patients [60]. They used EMR in 23 cases and achieved an en bloc resection rate of 87 % and all of these had tumor-free margins. The remaining 13 cases were ablated with argon plasma coagulation. Perforation occurred in one patient in the EMR group and was managed endoscopically without the need for surgery [61].

Matsumoto et al. reported a case series of five patients with carcinoid tumor in the duodenal bulb. Pre-ESD evaluation included an endoscopic ultrasound examination. Lesions ranged between 3 and 8 mm and all but one were successfully removed with ESD; the one patient required surgery for repair of perforation and excision of tumor. One additional perforation occurred but was managed endoscopically (perforation rate 40 %) [62]. Kim et al. reported endoscopic resection of 41 duodenal carcinoid tumors less than 10 mm in 38 patients with a variety of EMR and ESD techniques. Although endoscopic complete resection was accomplished in 98 % of cases, pathologic complete resection was observed in only 41 % of patients. Although the endoscopic complete resection rate did not differ according to the resection method, complete pathologic resection rates were higher in ESD cases than in EMR, as expected. Perforation did not occur and no recurrence of disease was noted during the 17 month follow-up period [63].

In summary, endoscopic resection of duodenal lesions is associated with a higher rate of complications, including bleeding and perforation, and technical difficulty both accessing lesions and removing lesions from the thin-walled duodenum. These factors make duodenal ESD more challenging and time-consuming for the gastroenterologist. Further experience in performing ESD in the duodenum is necessary for us to improve and perfect this technique.

Colon

Experimental Studies
Through-The-Scope Clips

A series of experimental studies were undertaken to systematically investigate and develop techniques for colon perforation closure.

In a pilot study to evaluate the feasibility and safety of closing colonic perforations with endoclips in a porcine model, small (1.5–2 cm) colon perforations were created in five pigs and closed with endoclips. All animals had an uneventful clinical course and none had any evidence of peritonitis or peri-colonic abscess at 1 week necropsy. Histopathology showed granulation tissue bridging the site of the perforation [64].

In order to develop techniques for closure of linear perforations, which develop from mechanical trauma during colonoscope insertion, and circular perforations, which develop after snare resection, further animal studies were undertaken. These studies demonstrated that a leak proof seal could be achieved with clip closure; linear perforations required longitudinal closure from the top end to the bottom end of perforation at 5 mm intervals, while circular perforations required transverse closure similar to surgical closure [65, 66].

In a placebo-controlled study using the multi-clip applicator device (InScope Multi Clip Applier, Ethicon Endosurgery, Cincinnati OH, USA) for closure of a 2 cm colon perforation, peritonitis, and adhesions were prominent on necropsy in the non-clip closure group, while the clip closure group revealed a clean peritoneal cavity. In addition, there was no difference in the outcomes between the two versus four clip closure groups [67].

Although clips are useful for closure of fresh perforations, animal studies revealed that clips fail to close perforations if the edges of the perforation are gaping and sloping [65, 66]. In such cases, suturing devices with T tag placement to bring the gaping edges together may be beneficial. In a study comparing the multi-clip applicator device (InScope Multi Clip Applier, Ethicon Endosurgery, Cincinnati OH, USA) with a through-the-scope full-thickness tissue approximation device (TAD, InScope, Ethicon Endo-Surgery Inc, Cincinnati OH, USA) in 4 cm colon perforations, T tag placement followed by suture closure was technically successful in all four pigs while clip closure failed in some [68].

In order to explore endoluminal full thickness of lesions tethered to the wall from prior incomplete resections as a concept, studies were undertaken to investigate and develop techniques to close large defects left after full-thickness resection of the colonic wall. Endoluminal closure was technically successful in closure of full-thickness colon resection in 19/20 animals. One animal developed clinical signs of peritonitis and necropsy revealed pericolic abscess and adhesions. This pilot study shows promising results for the use of through-the-scope devices to close colon defects [69].

Over-the-Scope Clips

Mathes et al. conducted an ex vivo study to determine the maximum closure capacity and burst pressure for a single OTSC [39]. They concluded that a single OTSC achieved excellent full-thickness closure of defects up to 25 mm in the colon, and adequate closure of defects up to 30 mm, but with bursting pressures lower for smaller defects. The investigators suggest more than one OTSC may be necessary or an OTSC may need to be supplemented with endoclips to achieve optimal closure of colonic defects larger than 30 mm [39].

In a survival study, Schurr et al. evaluated OTSC closure of 5–10 mm iatrogenic colon perforations in ten pigs. Closure was technically successful in all animals, with excellent healing [70].

In a study comparing OTSC closure with open surgical repair of 18 mm sigmoid perforations in 24 pigs, there was excellent sealing of perforations with no difference in the burst pressures between the two groups [71].

Voermans et al. conducted an ex vivo porcine study to evaluate the strength of six different closure techniques: surgical suture (gold standard), TTSC, T tags, OTSC, and two different stapler devices, with assessment by leak pressure [72]. Surgical and staple closure result in parallel closure, while TTSC and OTSC result in inverted closure; both are comparable in their robustness of closure, while T tags resulted in everted closure which is weaker at sustaining the leak pressures.

Over-the-Scope Suturing Device

In addition to closure with these recognized techniques, investigators have conducted feasibility studies with different devices. Pham et al. performed a feasibility study using a prototype endoscopic suturing device, the Eagle Claw (Apollo group with Olympus Medical Systems Corp, Tokyo Japan), in the closure of 2 cm colonic perforations in a pig model [73]. Endoscopic closure was successful in seven out of ten animals that also had uneventful clinical courses, and no complications were noted at necropsy. Closure was successful in one animal that subsequently had dehiscence of the closure at necropsy. Two animals did not have successful endoscopic closure [73].

Stents and Fillers

In a comparative study, biodegradable stent insertion was compared to primary hand sewn repair of colon perforation in 34 animals [74]. Four pigs in the surgical group died while there was no mortality in the stent group. Burst pressures were also higher in the animals that were stented.

Investigators have also successfully used bovine collagen wrap for closure of colon perforations. Nocca et al. affixed a belt of collagen sponge and collagen film around the outer part of the colon to cover the defect. This was technically successful and no complications occurred; one animal developed wound infection [75]. There may be a role for endoscopic closure of perforations with similar biomaterials in the future.

Clinical Studies

Yoshikane et al. reported the first case of successful clip closure of a perforation after EMR of a flat colonic lesion [76]. Subsequently, a group in Belgium reported successful clip closure of a sigmoid perforation caused by colonoscope trauma, which avoided surgery in an elderly patient [77].

Carvalho et al. conducted a prospective study to evaluate the success, complication rate and recurrence of sessile and flat colorectal polyps removed by EMR [78]. EMR was successfully performed on 73 large polyps (median size 30 mm) with a perforation rate of 1.4 % that was treated endoscopically [78]. In a prospective comparative study by Masci et al., the success and complication rates of EMR in the colon between high and low (<50 EMR) volume centers in Italy was comparable [79]. The perforation rate was also similar between the groups (2 %). Recurrence of disease was noted in 15 % of all patients regardless of the center where the procedure was performed. The authors conclude that EMR can be successfully performed in low volume centers [79].

A number of large retrospective studies on ESD of colonic lesions shed light on the incidence of colon perforation along with risk factors that predispose to perforation. The perforation rate varied from 7 % to 20 % [80–85]. Risk factors for ESD perforation include tumor size, laterally spreading tumor, and presence of fibrosis [80, 81, 84]. Submucosal injection of hyaluronic acid has been found to be protective against perforation [81]. The size of the perforation influences the outcome of the patient's recovery after the procedure. Patients with a macroperforation identified during endoscopy, compared to those with microperforation identified by post-procedure X-rays, required longer hospitalization and remained nothing by mouth and on antibiotic therapy for a greater period of time [83].

For tips and techniques specific to prevention and treatment of clinical perforation in the colon, please see Chap. 19. Please see Chap. 18 for those specific to the upper GI tract.

Management of Perforation

After successful clip closure of perforations, patients should be closely monitored for signs of mediastinitis or peritonitis in close collaboration with the surgical team. Patients should be kept nothing by mouth, started on broad-spectrum intravenous antibiotics with anaerobic and gram-negative organism coverage. Abdominal radiographs should be obtained for baseline evaluation. Serial blood counts as well inflammatory markers such as C-reactive protein assays should be performed. Oral intake can be resumed after the patient is asymptomatic and the bowel function returns.

Prevention of Perforation

In addition to proper endoscopic technique, a number of measures can be undertaken to limit the risk of perforation.

Unlike air, carbon dioxide is rapidly reabsorbed, making it the ideal gas for complicated endoscopic procedures such as EMR and ESD. In a retrospective comparative study, Maeda et al. reported significantly lower incidence of mediastinal emphysema in patients undergoing esophageal ESD with carbon dioxide compared to air insufflation [86].

Another critical element to limit complications related to perforation is excellent bowel preparation. If the colon preparation is not optimal, both EMR and ESD should be avoided. Stool interferes with EMR and ESD and escape of stool through a perforation can be a life-threatening disaster.

Limitations of Endoscopic Closure of Perforation

Despite significant strides in endoscopic closure of EMR and ESD perforations, clip closure may fail and result in serious complications. It is difficult to evaluate the completeness of endoscopic closure of colon perforations. With incomplete clip closure or early detachment of the clips, minor leakage can occur, which may delay the appearance of symptoms associated with peritonitis. It may be difficult to make a decision about surgery because the symptoms may not be clear-cut and gross contamination may require aggressive surgery including colon resection with diversion [87]. Premature detachment of clips could result in reopening of the perforation site, leakage of luminal contents, and peritonitis [25, 88]. Hence, it is important to inspect the closure site from all angles to ensure successful closure. In addition, these patients need intensive clinical observation for 24 h and immediate surgical intervention should be undertaken in cases of clinical deterioration. Another potential complication is that clips can interfere with laparoscopic closure of perforations [87].

Insertion of the endoscope loaded with the OTSC device should be done with caution under direct vision and only if no resistance is encountered. Therefore, the use of these devices may be limited by the location and orientation of the perforation/defect.

Conclusions

In summary, both EMR and ESD perforations can be closed successfully with clips and avoid the need for emergent surgery. One should be proficient in clip closure before embarking on EMR or ESD of gastrointestinal tumors, along with sound understanding of the principles of management after closure.

References

1. Pohl H, Srivastava A, Bensen SP, et al. Incomplete polyp resection during colonoscopy-results of the complete adenoma resection (CARE) study. Gastroenterology. 2013;144:74–80 e1.
2. Tanabe S, Koizumi W, Mitomi H, et al. Clinical outcome of endoscopic aspiration mucosectomy for early stage gastric cancer. Gastrointest Endosc. 2002;56: 708–13.
3. Saito Y, Fukuzawa M, Matsuda T, et al. Clinical outcome of endoscopic submucosal dissection versus endoscopic mucosal resection of large colorectal tumors as determined by curative resection. Surg Endosc. 2010;24:343–52.
4. Yokoi C, Gotoda T, Hamanaka H, Oda I. Endoscopic submucosal dissection allows curative resection of locally recurrent early gastric cancer after prior endoscopic mucosal resection. Gastrointest Endosc. 2006;64(2):212–8.
5. Cao Y, Liao C, Tan A, et al. Meta-analysis of endoscopic submucosal dissection versus endoscopic mucosal resection for tumors of the gastrointestinal tract. Endoscopy. 2009;41:751–7.
6. ASGE Technology Committee, Kantsevoy SV, Adler DG, et al. Endoscopic mucosal resection and endoscopic submucosal dissection. Gastrointest Endosc. 2008;68:11–8.
7. Toyonaga T, Man-i M, East JE, et al. 1,635 Endoscopic submucosal dissection cases in the esophagus, stomach, and colorectum: complication rates and long-term outcomes. Surg Endosc. 2013;27:1000–8.
8. Lee DW, Jeon SW. Management of complications during gastric endoscopic submucosal dissection. Diagn Ther Endosc. 2012;2012:624835.
9. Jeon SW, Jung MK, Kim SK, et al. Clinical outcomes for perforations during endoscopic submucosal dissection in patients with gastric lesions. Surg Endosc. 2010;24:911–6.
10. Binmoeller KF, Grimm H, Soehendra N. Endoscopic closure of a perforation using metallic clips after snare excision of a gastric leiomyoma. Gastrointest Endosc. 1993;39:172–4.
11. Raju GS, Gajula L. Endoclips for GI endoscopy. Gastrointest Endosc. 2004;59:267–79.
12. Jayaraman V, Hammerle C, Lo SK, et al. Clinical application and outcomes of over the scope clip device: initial US experience in humans. Diagn Ther Endosc. 2013;2013:381873.
13. Committee AT, Banerjee S, Barth BA, et al. Endoscopic closure devices. Gastrointest Endosc. 2012;76:244–51.
14. Kirschniak A, Kratt T, Stuker D, et al. A new endoscopic over-the-scope clip system for treatment of lesions and bleeding in the GI tract: first clinical experiences. Gastrointest Endosc. 2007;66:162–7.
15. Pohl J, Borgulya M, Lorenz D, et al. Endoscopic closure of postoperative esophageal leaks with a novel over-the-scope clip system. Endoscopy. 2010;42: 757–9.
16. Seebach L, Bauerfeind P, Gubler C. "Sparing the surgeon": clinical experience with over-the-scope clips for gastrointestinal perforation. Endoscopy. 2010;42: 1108–11.
17. Baron TH, Song LM, Ross A, et al. Use of an over-the-scope clipping device: multicenter retrospective results of the first U.S. experience (with videos). Gastrointest Endosc. 2012;76:202–8.
18. Weiland T, Fehlker M, Gottwald T, et al. Performance of the OTSC System in the endoscopic closure of iatrogenic gastrointestinal perforations: a systematic review. Surg Endosc. 2013;27:2258–74.
19. Reavis KM, Melvin WS. Advanced endoscopic technologies. Surg Endosc. 2008;22:1533–46.
20. Fritscher-Ravens A, Hampe J, Grange P, et al. Clip closure versus endoscopic suturing versus thoracoscopic repair of an iatrogenic esophageal perforation: a randomized, comparative, long-term survival study in a porcine model (with videos). Gastrointest Endosc. 2010;72:1020–6.
21. Fritscher-Ravens A, Patel K, Ghanbari A, et al. Natural orifice transluminal endoscopic surgery (NOTES) in the mediastinum: long-term survival animal experiments in transesophageal access, including minor surgical procedures. Endoscopy. 2007;39: 870–5.
22. Fritscher-Ravens A, Cuming T, Jacobsen B, et al. Feasibility and safety of endoscopic full-thickness esophageal wall resection and defect closure: a prospective long-term survival animal study. Gastrointest Endosc. 2009;69:1314–20.
23. Gomez-Esquivel R, Raju GS. Endoscopic closure of acute esophageal perforations. Curr Gastroenterol Rep. 2013;15:321.
24. Qadeer MA, Dumot JA, Vargo JJ, et al. Endoscopic clips for closing esophageal perforations: case report and pooled analysis. Gastrointest Endosc. 2007;66: 605–11.
25. Voermans RP, Le Moine O, von Renteln D, et al. Efficacy of endoscopic closure of acute perforations of the gastrointestinal tract. Clin Gastroenterol Hepatol. 2012;10:603–8.
26. Nishiyama N, Mori H, Kobara H, et al. Efficacy and safety of over-the-scope clip: including complications after endoscopic submucosal dissection. World J Gastroenterol. 2013;19:2752–60.

27. Fujishiro M, Yahagi N, Kakushima N, et al. Endoscopic submucosal dissection of esophageal squamous cell neoplasms. Clin Gastroenterol Hepatol. 2006;4:688–94.

28. Ono S, Fujishiro M, Koike K. Endoscopic submucosal dissection for superficial esophageal neoplasms. World J Gastrointest Endosc. 2012;4:162–6.

29. Oyama T, Tomori A, Hotta K, et al. Endoscopic submucosal dissection of early esophageal cancer. Clin Gastroenterol Hepatol. 2005;3:S67–70.

30. Repici A, Hassan C, Carlino A, et al. Endoscopic submucosal dissection in patients with early esophageal squamous cell carcinoma: results from a prospective Western series. Gastrointest Endosc. 2010;71: 715–21.

31. Ishihara R, Iishi H, Uedo N, et al. Comparison of EMR and endoscopic submucosal dissection for en bloc resection of early esophageal cancers in Japan. Gastrointest Endosc. 2008;68:1066–72.

32. Yamashina T, Ishihara R, Uedo N, et al. Safety and curative ability of endoscopic submucosal dissection for superficial esophageal cancers at least 50 mm in diameter. Dig Endosc. 2012;24:220–5.

33. Sato H, Inoue H, Ikeda H, et al. Clinical experience of esophageal perforation occurring with endoscopic submucosal dissection. Dis Esophagus. 2013;27: 617–22.

34. Hirasawa K, Kokawa A, Oka H, et al. Superficial adenocarcinoma of the esophagogastric junction: long-term results of endoscopic submucosal dissection. Gastrointest Endosc. 2010;72:960–6.

35. Kakushima N, Fujishiro M. Endoscopic submucosal dissection for gastrointestinal neoplasms. World J Gastroenterol. 2008;14:2962–7.

36. Yoshinaga S, Gotoda T, Kusano C, et al. Clinical impact of endoscopic submucosal dissection for superficial adenocarcinoma located at the esophagogastric junction. Gastrointest Endosc. 2008;67: 202–9.

37. von Renteln D, Vassiliou MC, Rothstein RI. Randomized controlled trial comparing endoscopic clips and over-the-scope clips for closure of natural orifice transluminal endoscopic surgery gastrotomies. Endoscopy. 2009;41:1056–61.

38. Voermans RP, van Berge Henegouwen MI, Bemelman WA, et al. Novel over-the-scope-clip system for gastrotomy closure in natural orifice transluminal endoscopic surgery (NOTES): an ex vivo comparison study. Endoscopy. 2009;41:1052–5.

39. Matthes K, Jung Y, Kato M, et al. Efficacy of full-thickness GI perforation closure with a novel over-the-scope clip application device: an animal study. Gastrointest Endosc. 2011;74:1369–75.

40. Zhang XL, Qu JH, Sun G, et al. Feasibility study of secure closure of gastric fundus perforation using over-the-scope clips in a dog model. J Gastroenterol Hepatol. 2012;27:1200–4.

41. Rajan E, Gostout CJ, Aimore Bonin E, et al. Endoscopic full-thickness biopsy of the gastric wall with defect closure by using an endoscopic suturing device: survival porcine study. Gastrointest Endosc. 2012;76:1014–9.

42. Park PO, Bergstrom M, Rothstein R, et al. Endoscopic sutured closure of a gastric natural orifice transluminal endoscopic surgery access gastrotomy compared with open surgical closure in a porcine model. A randomized, multicenter controlled trial. Endoscopy. 2010;42:311–7.

43. Dray X, Krishnamurty DM, Donatelli G, et al. Gastric wall healing after NOTES procedures: closure with endoscopic clips provides superior histological outcome compared with threaded tags closure. Gastrointest Endosc. 2010;72:343–50.

44. Sumiyama K, Gostout CJ, Rajan E, et al. Endoscopic full-thickness closure of large gastric perforations by use of tissue anchors. Gastrointest Endosc. 2007;65: 134–9.

45. Magno P, Giday SA, Dray X, et al. A new stapler-based full-thickness transgastric access closure: results from an animal pilot trial. Endoscopy. 2007;39:876–80.

46. Meireles OR, Kantsevoy SV, Assumpcao LR, et al. Reliable gastric closure after natural orifice transluminal endoscopic surgery (NOTES) using a novel automated flexible stapling device. Surg Endosc. 2008;22:1609–13.

47. Ersoy OF, Ozkan N, Celik A, et al. Effect of cyanoacrylate on closure of gastric perforation: a comparative study in a rat model. Minim Invasive Ther Allied Technol. 2009;18:225–31.

48. Cios TJ, Reavis KM, Renton DR, et al. Gastrotomy closure using bioabsorbable plugs in a canine model. Surg Endosc. 2008;22:961–6.

49. Hashiba K, Carvalho AM, Diniz Jr G, et al. Experimental endoscopic repair of gastric perforations with an omental patch and clips. Gastrointest Endosc. 2001;54:500–4.

50. Dray X, Giday SA, Buscaglia JM, et al. Omentoplasty for gastrotomy closure after natural orifice transluminal endoscopic surgery procedures (with video). Gastrointest Endosc. 2009;70:131–40.

51. Toyokawa T, Inaba T, Omote S, et al. Risk factors for perforation and delayed bleeding associated with endoscopic submucosal dissection for early gastric neoplasms: analysis of 1123 lesions. J Gastroenterol Hepatol. 2012;27:907–12.

52. Ohta T, Ishihara R, Uedo N, et al. Factors predicting perforation during endoscopic submucosal dissection for gastric cancer. Gastrointest Endosc. 2012;75: 1159–65.

53. Kim M, Jeon SW, Cho KB, et al. Predictive risk factors of perforation in gastric endoscopic submucosal dissection for early gastric cancer: a large, multicenter study. Surg Endosc. 2013;27:1372–8.

54. Watari J, Tomita T, Toyoshima F, et al. Clinical outcomes and risk factors for perforation in gastric endoscopic submucosal dissection: a prospective pilot study. World J Gastrointest Endosc. 2013;5:281–7.

55. Yoo JH, Shin SJ, Lee KM, et al. Risk factors for perforations associated with endoscopic submucosal dissection in gastric lesions: emphasis on perforation type. Surg Endosc. 2012;26:2456–64.

56. Li L, Wang F, Wu B, et al. Endoscopic submucosal dissection of gastric fundus subepithelial tumors originating from the muscularis propria. Exp Ther Med. 2013;6:391–5.

57. Minami S, Gotoda T, Ono H, et al. Complete endoscopic closure of gastric perforation induced by endoscopic resection of early gastric cancer using endoclips can prevent surgery (with video). Gastrointest Endosc. 2006;63:596–601.

58. Matsumoto S, Miyatani H, Yoshida Y. Endoscopic submucosal dissection for duodenal tumors: a single-center experience. Endoscopy. 2013;45:136–7.

59. Honda T, Yamamoto H, Osawa H, et al. Endoscopic submucosal dissection for superficial duodenal neoplasms. Dig Endosc. 2009;21:270–4.

60. Min YW, Min BH, Kim ER, et al. Efficacy and safety of endoscopic treatment for nonampullary sporadic duodenal adenomas. Dig Dis Sci. 2013;58:2926–32.

61. Hotagai K, Oono Y, Fu KI, et al. Unexpected endoscopic full-thickness resection of a duodenal neuroendocrine tumor. World J Gastroenterol. 2013;19:4267–70.

62. Matsumoto S, Miyatani H, Yoshida Y, et al. Duodenal carcinoid tumors: 5 cases treated by endoscopic submucosal dissection. Gastrointest Endosc. 2011;74:1152–6.

63. Kim GH, Kim JI, Jeon SW, et al. Endoscopic resection for duodenal carcinoid tumors: a multicenter, retrospective study. J Gastroenterol Hepatol. 2014;29:318–24.

64. Raju GS, Pham B, Xiao SY, et al. A pilot study of endoscopic closure of colonic perforations with endoclips in a swine model. Gastrointest Endosc. 2005;62:791–5.

65. Raju GS, Ahmed I, Brining D, et al. Endoluminal closure of large perforations of colon with clips in a porcine model (with video). Gastrointest Endosc. 2006;64:640–6.

66. Raju GS, Ahmed I, Shibukawa G, et al. Endoluminal clip closure of a circular full-thickness colon resection in a porcine model (with videos). Gastrointest Endosc. 2007;65:503–9.

67. Raju GS, Ahmed I, Xiao SY, et al. Controlled trial of immediate endoluminal closure of colon perforations in a porcine model by use of a novel clip device (with videos). Gastrointest Endosc. 2006;64:989–97.

68. Raju GS, Shibukawa G, Ahmed I, et al. Endoluminal suturing may overcome the limitations of clip closure of a gaping wide colon perforation (with videos). Gastrointest Endosc. 2007;65:906–11.

69. Raju GS, Malhotra A, Ahmed I. Colonoscopic full-thickness resection of the colon in a porcine model as a prelude to endoscopic surgery of difficult colon polyps: a novel technique (with videos). Gastrointest Endosc. 2009;70:159–65.

70. Schurr MO, Hartmann C, Ho CN, et al. An over-the-scope clip (OTSC) system for closure of iatrogenic colon perforations: results of an experimental survival study in pigs. Endoscopy. 2008;40:584–8.

71. von Renteln D, Schmidt A, Vassiliou MC, et al. Endoscopic closure of large colonic perforations using an over-the-scope clip: a randomized controlled porcine study. Endoscopy. 2009;41:481–6.

72. Voermans RP, Vergouwe F, Breedveld P, et al. Comparison of endoscopic closure modalities for standardized colonic perforations in a porcine colon model. Endoscopy. 2011;43:217–22.

73. Pham BV, Raju GS, Ahmed I, et al. Immediate endoscopic closure of colon perforation by using a prototype endoscopic suturing device: feasibility and outcome in a porcine model (with video). Gastrointest Endosc. 2006;64:113–9.

74. Liu K, Yu H, Zhang M, et al. Sutureless primary repair of colonic perforation with a degradable stent in a porcine model of fecal peritonitis. Int J Colorectal Dis. 2012;27:1607–17.

75. Nocca D, Aggarwal R, Deneve E, et al. Use of collagen wrap from bovine origin for the management of colic perforation. Preliminary study in a pig model. J Laparoendosc Adv Surg Tech A. 2009;19:79–83.

76. Yoshikane H, Hidano H, Sakakibara A, et al. Endoscopic repair by clipping of iatrogenic colonic perforation. Gastrointest Endosc. 1997;46:464–6.

77. Mana F, De Vogelaere K, Urban D. Iatrogenic perforation of the colon during diagnostic colonoscopy: endoscopic treatment with clips. Gastrointest Endosc. 2001;54:258–9.

78. Carvalho R, Areia M, Brito D, et al. Endoscopic mucosal resection of large colorectal polyps: prospective evaluation of recurrence and complications. Acta Gastroenterol Belg. 2013;76:225–30.

79. Masci E, Viale E, Notaristefano C, et al. Endoscopic mucosal resection in high- and low-volume centers: a prospective multicentric study. Surg Endosc. 2013;27:3799–805.

80. Kim ES, Cho KB, Park KS, et al. Factors predictive of perforation during endoscopic submucosal dissection for the treatment of colorectal tumors. Endoscopy. 2011;43:573–8.

81. Lee EJ, Lee JB, Choi YS, et al. Clinical risk factors for perforation during endoscopic submucosal dissection (ESD) for large-sized, nonpedunculated colorectal tumors. Surg Endosc. 2012;26:1587–94.

82. Coda S, Trentino P, Antonellis F, et al. A Western single-center experience with endoscopic submucosal dissection for early gastrointestinal cancers. Gastric Cancer. 2010;13:258–63.

83. Yoon JY, Kim JH, Lee JY, et al. Clinical outcomes for patients with perforations during endoscopic

submucosal dissection of laterally spreading tumors of the colorectum. Surg Endosc. 2013;27:487–93.

84. Ohata K, Nonaka K, Minato Y, et al. Endoscopic submucosal dissection for large colorectal tumor in a Japanese General Hospital. J Oncol. 2013;2013:218670.

85. Thorlacius H, Uedo N, Toth E. Implementation of endoscopic submucosal dissection for early colorectal neoplasms in Sweden. Gastroenterol Res Pract. 2013; 2013:758202.

86. Maeda Y, Hirasawa D, Fujita N, et al. A pilot study to assess mediastinal emphysema after esophageal endoscopic submucosal dissection with carbon dioxide insufflation. Endoscopy. 2012;44:565–71.

87. Cho SB, Lee WS, Joo YE, et al. Therapeutic options for iatrogenic colon perforation: feasibility of endoscopic clip closure and predictors of the need for early surgery. Surg Endosc. 2012;26:473–9.

88. Kim JS, Kim BW, Kim JI, et al. Endoscopic clip closure versus surgery for the treatment of iatrogenic colon perforations developed during diagnostic colonoscopy: a review of 115,285 patients. Surg Endosc. 2013;27:501–4.

Identification, Treatment, and Prevention of Complications: Perforation in the Upper Gastrointestinal Tract

Shigetaka Yoshinaga, Satoru Nonaka, and Ichiro Oda

Introduction

Endoscopic resection (ER) has been accepted as a minimally invasive method for local resection of superficial gastrointestinal tumors that have a negligible risk of lymph node metastasis [1–3]. Methods of ER vary from polypectomy and endoscopic mucosal resection (EMR) to endoscopic submucosal dissection (ESD). EMR procedures include inject and cut, strip biopsy, EMR with a cap-fitted endoscope, endoscopic aspiration mucosectomy and EMR with a ligating device. ESD is a relatively new endoscopic resection method that facilitates en bloc resection. The appropriate endoscopic resection technique should be safe, effective, and suitable to a variety of clinical situations. ER is associated with various complications, such as bleeding and perforation. In this chapter, ER-related perforation is described, with a focus on the prevention, identification, and treatment of perforation, separately in the esophagus, the stomach, and the duodenum.

Esophagus

Incidence

The reported rates of perforation induced by EMR and ESD in the esophagus are 0–2.5 and 0–10 %, respectively [4–14]. Though ESD generally has a higher incidence of perforation than EMR, some groups have reported no significant difference in the incidence of complications between EMR and ESD [7, 12]. Delayed perforation is extremely rare and almost all perforations occur during the procedure.

Prevention

In order to prevent perforation, it is important not to expose and injure the muscularis propria. For this reason, during EMR, sufficient submucosal injection should be performed to confirm a submucosal expansion before resection. In order to prevent muscle injury during ESD, excess pressure onto mucosa with the knife should be avoided during mucosal incision. During dissection of the submucosal fibers, one should recognize the muscularis propria and move the knife in a motion parallel to this layer. If bleeding occurs, it should be addressed as soon as possible; otherwise, it may be difficult to recognize blood vessels and the muscularis propria. Occasionally, it can be difficult to dissect submucosal fibers under direct visualization. In such cases, "countertraction" should be employed [15].

S. Yoshinaga, M.D., Ph.D. (✉) • S. Nonaka, M.D.
I. Oda, M.D.
Endoscopy Division, National Cancer Center Hospital,
5-1-1 Tsukiji, Chuo-ku, Tokyo 104-0045, Japan
e-mail: shiyoshi@ncc.go.jp

N. Fukami (ed.), *Endoscopic Submucosal Dissection: Principles and Practice*,
DOI 10.1007/978-1-4939-2041-9_18, © Springer Science+Business Media New York 2015

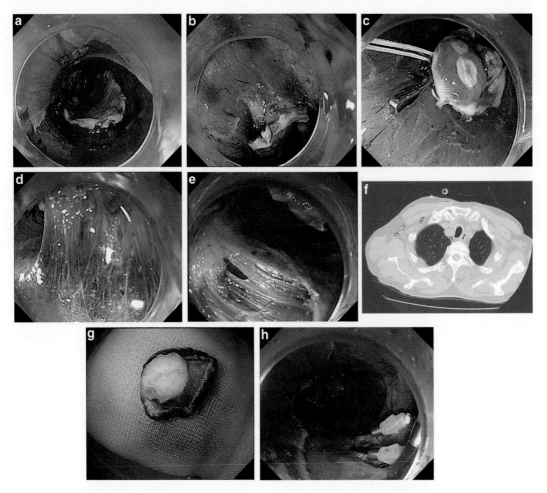

Fig. 17.1 (**a**) Before changing position. (**b**) After changing position. (**c**) Clipwith-line attached on the underside of the specimen. (**d**) After "Clip-with-line method". (**e**) Perforation occurrence during esophageal ESD. (**f**) CT showed mediastinal and subcutaneous emphysema. (**g**) "Target sign" of the resected specimen of esophageal EMR. (**h**) Perforation closed successfully using endoclips (same case as Fig. 17.1e)

There are two ways to use countertraction. One method is to change the patient's position in order to use gravity to provide countertraction. After changing position, gravity can pull down the target mucosa to reveal the submucosal fibers more directly (Fig. 17.1a, b). The other is the "clip-with-line" method. A clip attached to a line can be applied to the edge of the lesion to help provide traction during dissection (Fig. 17.1c, d). In addition, to minimize mediastinal emphysema and mediastinitis in case perforation occurs, use of carbon dioxide insufflation is recommended throughout the procedure, rather than air [16, 17].

Closure of the entire mucosal defect is not usually necessary, as delayed perforation is extremely rare. Additionally, prophylactic coagulation of visible vessels in the resection area after esophageal ESD is not usually necessary. Delayed bleeding is relatively rare in the esophagus and excess coagulation may instead cause undue delayed perforation.

Identification

During or after ER, the muscularis propria layer can be recognized as fibers that run transversely underneath the submucosal layer. This is likely because the esophagus does not have a serosa. Therefore, when a defect of such fibers is seen, a perforation must have occurred (Fig. 17.1e). Subsequently, subcutaneous emphysema can be recognized as "snow-ball crepitation" on the neck and/or chest if a substantial amount of air has escaped. Chest computed tomography (CT) or radiograph may show mediastinal or subcutaneous emphysema, with CT having a higher sensitivity of detection (Fig. 17.1f) [16, 18]. Even if the muscularis propria is not exposed, mediastinal emphysema can occur more than 50 % of the time due to air insufflation [18]. In EMR cases, a "target sign" on the resected specimens, indicating resection of the muscularis propria, may suggest a perforation (Fig. 17.1g) [19]. Though delayed perforation is rare, it can be a life-threatening event. Therefore, it is essential to appropriately suspect, identify and treat as soon as possible. Generally, patients are kept fasting for a few days after ESD. During this period, delayed perforation should be suspected if fever or chest pain occurs.

Treatment

Shimizu et al. reported 3 cases of successful closure of esophageal perforations after EMR with endoclips [5]. Perforations during esophageal ESD have also been managed by closure with endoscopic clips and conservative medical treatment [7]. However, this clipping method itself can injure the muscle and actually make the perforation larger. In such cases, the entire mucosal defect should be closed. Esophageal perforation may lead to life-threatening conditions such as severe mediastinal emphysema or mediastinitis.

When perforation does occur, the defect should be closed with endoclips (Fig. 17.1h). However, if the application of clips hinders the continuation of ER, such as would be the case in ESD, the resection should be continued. Once sufficient space has been created around the perforation, the clip(s) can be applied to the defect and submucosal dissection can then be continued. In some cases, ESD can be converted to EMR in order to complete the procedure. After the procedure, the patient should be kept fasting with antibiotics administered intravenously for several days.

In cases of delayed perforation, mediastinal emphysema and mediastinitis can occur. It is still a controversial issue that surgical interventions are needed immediately. If conservative treatments are not effective, surgical interventions should be considered.

Stomach

Incidence

The rates of perforation during gastric EMR and ESD have been reported as 0.5–5.3 and 1.2–9.6 %, respectively [20–32]. The risk factors for perforation during gastric ESD are the following: lesions in the upper third of the stomach, larger lesions, and lesions with ulceration [25, 31, 32]. Delayed perforation after gastric ESD has been reported to occur in approximately 0.5 % [33].

Prevention

Preventions of perforation in gastric ESD are similar to the previously mentioned methods for esophageal ESD. If the lesion is located on the greater curvature of the gastric body, identification of the muscularis propria may be difficult due to frequent bleeding (Fig. 17.2a); thus, adequate hemostasis is essential in order to avoid perforation. If there is severe fibrosis beneath the lesion, dissection of submucosal fibers can be difficult, and occasionally, injury of the muscularis propria can occur. In the setting of severe fibrosis, the endoscopist should imagine the curve of the proper muscle layer and dissect little-by-little, using the knife in a very careful manner (Fig. 17.2b). The "clip-with-line" countertraction method is also useful in assisting dissection in these cases (Fig. 17.2c–e). However, one should dissect carefully, because the curve of the muscle layer may change due to excess tension on the clip.

Closure of the entire mucosal defect is not always necessary, as delayed perforation is a rare event.

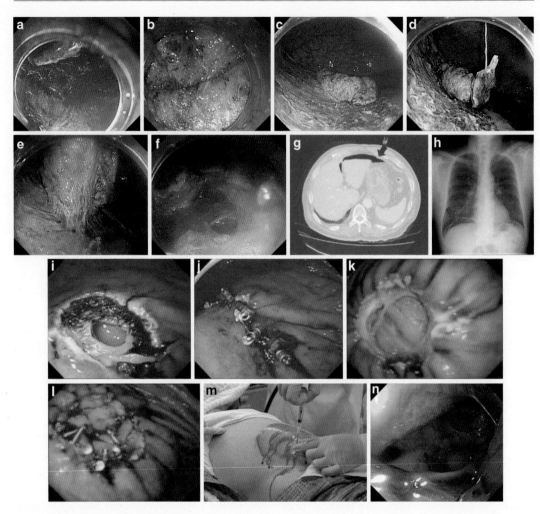

Fig. 17.2 (**a**) Blood made confirmation of the submucosal layer difficult. (**b**) The imaginary curve of the proper muscle layer with severe fibrosis (*red dotted line*). (**c**) Before "Clip-with-line method". (**d**) Clip-with-line attached on the underside of the specimen. (**e**) After "Clip-with-line method". (**f**) Perforation occurrence during gastric ESD. (**g**) CT shows "free air" in abdominal cavity (*arrow*). (**h**) Abdominal radiography shows "free air" under diaphragm (*arrow*). (**i**) Perforation occurrence after gastric EMR. (**j**) Perforation closed successfully with "single-closure method". (**k**) Perforation occurrence after gastric EMR. (**l**) Perforation closed successfully with "omental-patch method". (**m**) Paracentesis for aspiration of intraabdominal air. (**n**) A large delayed perforation (defect of the entire resected area)

Identification

During or after ER, the muscularis propria can be recognized as fibers that run transversely or longitudinally underneath the submucosal layer. The stomach has a thicker muscularis propria, especially in the antrum. The stomach also has serosa; therefore, even if the muscularis propria is injured, perforation does not always occur (Fig. 17.2f). However, if both the muscularis propria and the serosa are injured, this likely leads to pan-peritonitis. Abdominal CT and abdominal/chest radiography may reveal "free air," confirming leakage of air into the abdominal cavity (Fig. 17.2g, h).

Though delayed perforation is relatively rare, it may require surgical intervention. Therefore, it should be recognized as soon as possible. Generally, patients are kept fasting for a few days after ESD. During this period, delayed perforation should be suspected if the patient is suffering from fever or abdominal pain. Abdominal CT and abdominal/chest radiography are also useful in confirming perforation by free air and/or contrast leak.

Treatment

Closure of perforation using endoscopic clips after snare excision of a gastric leiomyoma was first reported by Binmoeller et al. in 1993 [34]. In 2006, closure with endoscopic clips for EMR/ESD-related gastric perforation was reported to be effective in a large series of consecutive cases [22]. Two methods of endoscopic closure using endoclips have been reported, including the "single-closure method" and the "omental-patch method" [22]. The single-closure method is performed to treat small defects and starts from the edge of the perforation rather than the center (Fig. 17.2i, j). The omental-patch method is performed on relatively larger defects by suctioning either the greater omentum or the lesser omentum into the stomach lumen and then clipping the omentum as a patch to the edges of the perforation (Fig. 17.2k, l). However, if the clips make the continuation of ER difficult (such as in ESD), and the patient's condition is stable, the procedure should be continued before clips are applied. The clips can then be placed once sufficient dissection has been performed. In some cases, ESD should be converted to EMR in order to complete the procedure. If there is leakage of a large amount of air, the increase in intraabdominal pressure can result in potentially fatal hypotension—so called "abdominal compartment syndrome or tension pneumoperitoneum." In such cases, the pressure of the intraabdominal cavity must be reduced immediately. This can be achieved by performing paracentesis to aspirate intraabdominal air. After testing for pneumoperitoneum with a 23-G needle attached to a syringe filled with water, decompression of the pneumoperitoneum must be performed with a 14- or 16-G puncture needle with side slits (Fig. 17.2m). Then, the patient is kept fasting and an antibiotic is administered intravenously for a few days. If the patient suffers from fever over 38 °C or chest pain, an endoscopic examination with CO_2 insufflation should be performed to evaluate that the defect still is closed or reopened.

When delayed perforation is diagnosed, panperitonitis must have occurred due to leakage of gastric acid, bile and pancreatic juices; therefore, surgical intervention may be necessary even if endoscopic closure has been performed successfully. In some cases, large delayed perforations occur, which may encompass the entire resected area (Fig. 17.2n). In such cases, surgical treatment is most definitely necessary.

Duodenum (Non-ampullary)

Incidence

There are few reports of ER in the duodenum. In these limited reports, the rates of perforation during EMR and ESD have been reported as 0–3.8 and 0–21.4 %, respectively [35–47]. The corresponding rates of delayed perforation have been reported as 0–3.8 and 0–20 %, respectively. Compared with the stomach and the esophagus, the incidences of immediate and delayed perforation seem to be relatively higher in the duodenum, particularly in ESD cases. The reasons may be that the duodenal wall is the thinnest among these three organs. Additionally, it is especially difficult to manipulate and stabilize the endoscope in the duodenum. Inoue et al. proposed that extensive piecemeal EMR for large lesions and the high concentration of digestive enzymes in the duodenal lumen are also reasons for the high incidence of delayed perforation [44]. In this study, all cases of delayed perforation were associated with lesions located distal to the major ampulla. The authors concluded that lesions treated with piecemeal EMR or ESD and located distal to the major ampulla are especially prone to delayed perforation.

Prevention

Though the methods of preventing perforation are the same in duodenal as in esophageal and gastric cases, as previously described, it is especially difficult to operate and stabilize the scope in the duodenum. Therefore, duodenal ESD should be performed with great care, and it may be necessary to terminate the procedure if significant difficulty is encountered.

Inoue et al. reported two cases of delayed perforation after prophylactic clipping [44]; therefore, there is no evidence that clipping decreases the incidence of delayed perforation. However, in our opinion, in order to prevent delayed perforation, closure of the mucosal defect by prophylactic clipping should always be performed if possible. Recently, Mori et al. reported two cases of complete closure of post-ESD duodenal ulcer using an over-the-scope-clip (OTSC) [48]. This technique may be effective for prevention of delayed perforation.

Identification

The very thin muscularis propria in the duodenum can be recognized as fibers that run transversely underneath the submucosal layer. If a defect of these layers is noticed, perforation must be considered. Because the duodenum is a retroperitoneal organ, a delayed perforation located on the posterior wall will not present with pneumoperitoneum. Patients may present with fever, but, unlike gastric perforation, symptoms of retroperitoneal perforation are generally mild [44]. Therefore, delayed perforation should be suspected and abdominal CT performed for confirmation even if patients' symptoms are mild.

Treatment

If duodenal perforation occurs, endoscopic closure should be performed, similar to cases of esophageal and gastric perforation, if the patient's condition is stable. Kaneko et al. reported two cases of successful closure of duodenal perforations after EMR for duodenal carcinoid tumors with endoclips [49]. However, endoscopic clipping of duodenal perforation is difficult because the lumen is narrow and tortuous [47]. Failure to close the perforation endoscopically may lead to severe complications due to leakage of bile and pancreatic juice. In such cases, surgical treatment would likely be necessary.

In cases of delayed perforation, the defect should be closed if possible; however, it may

result in a formation of retroperitoneal abscess [44]. This is difficult to manage conservatively and an invasive surgical intervention may be necessary due to anatomical proximity to the pancreas. Therefore, retroperitoneal perforation should be addressed as early as possible.

References

1. Rembacken BJ, Gotoda T, Fujii T, et al. Endoscopic mucosal resection. Endoscopy. 2001;33:709–18.
2. Soetikno R, Gotoda T, Nakanishi Y, et al. Endoscopic mucosal resection. Gastrointest Endosc. 2003;57:567–79.
3. Soetikno R, Kaltenbach T, Yeh R, et al. Endoscopic mucosal resection for early cancers of the upper gastrointestinal tract. J Clin Oncol. 2005;23:4490–8.
4. Inoue H, Tani M, Nagai K, et al. Treatment of esophageal and gastric tumors. Endoscopy. 1999;31:47–55.
5. Shimizu Y, Kato M, Yamamoto J, et al. Endoscopic clip application for closure of esophageal perforations caused by EMR. Gastrointest Endosc. 2004;60:636–9.
6. Tomizawa Y, Iyer PG, Wong Kee Song LM, et al. Safety of endoscopic mucosal resection for Barrett's esophagus. Am J Gastroenterol. 2013;108(9):1440–7.
7. Takahashi H, Arimura Y, Masao H, et al. Endoscopic submucosal dissection is superior to conventional endoscopic resection as a curative treatment for early squamous cell carcinoma of the esophagus. Gastrointest Endosc. 2010;72:255–64.
8. Ono S, Fujishiro M, Niimi K, et al. Long-term outcomes of endoscopic submucosal dissection for superficial esophageal squamous cell neoplasms. Gastrointest Endosc. 2009;70:860–6.
9. Oyama T, Tomori A, Hotta K, et al. Endoscopic submucosal dissection of early esophageal cancer. Clin Gastroenterol Hepatol. 2005;3:S67–70.
10. Hirasawa K, Kokawa A, Oka H, et al. Superficial adenocarcinoma of the esophagogastric junction: long-term results of endoscopic submucosal dissection. Gastrointest Endosc. 2010;72:960–6.
11. Ishii N, Horiki N, Itoh T, et al. Endoscopic submucosal dissection with a combination of small-caliber-tip transparent hood and flex knife is a safe and effective treatment for superficial esophageal neoplasias. Surg Endosc. 2010;24:335–42.
12. Ishihara R, Iishi H, Uedo N, et al. Comparison of EMR and endoscopic submucosal dissection for en bloc resection of early esophageal cancers in Japan. Gastrointest Endosc. 2008;68:1066–72.
13. Repici A, Hassan C, Carlino A, et al. Endoscopic submucosal dissection in patients with early esophageal squamous cell carcinoma: results from a prospective Western series. Gastrointest Endosc. 2010;71:715–21.
14. Isomoto H, Yamaguchi N, Minami H, et al. Management of complications associated with endo-

scopic submucosal dissection/ endoscopic mucosal resection for esophageal cancer. Dig Endosc. 2013;25 Suppl 1:29–38.

15. Oyama T. Counter traction makes endoscopic submucosal dissection easier. Clin Endosc. 2012;45:375–8.

16. Maeda Y, Hirasawa D, Fujita N, et al. A pilot study to assess mediastinal emphysema after endoscopic submucosal dissection with carbon dioxide insufflation. Endoscopy. 2012;44:565–71.

17. Nonaka S, Saito Y, Takisawa H, et al. Safety of carbon dioxide insufflation for upper gastrointestinal tract endoscopic treatment of patients under deep sedation. Surg Endosc. 2010;24:1638–45.

18. Tamiya Y, Nakahara K, Kominato K, et al. Pneumomediastinum is a frequent but minor complication during esophageal endoscopic submucosal dissection. Endoscopy. 2010;42:8–14.

19. Swan MP, Bourke MJ, Moss A, et al. The target sign: an endoscopic marker for the resection of the muscularis propria and potential perforation during colonic endoscopic mucosal resection. Gastrointest Endosc. 2011;73:79–85.

20. Oka S, Tanaka S, Kaneko I, et al. Advantage of endoscopic submucosal dissection compared with EMR for early gastric cancer. Gastrointest Endosc. 2006;64:877–83.

21. Oda I, Saito D, Tada M, et al. A multicenter retrospective study of endoscopic resection for early gastric cancer. Gastric Cancer. 2006;9:262–70.

22. Minami S, Gotoda T, Ono H, et al. Complete endoscopic closure of gastric perforation induced by endoscopic resection of early gastric cancer using endoclips can prevent surgery. Gastrointest Endosc. 2006;63:596–601.

23. Hoteya S, Iizuka T, Kikuchi D, et al. Benefits of endoscopic submucosal dissection according to size and location of gastric neoplasm, compared with conventional mucosal resection. J Gastroenterol Hepatol. 2009;24:1102–6.

24. Ahn JY, Jung HY, Choi KD, et al. Endoscopic and oncologic outcomes after endoscopic resection for early gastric cancer: 1370 cases of absolute and extended indications. Gastrointest Endosc. 2011;74:485–93.

25. Oda I, Gotoda T, Hamanaka H, et al. Endoscopic submucosal dissection for early gastric cancer: technical feasibility, operation time and complications from a large consecutive series. Dig Endosc. 2005;17: 54–8.

26. Jung HY, Choi KD, Song HJ, et al. Risk management in endoscopic submucosal dissection using needle knife in Korea. Dig Endosc. 2007;19 Suppl 1:S5–8.

27. Ono H, Hasuike N, Inui T, et al. Usefulness of a novel electrosurgical knife, the insulation-tipped diathermic knife-2, for endoscopic submucosal dissection of early gastric cancer. Gastric Cancer. 2008;11:47–52.

28. Chung IK, Lee JH, Lee SH, et al. Therapeutic outcomes in 1000 cases of endoscopic submucosal dissection for early gastric neoplasms: Korean ESD Study Group multicenter study. Gastrointest Endosc. 2009;69:1228–35.

29. Mannen K, Tsunada S, Hara M, et al. Risk factors for complications of endoscopic submucosal dissection in gastric tumors: analysis of 478 lesions. J Gastroenterol. 2010;45:30–6.

30. Akasaka T, Nishida T, Tsutsui S, et al. Short-term outcomes of endoscopic submucosal dissection (ESD) for early gastric neoplasm: multicenter survey by osaka university ESD study group. Dig Endosc. 2011;23:73–7.

31. Ohta T, Ishihara R, Uedo N, et al. Factors predicting perforation during endoscopic submucosal dissection for gastric cancer. Gastrointest Endosc. 2012;75:1159–65.

32. Yoo JH, Shin SJ, Lee KM, et al. Risk factors for perforations associated with endoscopic submucosal dissection in gastric lesions: emphasis on perforation type. Surg Endosc. 2012;26:2456–64.

33. Hanaoka N, Uedo N, Ishihara R, et al. Clinical features and outcomes of delayed perforation after endoscopic submucosal dissection for early gastric cancer. Endoscopy. 2010;42:1112–5.

34. Binmoellar KF, Grimm H, Soehendra N. Endoscopic closure of a perforation using metallic clips after snare excision of gastric leiomyoma. Gastrointest Endosc. 1993;39:172–4.

35. Ahmad NA, Kochman ML, Long WB, et al. Efficacy, safety, and clinical outcomes of endoscopic mucosal resection: a study of 101 cases. Gastrointest Endosc. 2002;55:390–6.

36. Oka S, Tanaka S, Nagata S, et al. Clinicopathologic features and endoscopic resection of early primary nonampullary duodenal carcinoma. J Clin Gastroenterol. 2003;37:381–6.

37. Lepilliez V, Chemaly M, Ponchon T, et al. Endoscopic resection of sporadic duodenal adenomas: an efficient technique with a substantial risk of delayed bleeding. Endoscopy. 2008;40:806–10.

38. Kedia P, Brensinger C, Ginsberg G. Endoscopic predictors of successful endoluminal eradication in sporadic duodenal adenomas and acute complications. Gastrointest Endosc. 2010;72:1297–301.

39. Abbass R, Rigaux J, Al-Kawas H. Nonampullary duodenal polyps: characteristics and endoscopic management. Gastrointest Endosc. 2010;71:754–9.

40. Sohn JW, Jeon SW, Cho CM, et al. Endoscopic resection of duodenal neoplasms: a single-center study. Surg Endosc. 2010;24:3195–200.

41. Fanning SB, Bourke MJ, Williams SJ, et al. Giant laterally spreading tumors of the duodenum: endoscopic resection outcomes, limitations, and caveats. Gastrointest Endosc. 2012;75:805–12.

42. Maruoka D, Arai M, Kishimoto T, et al. Clinical outcomes of endoscopic resection for nonampullary duodenal high-grade dysplasia and intramucosal carcinoma. Endoscopy. 2013;45:138–41.

43. Endo M, Abiko Y, Oana S, et al. Usefulness of endoscopic treatment for duodenal adenoma. Dig Endosc. 2010;22:360–5.

44. Inoue T, Uedo N, Yamashita T, et al. Delayed perforation: a hazardous complication of endoscopic resection for non-ampullary duodenal neoplasm. Dig Endosc. 2014;26(2):220–7.

45. Honda T, Yamamoto H, Osawa H, et al. Endoscopic submucosal dissection for superficial duodenal neoplasms. Dig Endosc. 2009;21:270–4.

46. Matsumoto S, Miyatani H, Yoshida Y. Endoscopic submucosal dissection for duodenal tumors: a single-center experience. Endoscopy. 2013;45:136–7.

47. Jung JH, Choi KD, Ahn JY, et al. Endoscopic submucosal dissection for sessile, nonampullary duodenal adenomas. Endoscopy. 2013;45:133–5.

48. Mori H, Fujihara S, Kobara H, et al. Successful closing of duodenal ulcer after endoscopic submucosal dissection with over-the-scope clip to prevent delayed perforation. Digest Endosc. 2013;25:459–61.

49. Kaneko T, Akamatsu T, Shimodaira K, et al. Nonsurgical treatment of duodenal perforation by endoscopic repair using a clipping device. Gastrointest Endosc. 1999;50:410–4.

Prevention, Identification, and Treatment of Perforation in the Lower Gastrointestinal Tract

19

Takashi Toyonaga

Introduction

The walls of the colon are susceptible to perforation due to their inherent thinness and natural curvature. Electric discharge for electrocautery on the musclaris propia is the main cause of perforation. The intestine's vulnerability to perforation is dependent on its nature—such as fibrosis of the target area or risk of bleeding—as well as its location and the presence of adhesions that cause difficulty in scope manipulation; this vulnerability can make endoscopic procedures increasingly challenging. Any amount of electric discharge, regardless of degree, could directly induce intraprocedural perforation and should be considered a risk. Technically, damage confined to the internal layer of the muscularis propria or that which does not extend beyond the subserosa is not considered a perforation; however, it should be noted that this holds sufficient potential to later develop into a delayed, postprocedural perforation.

Prevention

Even when meticulous care is taken, perforations can occur. Therefore, thorough and complete pre-procedural planning is critical to ESD. In cases where extra colonic fluid is present, delay of the procedure and additional colonic cleansing (i.e. PEG solution) should be considered. Direct administration of PEG under endoscopy may facilitate the completion of preparation for ESD.

Intraprocedural Perforation

Prevention of intraprocedural perforation hinges on the extent of care invested in maneuvering the scope and conducting all procedures under direct observation. Positively identifying which layer is to be dissected, and from what direction, is the most critical component for success [1]. During this process, it is imperative to prevent bleeding, as it obscures the submucosa and, hence, increases the difficulty of layer recognition. The vasculature of the gastrointestinal tract penetrates through the muscularis propria as branches, then horizontally within the mid-layer of the submucosa [2]. These transverse vessels and muscle fibers are the most important landmarks for dissection; dissection should be performed exactly between the two. First, the initial endoscopic incision should not extend beyond the level directly below the muscularis mucosae in order

T. Toyonaga, M.D. (✉)
Kobe University Hospital,
7-5-1 Kusunoki, Chuo, Kobe, Hyogo, Japan
e-mail: toyonaga@med.kobe-u.ac.jp

N. Fukami (ed.), *Endoscopic Submucosal Dissection: Principles and Practice*,
DOI 10.1007/978-1-4939-2041-9_19, © Springer Science+Business Media New York 2015

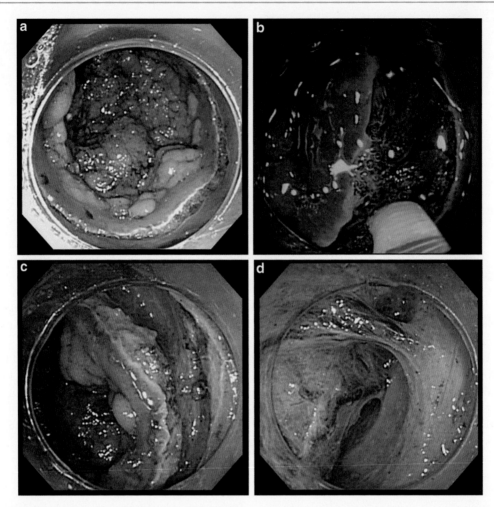

Fig. 19.1 Granular-type laterally spreading tumor in the rectum. (**a**) After incision of the mucosa. Bleeding from the incision was prevented by controlling the depth of the incision to directly below the muscularis mucosae. A number of transverse vessels are observed in the submucosa within the periphery of the incision. (**b**) Hemostatic processing of the vasculature. (**c**) The layers below the transverse vessels and above the muscularis were dissected, and a mucosal flap was formed. (**d**) Dissection was performed, leaving the perforating branches. In the absence of bleeding, the vessels and the muscle fibers are distinctly visible, and dissection can be performed safely

to prevent hemorrhaging at the mucosal incision. Second, one should induce the formation of a submucosal groove around the margins at the incision line by appropriately and timely coagulating the transverse vessels below the incision, then dissect below the transverse vessels and extend the mucosal flap to reach the appropriate depth for dissection. If bleeding has not occurred, a clear, semi-transparent submucosal layer should be recognizable. Finally, avoidance of cutting thick vessels and appropriate pre-cut coagulation of these vessels in the subsequent repetitive steps

should theoretically allow for completion of the procedure without any problematic hemorrhage (Fig. 19.1) [3].

Hemostasis should be achieved as soon as unforeseeable bleeding or oozing occurs [4]. Hemostasis should be attempted first using the knife with coagulation current [5]. If the bleeding does not stop after two or three attempts at coagulation by knife, hemostatic forceps should be used. Caution is required, as repeated coagulation poses the risk of perforation. Once hemostasis is achieved, dissection should be resumed.

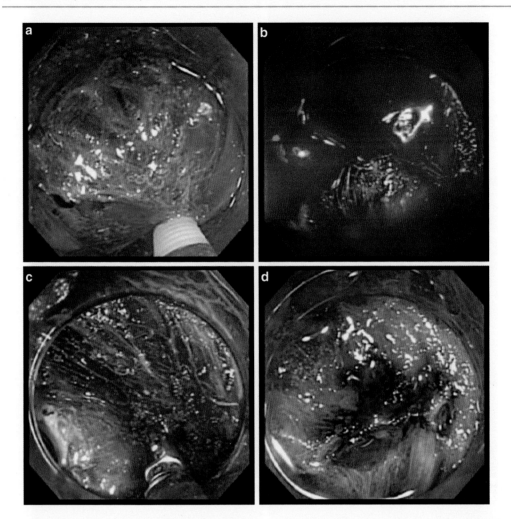

Fig. 19.2 Problems with and countermeasures against intraprocedural bleeding. (**a**, **b**) Bleeding immediately compromises visibility. (**c**) Perform hemostasis as quickly as possible. Delay in hemostasis leads to formation of hematoma in the submucosa, significantly impeding its visualization. (**d**) Hemostasis was successful, though discoloration of the blood into brown is impeding the identification of the layers. Resume dissection from areas where layers are clearly identifiable (*arrow*), not from areas with obscured visibility (*asterisk*)

However, dissection should never be performed forcefully when bleeding has obscured the tissue layers. Dissection should only be resumed at areas where the muscle layer and vascular plexus are distinctly identifiable, and the indistinct areas should be carefully dissected from both sides of the lesion, where the submucosal layer is clearly visible. At all times, prevent misidentification of layers and ensure dissection is performed at the level between the transverse vascular plexus and muscle fibers (Fig. 19.2). Oftentimes in the colon, especially in the lower rectum, a loose,

submucosa-like layer lies between the bundles of the muscle fibers. Mistakes can be avoided if the operator understands this and is aware of this similarity (Fig. 19.3).

Prevention of Postprocedural Perforation

In the colon, the risk of transmural coagulation necrosis and, hence, the risk of postprocedural perforation is set high when coagulation is per-

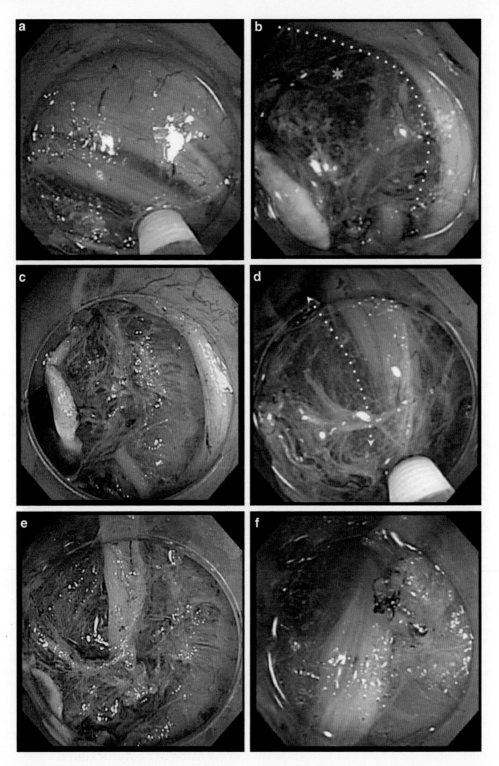

Fig. 19.3 Points of caution in the rectum. (**a**) There are loose layers of muscle in the rectum (especially in the lower rectum). (**b**, **c**) Perforating branches (*asterisk*) of the rectum are thick and often flow in bundles of 2–3. The sides of the vessels lack the muscularis in a wedge-shaped configuration. If only the muscularis and the loose, submucosa-like tissue are used as landmarks for dissection, there is a risk of losing visual identification of the vascu-latures as they tend to get lost in the vast network of muscle fibers. (**c**, **d**) Scan the surrounding area and maintain an appropriate dissection depth by noting the space already dissected, the area between the plexus of the transverse vessels and the muscularis. (**e**, **f**) Tissue was detached once the area surrounding the perforating branches (*asterisk*) was dissected in the correct layer. The dissection depth has returned to an appropriate level

formed adjacent to or on the thin muscle layers. This phenomenon is equivalent to that observed in perforation cases after the use of hot biopsy and those reported as postpolypectomy coagulation syndrome. It is necessary to avoid coagulation that has the potential to extend to the muscle layer when performing hemostasis, such as by forcefully gripping the point of hemorrhage. Postprocedural perforation has been experienced in a case where coagulation was performed adjacent to the muscle layer in an effort to prevent bleeding after resection (Fig. 19.4). Once we modified the method of preemptive coagulation at the completion of resection, limiting the application of coagulation current only to the transected vessel with pulsatile movement and only holding at the tip of vessel and coagulating while pulling off of the muscle layer, no further delayed perforation occurred. However, in some of those lesions with severe fibrosis due to past piecemeal resections or argon plasma coagulation therapy, we have experienced delayed perforation. Preemptive clip closure of post-ESD defect is recommended if there is any suspicion of injury to the muscularis propria, even without clear evidence of perforation [2]. Furthermore, we have experienced delayed perforation that was most likely caused by the increased intraluminal pressure due to air insufflation (Fig. 19.5). Currently, we use CO_2 gas for insufflation for all cases undergoing ESD procedure. This reduces the duration of dead space caused by perforation and accumulation of gas, and also reduces any symptoms associated with rapid resorption of gas (Fig. 19.6).

Identification of Deep Muscle Injury

Intraprocedural perforation is visually detectable as a tear in the muscle fibers, and is extremely important to treat as quickly as possible to ensure better patient outcome. However, adhesions of blood clots to the tear after repeated bleeding, or lesions in unavoidable blind locations may delay the detection of perforations. Post-ESD perforation is relatively easy to recognize, as patients present with abdominal pain, fever, and symptoms consistent with peritonitis. Upon confirmation of

pneumoperitoneum by either x-ray or computed tomography (CT), diagnosis is made. Under normal circumstances, endoscopy is not necessary to confirm a diagnosis of post-ESD perforation.

Treatment

Intraprocedural Perforation

Clip closure is an effective means of treating perforation. Time is of the essence, though, and it is imperative that the perforation be repaired as quickly as possible. Yet, repairs should be exercised with great caution and in a manner that will not interfere with subsequent resection procedures. First and foremost, the immediate periphery of the perforation should be opened with dissection of the submucosa in order to secure ample space. It is important to note that the prevention of any intestinal content leakage throughout this procedure is absolutely critical for clip closure. One clip is usually sufficient to close a pinhole-sized perforation (Fig. 19.7). Due to the lack of serosal membrane and the characteristic thinness of the tunica muscularis, the esophagus is exceptionally vulnerable to laceration upon direct grasping of the muscle layer with endoscopic clips. In contrast, the serosal membrane is present along the entire length of the colon (except in the rectum) and its muscularis is more durable than that of the esophagus, and, therefore, direct clamping of the muscle layer does not readily cause any separation of muscle. Nevertheless, the use of large clips and the grasping of the tissues at both ends of the perforation are recommended to avoid the aggregation of force in a concentrated area and to evenly disperse pressure around the perforation (Fig. 19.8). Clamping of the mucosa together with the deeper layers, as well as double-layered suturing [6] (Fig. 19.9), may be considered in patients presenting with a thinner muscularis or lesions involving the cecum in order to avoid having the clamping force concentrating within the muscularis propria. If the perforation is effectively repaired, conservative management is sought instead of surgery. The patient should be treated appropriately with NPO and bed rest, and

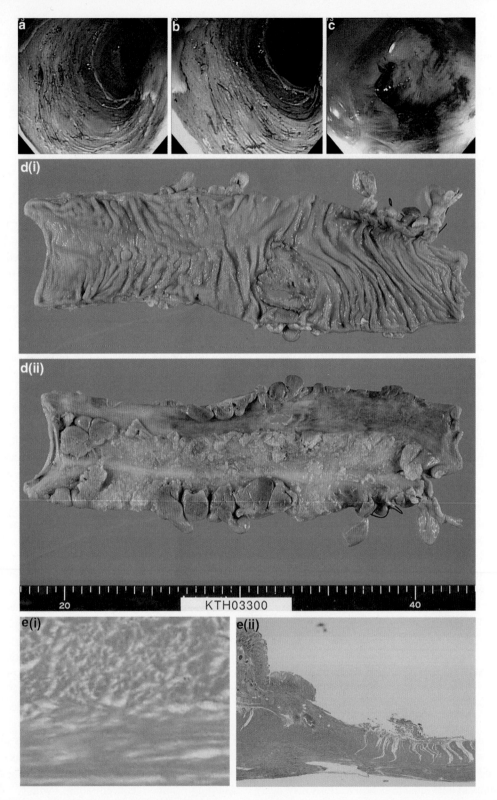

Fig. 19.4 A case of postprocedural perforation of the sigmoid colon. (**a**) Resection bed after an ESD procedure. (**b**) Contact coagulation was performed on exposed vessels using the soft coagulation mode on the hot biopsy forceps. (**c**) On the day following the ESD procedure, pneumoperitoneum was confirmed with a CT after a sudden onset of a abdominal pain. Endoscopy was performed in an attempt to reef the wound. Large, flap-shaped perforation and leakage of opaque intestinal fluid was confirmed. (**d**) Excised sample. Conservative treatment was deemed extremely risky and an emergency laparotomy was performed. (**e**) Histopathological image. Widespread coagulation necrosis has extended to the periphery of the dislodged muscularis

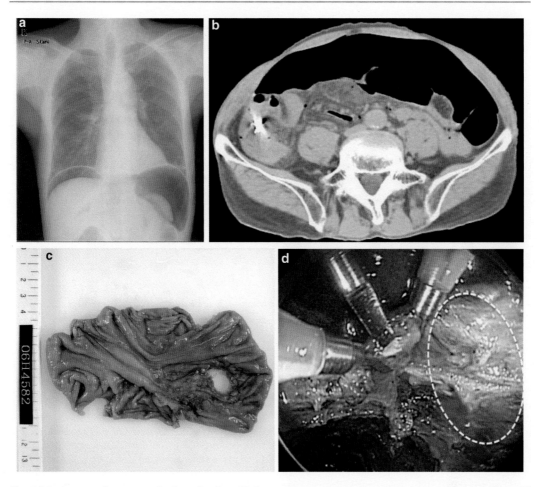

Fig. 19.5 A case of postprocedural perforation, likely caused by the air supply. (**a, b**) Chest XP and CT performed in the morning following an ESD procedure in the case shown in Fig. 19.7. Significant pneumoperitoneum and intestinal gas are visible. (**c**) No notable clinical symptoms other than abdominal distension. Abdominal pain increased in the evening, and signs of peritoneal irritation emerged. Sharp increase in WBC was noted and an emergency lapa-rotomy was performed. Excised sample from surgery; all three clips remained in place, but a widespread loss of the muscularis was noted in their immediate vicinity. (**d**) Endoscopic image at the end of ESD. The area within the *dotted line* is the estimated location of the perforation. Some damage to the muscularis is noted, but there was no obvious perforation. Air pressure was thought to have caused a rupture in this area

closely monitored for clinical symptoms including fever and abdominal pain. Antibiotics should be administered to prevent or treat peritonitis. If C-reactive protein (CRP) levels have leveled out and the clinical course is stable, the patient can finish a course of antibiotics and may even resume diet, while carefully monitoring progress. Usually, patients are monitored closely for 3 days before they reach this stage.

Postprocedural Perforation

Patients would require urgent care, and surgery must be performed as soon as possible. In delayed perforation, leakage of contaminated intestinal fluid into the peritoneal cavity may induce sepsis and endotoxic shock. The decision to perform surgery should be made promptly, as any delay in treatment can be fatal. Endoscopic treatment

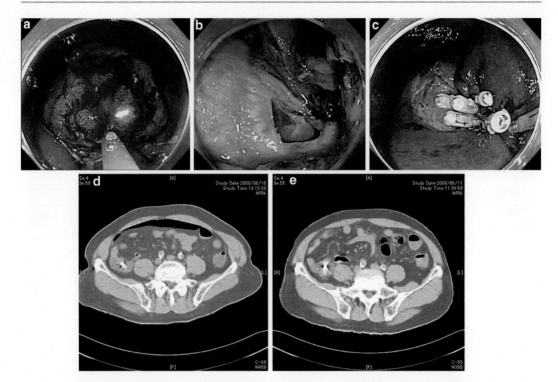

Fig. 19.6 A case of perforation during simplified ESD (CO_2 air supply) [7]. (**a**) Once the vascular plexus around the entire circumference of the incision was processed and a submucosal groove was formed, en bloc resection was performed with snare. (**b**) The lesion was resected en bloc, but resection caused a perforation. (**c**) Given that complete repair was possible via clipping, conservative treatment was elected. (**d**) CT taken immediately after ESD. Pneumoperitoneum is seen, though insignificant. Intestinal gas has disappeared almost entirely. (**e**) CT taken the day after ESD was performed. Pneumoperitoneum has already disappeared. Neither fever nor abdominal pain developed, and CRP decreased to 1.87 on day 3 postop, after peaking at 7.67 on day 2. Dietary restriction was lifted in the afternoon of day 3, and the patient continued to make an otherwise uncomplicated recovery. This is an exemplary case illustrating the utility of the CO_2 air supply

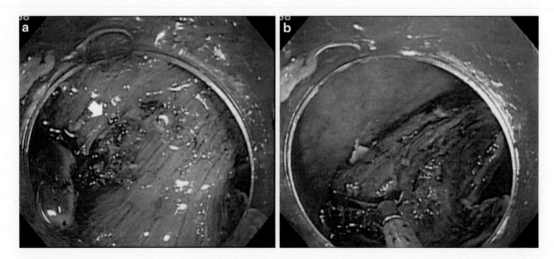

Fig. 19.7 Small perforation in colorectal ESD. (**a**) Pinhole perforation during dissection (*arrow*). (**b**) One clip was sufficient for repair

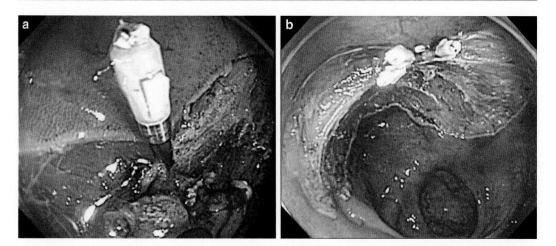

Fig. 19.8 Intraprocedural perforation in the ascending colon. (**a**) Upon detection of the perforation, clipping was performed after additional dissection was conducted in order to secure ample space. (**b**) Clips were added to the sides of the wound upon completion of dissection

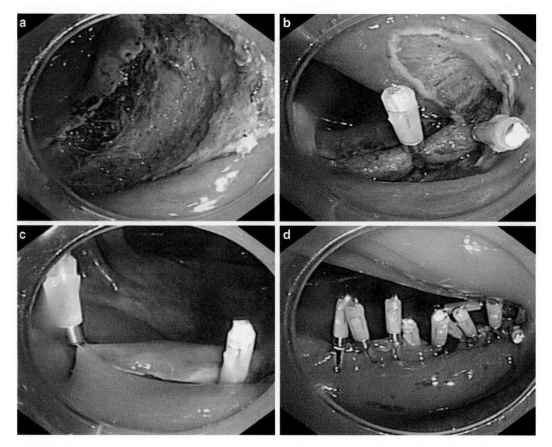

Fig. 19.9 One example of double-layered suturing. (**a**) Endoscopic image at the end of ESD. (**b**) First, clipping is performed in the muscularis. This results in a reduced width of the floor of the ulcer. (**c**) Mucosa is subsequently clipped, guarding against the muscularis clip from being buried. (**d**) After repair has been completed

should not be considered as this only results in a loss of time and, ultimately, a delay in definitive treatment (Fig. 19.4).

Conclusions

Perforation that occurs during colonic ESD can be conservatively treated once primary endoscopic closure with clips or suturing methods is completed. However, perforation in the colon may also result in bacteremia or endotoxic shock, which can be fatal when proper treatment is delayed. Decision-making regarding surgical therapy must be timely and without delay. Prevention is the best treatment for perforation, and it is of upmost importance to perform precise, step-by-step maneuvers under direct visualization with proper identification of submucosal vasculature and the muscle layer.

References

1. Toyonaga T, Nishino E, Man-i M, East JE, Azuma T. Principles of quality controlled endoscopic submucosal dissection with appropriate dissection level and high quality resected specimen. Clin Endosc. 2012;45:362–74.
2. Toyonaga T, Azuma T. How to prevent complications at ESD of colorectal lesions. Video J Encycl GI Endosc. 2013;1(2):365–6.
3. Toyonaga T, Man-i M, East JE, et al. 1,635 Endoscopic submucosal dissection cases in the esophagus, stomach and colorectum: complication rates and long-term outcomes. Surg Endosc. 2013;27(3):1000–8.
4. Toyonaga T, Man-i M, Fujita T, East JE, Nishino E, Ono W, Morita Y, Sanuki T, Yoshida M, Kutsumi H, Inokuchi H, Azuma T. Retrospective study for technical aspects and complications of endoscopic submucosal dissection for laterally spreading tumors of the colorectum. Endoscopy. 2010;42:714–22.
5. Toyonaga T, Man-i M, Fujita T, East JE, Coumaros D, Morita Y, Yoshida M, Hayakumo T, Inokuchi H, Azuma T. Endoscopic submucosal dissection using the Flush knife and the Flush knife BT. Tech Gastrointest Endosc. 2011;13:84–90.
6. Tanaka S, Toyonaga T, Obata D, Ishida T, Morita Y, Azuma T. Endoscopic double-layered suturing: a novel technique for closure of large mucosal defects after endoscopic mucosal resection (EMR) or endoscopic submucosal dissection (ESD). Endoscopy. 2012;44:E153–4.
7. Toyonaga T, Man-i M, Morita Y, Sanuki T, Yoshida M, Kutsumi H, Inokuchi H, Azuma T. The new resources of treatment for early stage colorectal tumors: EMR with small incision and simplified endoscopic submucosal dissection. Dig Endosc. 2009;21:S31–7.

Jun-Hyung Cho, Bong Min Ko, and Joo Young Cho

Esophagus

Esophageal squamous cell carcinoma invading the muscularis mucosae or deeper is associated with increased risk of lymph node and distant metastasis [1, 2]. Metastatic lesions are usually detected within 2 years after endoscopic resection. Usually, computed tomography (CT) examinations of the neck, chest, and abdomen are performed at 6- to 12-month intervals. Also, the Japan Esophageal Society (JES) recommends that ultrasonography of the neck, as well as endoscopic ultrasonography (EUS), are carried out during endoscopic follow up after ESD [3].

Incidence rates of metachronous esophageal squamous cell carcinoma range from 7.8 to 20 % [4]. During surveillance endoscopy, Lugol's iodine chromoendoscopy is useful for detection of metachronous esophageal lesions. Several studies have reported that a higher risk of metachronous esophageal carcinoma is associated with multiple Lugol-voiding lesions, and that such lesions require more meticulous follow-up examination [5, 6]. A multicenter cohort study by the JES is currently ongoing to investigate the risk of metachronous cancers and to assess surveillance interval time after endoscopic resec-

tion. To date, endoscopic examinations can be scheduled at 3-month intervals for 6 months after initial ESD, then every 6 months thereafter. As well, it is recommended that the head and neck region be examined by an otolaryngologist every 1 year after ESD [7].

Stomach

Although ESD may achieve curative resection of early gastric cancer (EGC), remnant background mucosa still has a high risk of metachronous gastric cancer (MGC). During follow-up period after ESD, MGC has been reported to range from 7.9 to 14 %. In patients with difficult tumor locations or submucosal fibrosis, non-curative resection or piecemeal resection may be unavoidable. Such resections are associated with higher local recurrence and regional metastasis.

Missed Synchronous Neoplasm

Synchronous gastric neoplasm (SGN) is defined as an additional lesion observed simultaneously, before initial ESD. Previous studies have shown an incidence of synchronous multiple gastric cancers ranging from 4.8 to 20.9 % in surgically resected specimens [8]. Epidemiologically, multiple gastric cancers tend to occur in the elderly and in men [9]. Histologically, they also arise in gastric mucosa with chronic gastritis, particularly

J.-H. Cho, M.D. • B.M. Ko, M.D.
J.Y. Cho, M.D., Ph.D. (✉)
Digestive Disease Center, Soonchunhyang University Hospital, Bucheon, Korea
e-mail: cjy6695@dreamwiz.com

N. Fukami (ed.), *Endoscopic Submucosal Dissection: Principles and Practice*,
DOI 10.1007/978-1-4939-2041-9_20, © Springer Science+Business Media New York 2015

intestinal metaplasia. Both the degree of intestinal metaplasia in the background mucosa (severe) and age (≥65 years) were significant independent risk factors for multiple gastric cancers (odds ratio = 2.19, $P = 0.02$; OR = 2.75, $P = 0.004$, respectively). In one study, 5.1 % (117/2,299) had multiple EGC lesions [10]. Multiple EGCs occurred more frequently in patients with adenoma, atrophic gastritis, or a family history of gastric cancer.

When a second neoplasm is detected within 1 year after ESD, it is defined as missed SGN. During endoscopic follow up, overall incidence of missed SGN can reportedly reach 1.0–5.6 % [9]. In another study, missed SGNs were found in 11.6 % (29/250) of patients with EGC or gastric adenoma [11], and two predictive factors were found to be significantly associated with missed SGN. Older patients (>65 years) had a higher risk of missed SGN than younger patients (OR = 2.315, $P = 0.040$). Tumor number at the time of ESD was an independent predictive factor for presence of missed SGN (OR = 5.302, $P = 0.006$). In one center, 2.0 % patients (12/602) had missed SGN [12]. Among them, all seven cases with carcinomas were found to be located in the posterior wall of the upper and mid gastric body. Missed SGN was more frequently observed when the primary gastric neoplasm was adenoma (4.0 vs. 1.0 %; OR = 4.114). Therefore, the whole stomach should always be examined in a meticulous manner before ESD is to be performed.

Simultaneous ESD for synchronous EGCs can be a feasible and safe option, and it can reduce hospital stay. In a study examining the safety and efficacy of simultaneous ESD, 124 synchronous double cancers from 62 patients were treated by simultaneous ESD [13]. In comparison with the single lesion group, there was no difference in length of the post-procedure fasting period (1.4 ± 1.1 vs. 1.1 ± 0.5 days, $P = 0.082$). Procedure-related complication rates per one lesion did not differ between the two groups (5.6 vs. 5.4 %, $P = 0.914$). Hence, simultaneous ESD can be considered a viable option in patients with multiple gastric neoplasias.

Metachronous Neoplasm

Many studies have suggested that patients with EGC treated by endoscopic resection are likely to be at high risk of subsequent cancers. The annual incidence rate of metachronous gastric cancer (MGC) has been reported to be 3.3 %. In one study, MGCs developed in 5.1 % (9/176) during the follow-up period (median 30 months, range 18–42 months) [14]. On multivariate analysis with occurrence of MGC, age and degree of antral atrophy had significant correlation. Especially, antrum atrophy was significantly associated with the incidence of MGCs (OR = 1.323, $P = 0.011$).

A total of 143 patients with EGC underwent endoscopic resection and were followed up for 24 months or longer [15]. Of the 20 patients with MGCs (14 %), 15 were also treated by endoscopic resection. In another study, MGCs were observed in 8.2 % (52/633) of patients whom underwent endoscopic resection [16]. The annual incidence was constant, and the cumulative 3 year incidence was 5.9 %. The average time to first detection of MGC was 3.1 ± 1.7 years (range 1–8.6 years).

In a large-scale study, the detection rate of MGC was 5.2 % (65/1,258) during a mean of 26.8 months after curative ESD of EGC [17]. The cumulative incidence increased linearly (2, 3, 4, and 5 years; 3.7, 6.9, 10, and 16 %) and the mean annual incidence rate was 3.5 %. Almost all of the MGCs were treated curatively with repeat endoscopic resection (96.2 %, $n = 50/52$). As surveillance after initial endoscopic resection, endoscopic examination was both practical and effective for a treatment opportunity of newly detected MGCs.

Local Recurrence

Compared to EMR, ESD has the advantage of minimizing local recurrence during the follow-up period. In a study of 510 EGCs, the local recurrence rate was 0.8 % (4/510). One out of 481 (0.2 %) was from a curative but piecemeal resection, and the other three (10.3 %, 3/29) were

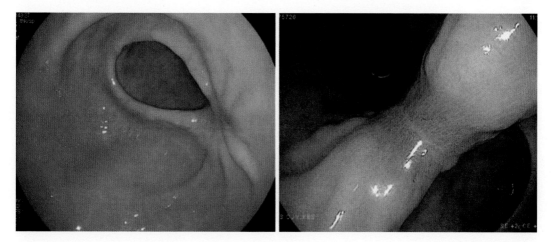

Fig. 20.1 Post-ESD scars (after curative resection of EGC)

from non-curative resection. There was a significant difference in the recurrence rate between the curative and non-curative groups ($P < 0.001$) [18]. In another study, locally recurrent carcinoma occurred in 2 of 212 lesions (0.9 %) during a median endoscopic follow up of 36 months (range 2–93 months). In incomplete resection group, local recurrence was significantly more frequent than complete resection group (8.7 % [2/23] vs. 0 % [0/189]; $P = 0.011$) [19]. Several studies have also shown that tumor size (>20 mm), piecemeal resection, and incomplete resection were associated with local recurrence [20, 21]. According to ESD indications, local recurrence rate was higher in the expanded group than that in the standard group (7.0 vs. 1.8 %; $P = 0.025$) [21].

Endoscopic Follow Up

In Korea and Japan, annual endoscopy surveillance has been accepted for patients who underwent ESD of EGC [22, 23]. Many studies have reported that almost all MGCs detected during annual follow up met ESD criteria, resulting in repeat ESD. After curative resection, local recurrence rates were low (<1.0 %) in both the standard and expanded indication groups [18, 19, 24, 25].

However, in clinical practice, curative endoscopic resection cannot be achieved in all cases.

If a positive horizontal margin or piecemeal resection of differentiated-type adenocarcinoma is the only non-curative factor, endoscopic follow up may be an acceptable option rather than additional gastrectomy [23]. Usually, surveillance follow-up endoscopy is performed 2, 6, and 12 months after ESD. If the local recurrence risk is not negligible, due to lateral margin positivity of resected specimen, close observation of ESD scar is important within 1 year after ESD (Figs. 20.1 and 20.2). During the follow-up period, irregular ulcer shapes or delayed healing can often be associated with local tumor recurrence (Fig. 20.3). For early diagnosis of recurrence after ESD, a biopsy specimen from the endoscopic examination may be necessary at regular intervals. In addition, abdominal ultrasonography or CT scan for detection of regional tumor recurrence is recommended alongside endoscopic follow up.

Colorectum

The objectives of surveillance after EMR or ESD for colorectal tumors are: (1) early detection and treatment of recurrence; and (2) early detection and treatment of metachronous colorectal cancer (CRC). ESD is the most useful method for resection of large colorectal neoplasms when complete resection by EMR would not be possible. Although ESD has the potential to cure CRC,

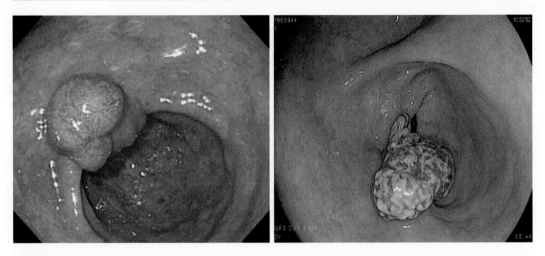

Fig. 20.2 Granulation tissue after ESD of EGC (surveillance biopsy showed no local tumor recurrence)

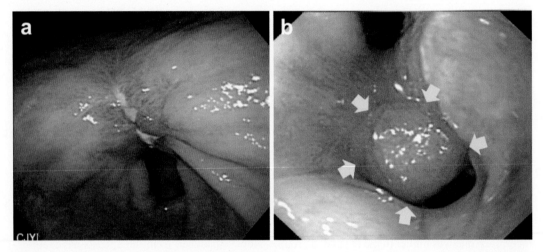

Fig. 20.3 Local recurrence at previous ESD site (after non-curative resection). (**a**) Irregular ulcer margin and delayed healing state (2 months after ESD). (**b**) Nodular lesion at ESD scar (*yellow arrows*)

patients who undergo resection for CRC are at high risk for developing metachronous neoplasia in the remnant colorectum. Non-curative resection, tumor location, submucosal fibrosis, and piecemeal resection are associated with higher local recurrence rates. Therefore, surveillance after ESD procedure is absolutely required.

Local Recurrence

Conventional EMRs usually results in endoscopic piecemeal resections (EPMRs), particularly for large laterally spreading tumor (LST) ≥ 20 mm,

with reports of local recurrence rates ranging from 7.4 to 17 % [26–28]. A case series of 67 colorectal neoplasia removed by ESD was reported [29]. The rate of en bloc resection and complete resection were 66/67 (98.5 %) and 39/67 (58.2 %), respectively. Patients who had successful en bloc resection successfully did not require additional therapy. The average duration of follow up in 48 cases was 256.1 ± 184.7 days, and no local tumor residue, metastasis, or recurrence was observed. Surgical resection and lymphadenectomy were performed for 14 lesions that indicated additional treatment, one case of local tumor residue and one case of tumor nodule in pericolic fat tissue without lymph node metastasis and local tumor residue were observed in the corresponding specimens.

Ikematsu et al. reported that for patients with early colorectal cancer, approximately 10 % of recurrences were detected within 1 year after resection, approximately 32 % within 2 years, and approximately 15 % of the recurrences after 5 years after resection [30]. Saito et al. reported 145 colorectal neoplasia cases removed by ESD. The rate of en bloc resection was 84 % (122/145), while recurrence rate was 2 %. Mean duration of recurrence detection was 6 months (2–18 months) in the EMR group and 6 months (4–6 months) in the ESD group [31]. In a systematic review, 13 series including 1,397 R0 ESD resections provided information on post-ESD follow up. Median follow up across the series was 22 months (range 6–43 months). Only one case of recurrence was reported, corresponding to a pooled risk of 0.07 % (95 % CI 0–0.2 %) [32]. ESD resulted in a significantly higher en bloc resection rate and, consequently, a significantly lower recurrence rate.

Lymph Node and Distant Metastasis

Lymph node metastasis (LNM) occurs in approximately 6–12 % of patients with submucosal invasive colorectal cancer [33–35]. According to the Paris classification and Japanese guidelines, submucosal invasive colorectal cancer lesions with well-differentiated or moderately differentiated adenocarcinoma, no evidence of vascular or lymphatic invasion, and an invasion depth of less than 1,000 μm are classified as low-risk submucosal invasive colorectal cancer, while a positive observation for any of these risk factors results in a high-risk classification of the lesion [30]. Therefore, endoscopic resection is commonly performed for low-risk submucosal invasive colorectal cancer and surgical resection with lymph node dissection is commonly performed for high-risk submucosal invasive colorectal cancer [36]. If any of the high-risk findings are observed during histopathologic examination of

the endoscopic resected specimen, surgical resection with lymph node dissection is considered as an additional treatment. However, it was noted that approximately 90 % of patients with submucosal colorectal cancer with a depth of invasion of ≥1,000 μm did not have LNM. Therefore, it is important to determine whether additional treatment is indicated after sufficiently considering the depth of SM invasion in addition to whether other risk factors for lymph node metastasis are present, the physical and social background of the patient, as well as the patient's wishes [37]. Follow-up examinations should therefore include confirmation of the presence or absence of lymph node metastasis and distant metastasis.

Metachronous Colorectal Cancer

Few reports have compared the long-term outcomes of colorectal neoplasms treated by ESD. Although both surgical and endoscopic resections have the potential to cure colorectal neoplasms, patients who undergo endoscopic resection for CRC are at a higher risk for developing metachronous neoplasia in the remnant colorectum [38, 39]. The value of intensive follow up of patients after resection of colorectal cancer remains under debate because of a lack of data. Meta-analyses of randomized controlled trials on follow up programs for patients with curatively resected colorectal cancer, however, have indicated improved overall survival and a better resection success rate for recurrent disease. Colorectal cancer surveillance colonoscopies were conducted for patients despite the long-term interval without recurrence [40, 41].

Endoscopic Follow Up

For adenomatous polyps that have been completely resected, current guidelines recommend surveillance colonoscopy 3–5 years after initial treatment. The interval is adapted in relation to the risk of developing new lesions or a late recurrence. An interval of 1–2 years is recommended for high-risk lesions which have been completely resected (high-grade intraepithelial neoplasia, villous and tubulovillous adenoma). An interval of 3 years is recommended for low-risk lesions (low-grade intraepithelial neoplasia) [42, 43]. According to data analysis between ESD and EMR, follow-up colonoscopy is recommended after 1 year for curative en bloc ESD cases considering local recurrence rates [29, 31, 32]. However, larger polyps are more likely to be incompletely resected than smaller polyps, and therefore, the US Multi-Society Task Force recommends consideration of a shorter interval for repeat colonoscopy if there is any question about completeness of resection of neoplastic tissue [44]. In clinical practice, if incomplete resection is suspected, follow-up colonoscopy can be performed 6 months after the initial ESD.

Conclusions

In patients with atrophy and intestinal metaplasia, SGNs are more frequently detected. These patients are also at higher risk for metachronous lesions. Therefore, intensive surveillance is preferred in the first year after endoscopic resection. For post-procedure surveillance, annual endoscopic examination is recommended for at least 5 years. If newly detected tumors are adequately indicated, repeat ESD can be performed. After successful ESD, the whole stomach can be preserved in many patients. In cases with noncurative resection, even closer observation, along with more surveillance biopsies, are required during endoscopic follow up.

ESD achieves a high rate of en bloc resection in patients with colorectal neoplasms. Because histopathologic diagnosis can be conducted sufficiently, the suitability of additional surgical resection can be correctly judged. Therefore, ESD is a useful method of treatment for large colorectal tumors. More outcome research and technical advances are needed, as they will play an important role in the therapeutic strategy for colorectal tumors in the future.

References

1. Shimizu Y, Tsukagoshi H, Fujita M, et al. Long-term outcome after endoscopic mucosal resection in patients with esophageal squamous cell carcinoma invading the muscularis mucosae or deeper. Gastrointest Endosc. 2002;56:387–90.
2. Katada C, Muto M, Momma K, et al. Clinical outcome after endoscopic mucosal resection for esophageal squamous cell carcinoma invading the muscularis mucosae – a multicenter retrospective cohort study. Endoscopy. 2007;39:779–83.
3. The Japan Esophageal Society. The clinical practice guidelines for esophageal cancer (in Japanese). 3rd ed. Tokyo: Kanehara Shuppan; 2012.
4. Ono S, Fujishiro M, Niimi K, et al. Long-term outcomes of endoscopic submucosal dissection for superficial esophageal squamous cell neoplasms. Gastrointest Endosc. 2009;70:860–6.
5. Shimizu Y, Tukagoshi H, Fujita M, et al. Metachronous squamous cell carcinoma of the esophagus arising after endoscopic mucosal resection. Gastrointest Endosc. 2001;54:190–4.
6. Urabe Y, Hiyama T, Tanaka S, et al. Metachronous multiple esophageal squamous cell carcinomas and Lugol-voiding lesions after endoscopic mucosal resection. Endoscopy. 2009;41:304–9.
7. Katada C, Muto M, Tanabe S, et al. Surveillance after endoscopic mucosal resection or endoscopic submucosal dissection for esophageal squamous cell carcinoma. Dig Endosc. 2013;25 Suppl 1:39–43.
8. Kodera Y, Yamamura Y, Torii A, et al. Incidence, diagnosis and significance of multiple gastric cancer. Br J Surg. 1995;82:1540–3.
9. Nitta T, Egashira Y, Akutagawa H, et al. Study of clinicopathological factors associated with the occurrence of synchronous multiple gastric carcinomas. Gastric Cancer. 2009;12:23–30.
10. Lee IS, Park YS, Kim KC, et al. Multiple synchronous early gastric cancers: high-risk group and proper management. Surg Oncol. 2012;21:269–73.
11. Yoo JH, Shin SJ, Lee KM, et al. How can we predict the presence of missed synchronous lesions after endoscopic submucosal dissection for early gastric cancers or gastric adenomas? J Clin Gastroenterol. 2013;47:e17–22.
12. Kim HH, Cho EJ, Noh E, et al. Missed synchronous gastric neoplasm with endoscopic submucosal dissection for gastric neoplasm: experience in our hospital. Dig Endosc. 2013;25:32–8.
13. Kasuga A, Yamamoto Y, Fujisaki J, et al. Simultaneous endoscopic submucosal dissection for synchronous double early gastric cancer. Gastric Cancer. 2013;16:555–62.
14. Han JS, Jang JS, Choi SR, et al. A study of metachronous cancer after endoscopic resection of early gastric cancer. Scand J Gastroenterol. 2011;46:1099–104.

15. Nasu J, Doi T, Endo H, et al. Characteristics of metachronous multiple early gastric cancers after endoscopic mucosal resection. Endoscopy. 2005;37:990–3.

16. Nakajima T, Oda I, Gotoda T, et al. Metachronous gastric cancers after endoscopic resection: how effective is annual endoscopic surveillance? Gastric Cancer. 2006;9:93–8.

17. Kato M, Nishida T, Yamamoto K, et al. Scheduled endoscopic surveillance controls secondary cancer after curative endoscopic resection for early gastric cancer: a multicenter retrospective cohort study by Osaka University ESD study group. Gut. 2013;62:1425–32.

18. Isomoto H, Shikuwa S, Yamaguchi N, et al. Endoscopic submucosal dissection for early gastric cancer: a large-scale feasibility study. Gut. 2009;58:331–6.

19. Goto O, Fujishiro M, Kodashima S, et al. Outcomes of endoscopic submucosal dissection for early gastric cancer with special reference to validation for curability criteria. Endoscopy. 2009;41:118–22.

20. Jang JS, Choi SR, Qureshi W, et al. Long-term outcomes of endoscopic submucosal dissection in gastric neoplastic lesions at a single institution in South Korea. Scand J Gastroenterol. 2009;44:1315–22.

21. Choi MK, Kim GH, Park do Y. Long-term outcomes of endoscopic submucosal dissection for early gastric cancer: a single-center experience. Surg Endosc. 2013;27:4250–8.

22. Korean Academy of Medical Science. Korean clinical practice guideline for gastric cancer. Seoul: Korean Academy of Medical Science; 2012.

23. Japanese Gastric Cancer Association. Japanese gastric cancer treatment guidelines 2010 (ver. 3). Gastric Cancer. 2011;14:113–23.

24. Yamaguchi N, Isomoto H, Fukuda E, et al. Clinical outcomes of endoscopic submucosal dissection for early gastric cancer by indication criteria. Digestion. 2009;80:173–81.

25. Lee TH, Cho JY, Chang YW, et al. Appropriate indications for endoscopic submucosal dissection of early gastric cancer according to tumor size and histologic type. Gastrointest Endosc. 2010;71:920–6.

26. Walsh RM, Ackroyd FW, Shellito PC. Endoscopic resection of large sessile colorectal polyps. Gastrointest Endosc. 1992;38:303–9.

27. Saito Y, Fujii T, Kondo H, et al. Endoscopic treatment for laterally spreading tumors in the colon. Endoscopy. 2001;33:682–6.

28. Uraoka T, Fujii T, Saito Y, et al. Effectiveness of glycerol as a submucosal injection for EMR. Gastrointest Endosc. 2005;61:736–40.

29. Ko BM, Lee MS, Choi HJ, et al. Outcomes of endoscopic submucosal dissection (ESD) in colorectal neoplasms over 3 years in Korea. Gastrointest Endosc. 2008;67:AB249–50.

30. Ikematsu H, Yoda Y, Matsuda T, et al. Long-term outcomes after resection for submucosal invasive colorectal cancers. Gastroenterology. 2013;144:551–9.

31. Saito Y, Fukuzawa M, Matsuda T, et al. Clinical outcome of endoscopic submucosal dissection versus endoscopic mucosal resection of large colorectal tumors as determined by curative resection. Surg Endosc. 2010;24:343–52.

32. Repici A, Hassan C, De Pessoa Paula D, et al. Efficacy and safety of endoscopic submucosal dissection for colorectal neoplasia: a systematic review. Endoscopy. 2012;44:137–50.

33. Kyzer S, Begin LR, Gordon PH, et al. The care of patients with colorectal polyps that contain invasive adenocarcinoma. Endoscopic polypectomy or colectomy? Cancer. 1992;70:2044–50.

34. Minamoto T, Mai M, Ogino T, et al. Early invasive colorectal carcinomas metastatic to the lymph node with attention to their nonpolypoid development. Am J Gastroenterol. 1993;88:1035–9.

35. Nusko G, Mansmann U, Partzsch U, et al. Invasive carcinoma in colorectal adenomas: multivariate analysis of patient and adenoma characteristics. Endoscopy. 1997;29:626–31.

36. Watanabe T, Itabashi M, Shimada Y, et al. Japanese Society for Cancer of the Colon and Rectum (JSCCR) guidelines 2010 for the treatment of colorectal cancer. Int J Clin Oncol. 2012;17:1–29.

37. Ikematsu H, Singh R, Yoda Y, et al. Follow up after endoscopic resection in submucosal invasive colorectal cancers. Dig Endosc. 2013;25:6–10.

38. Rao AR, Kagan AR, Chan PM, et al. Patterns of recurrence following curative resection alone for adenocarcinoma of the rectum and sigmoid colon. Cancer. 1981;48:1492–5.

39. Castells A, Bessa X, Daniels M, et al. Value of postoperative surveillance after radical surgery for colorectal cancer: results of a cohort study. Dis Colon Rectum. 1998;41:714–23.

40. Figueredo A, Rumble RB, Maroun J, et al. Follow up of patients with curatively resected colorectal cancer: a practice guideline. BMC Cancer. 2003;3:26.

41. Tjandra JJ, Chan MK. Follow up after curative resection of colorectal cancer: a meta-analysis. Dis Colon Rectum. 2007;50:1783–99.

42. Froehlich F, Pache I, Burnand B, et al. Performance of panel-based criteria to evaluate the appropriateness of colonoscopy: a prospective study. Gastrointest Endosc. 1998;48:128–36.

43. Kahi CJ, Rex DK, Imperiale TF. Screening, surveillance, and primary prevention for colorectal cancer: a review of the recent literature. Gastroenterology. 2008;135:380–99.

44. Lieberman DA, Rex DK, Winawer SJ, et al. Guidelines for colonoscopy surveillance after screening and polypectomy: a consensus update by the US Multi-Society Task Force on Colorectal Cancer. Gastroenterology. 2012;143:844–57.

Part VI

ESD Expansion

Haruhiro Inoue, Esperanza Grace Santi, Haruo Ikeda, Manabu Onimaru, and Hiroaki Itoh

Introduction

Per-oral endoscopic myotomy (POEM) [1] is an evolving minimally invasive endoscopic surgery with no skin incision, intending long-term recovery from symptoms of esophageal achalasia. POEM is considered one of the best applications of natural orifice translumenal endoscopic surgery (NOTES) [2]. The first case was performed on 8 September 2008 at the Showa University Northern Yokohama Hospital [3]. Since then more than 690 achalasia cases have received the POEM procedure in our hospital with no major complications. POEM was developed based on the already established surgical principles of esophageal myotomy as well as advanced endoscopic techniques of endoscopic submucosal dissection (ESD). In this article, how POEM was developed will be reported and discussed. Furthermore, as an extension of the POEM technique, per-oral endoscopic tumor resection (POET) was developed [4].

H. Inoue, M.D., Ph.D., F.A.S.G.E. (✉)
E.G. Santi, M.D. • H. Ikeda, M.D.
M. Onimaru, M.D. • H. Itoh, M.D., Ph.D.
Digestive Disease Center, Showa University
Koto-Toyosu Hospital, Koto-ku, Tokyo
135-0061, Japan
e-mail: haruinoue777@yahoo.co.jp

Advancement in Technology from EMR/ESD to POEM

Development of snare polypectomy with electrocautery opened the door of therapeutic endoscopy in the gastrointestinal tract. Snare polypectomy became the standard treatment for polypoid lesions with less risk of bleeding. But application of snare polypectomy to non-polypoid lesion was technically difficult and remained to be solved. Then, endoscopic mucosal resection (EMR) was developed for resection of flat mucosal lesion. Deyhle et al. [5] reported endoscopic resection of mucosa combined with submucosal injection. Submucosal injection creates a mucosal bleb and is followed by snare resection. Later, EMR using a suction cap (EMR-C) was developed [6]. Further modification of the suction cap technique is EMR with a band ligator [7, 8], which accelerated the popularization of EMR. EMR enables resection of flat mucosal lesions, but the size of resected specimens is still limited to those that are quite small. Large mucosal lesions can be successfully excised by repeated EMRs, although the acquired specimens are fragmented [9, 10]. In order to acquire one-piece large specimen for accurate histopathological evaluation, a novel method of ESD was developed using an insulation-tip knife by Ono et al. [11]. In order to complete ESD, various basic techniques are used;

submucosal injection, mucosal cutting, submucosal dissection, hemostasis, and so on. Currently, ESD is regarded as endoscopic microsurgery using a flexible endoscope. Fundamental techniques used in POEM (submucosal injection, mucosal incision, submucosal tunneling, and hemostasis) are very similar to the techniques of ESD.

Background of Achalasia Treatment

Achalasia (the word itself a Greek term that means "does not relax") is a chronic benign disease with a subtle onset and symptoms that may progress gradually for years before exact diagnosis can be made [12]. It is the most common primary motility disorder of the esophagus; however, it occurs rarely, with an annual incidence of approximately 0.03–1/100,000 per year. Achalasia affects men and women equally and may occur at any age. Despite increasing understanding of its pathophysiology, the etiology of achalasia remains largely unknown [13].

All current treatments have different advantages and drawbacks [14–17]. Therapy has focused mainly on the forced relaxation of the lower esophageal sphincter (LES) by endoscopic or surgical means. As few randomized controlled trials have tried to determine the optimal strategy, treatment still varies widely. First-line endoscopic treatments are botulinum toxin ("Botox") injection and esophageal balloon dilatation [18]. Endoscopic pneumatic balloon dilatation temporarily relieves dysphagia in up to 70 % of cases and is still widely performed because of its relative noninvasiveness. However, it is associated with a potential risk of esophageal perforation (2.5 %) and frequent recurrences. The cumulative 5 year remission rate of pneumatic dilatation for achalasia is reported to be between 50 and 70 %. If these interventions are ineffective, surgical myotomy is generally indicated.

Surgical myotomy was originally reported by Heller et al. in 1913. The myotomy consists of two longitudinal cuts of approximately 8 cm, on the anterior and posterior esophageal wall, that includes about 2 cm of the dilated part (esophagus) and a short cut over the cardia into the fundus. This suggests that complete release of LES is mandatory to achieve excellent relief from the symptoms. Later, bilateral myotomy was modified to single myotomy, but the basic principles have not changed. Although surgical myotomy provides a better solution for esophageal achalasia, it still has limitations and failures. In particular, gastroesophageal reflux disease (GERD) may occur in 30 % of cases after Heller myotomy, and, therefore, it is generally accompanied by an additional antireflux procedure, such as Dor fundoplication.

Laparoscopic myotomy is a less invasive technique that significantly reduces the morbidity of open surgery [19]. However, it still requires several abdominal incisions and also involves dissection of normal esophageal hiatus which may cause potential hiatal hernia.

Endoscopic Myotomy

The concept of endoscopic myotomy for the treatment of achalasia was first reported in a case series in 1980 [20]. However, the direct incision method through mucosal layer described was not considered a safe and reliable approach, and therefore this method was not further followed. Pasricha et al. [21] recently reported the possibility of endoscopic myotomy through a submucosal tunnel in a porcine model. Sumiyama et al. [22] also reported the technical feasibility of submucosal tunneling in a porcine model, while Perretta et al. [23] reported on the safety and effectiveness of endoscopic submucosal esophageal myotomy in a pig model. Based on this experimental background, the present authors refined the techniques for clinical application in order to perform endoscopic myotomy in humans, namely POEM (per-oral endoscopic myotomy) [24, 25].

What Are the Theoretical Differences Between ESD and POEM?

ESD was firstly developed by Ono et al. [11] to resect intramucosal cancer endoscopically with a one-piece, non-fragmented specimen. Mucosal lesions (high-grade dysplasia or intramucosal carcinoma) resected in a single piece allows complete histopathological assessment, including horizontal spread and vertical infiltration of tumor. In ESD, the mucosal layer was resected together with a major part of the submucosal layer, while muscle layer is absolutely preserved. Muscle layer and serosa (or adventitia) facilitates as a barrier against a leakage of gastrointestinal fluid toward the mediastium and peritoneal cavity. Once the muscle layer is incidentally disrupted, that means perforation of the gastrointestinal wall, that is a definite cause of mediastinitis or peritonitis. Perforation should be closed with endoscopic clips.

In the POEM procedure, the muscle layer is intentionally dissected and divided. As a result, the mediastinum is eventually open to the submucosal space. In the POEM procedure, the preserved mucosa works as a strong barrier to isolate the GI lumen from the mediastinum or peritoneum. Advanced endoscopic technology of POEM enables dissection of the muscle layer through submucosal tunneling without tearing the overlying mucosa. Endoscopic complete myotomy had never been clinically experienced before the development of POEM.

Finally, what we learn from both ESD and POEM is that if we keep either mucosa or muscle layer intact, neither peritonitis nor mediastinitis may occur, because either mucosa or muscle layer works as a strong barrier (see Fig. 21.1).

The POEM Procedure

Equipment Required for POEM

Endoscope and Distal Attachment
A standard forward-viewing diagnostic gastroscope can be used for the POEM procedure. But if it is available, a large working channel (3.2 mm) endoscope with water jet function is more useful. A transparent distal small "tapered" cap (ST Hood; Fujifilm, Tokyo, Japan) is preferably attached at the tip of the endoscope. An oblique cap (MH-588; Olympus, Tokyo, Japan) can be used as an alternative. The oblique cap is particularly necessary for clipping the esophageal opening. An overtube is used for stabilization of the endoscope which effectively avoids mucosal laceration at the mucosal incision site during the POEM procedure. This equipment used for POEM is similar to that used for ESD.

Carbon Dioxide (CO_2) Insufflator
CO_2 as insufflation is essential to achieve a safe POEM. Endoscopic CO_2 insufflation with a controlled gas feed of 1.2 L/min is beneficial for reducing the risk of both mediastinal emphysema and pneumoperitoneum. Air supply button should definitely be closed during the POEM procedure, even when CO_2 insufflator is turned on. In contrast, ESD can be carried out even under air insufflation, because the muscle layer is definitely kept intact.

Triangle-Tip Knife
A triangle-tip knife (TT knife) (KD-640L; Olympus) is used for submucosal tunneling and myotomy. The TT knife has a triangle plate at its tip. The Triangle plate has three angulations that allow spraying of energy toward a wide circumferential range. Submucosal dissection is effectively carried out without making direct contact with the tissue to be dissected.

Electrocautery Generator
A high-frequency electrosurgical energy generator (VIO300D; ERBE Elektromedizin GmbH, Tubingen, Germany, or ESG400; Olympus, Tokyo) that has a spray coagulation mode with non-contact tissue dissection is effectively used in combination with the TT knife. Spray coagulation mode, effect 2, 50 W is the best match with the TT knife for both submucosal dissection and myotomy. Settings should be individually adjusted during the operation.

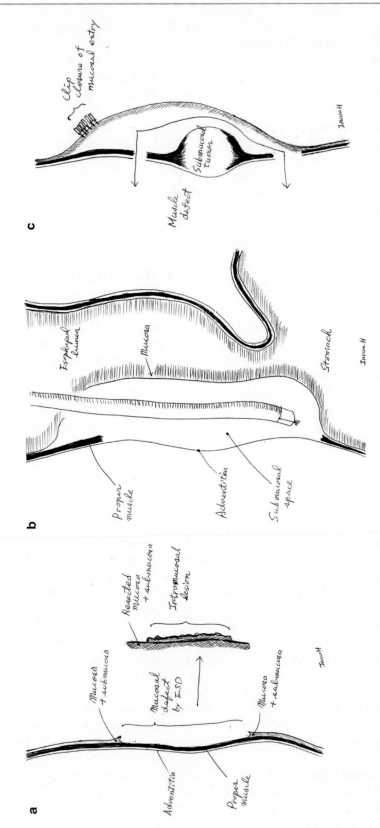

Fig. 21.1 (a) ESD: Mucosa, with some submucosal tissue, is resected, and the exposed muscle layer facilitates as a barrier to esophageal content. (b) POEM: Muscle layer was dissected in submucosal tunnel. Mucosa works as a barrier between esophageal lumen and mediastinum. (c) POET: Tumor from muscle layer was resected through submucosal tunnel. Mucosa acts as a barrier to avoid mediastinitis

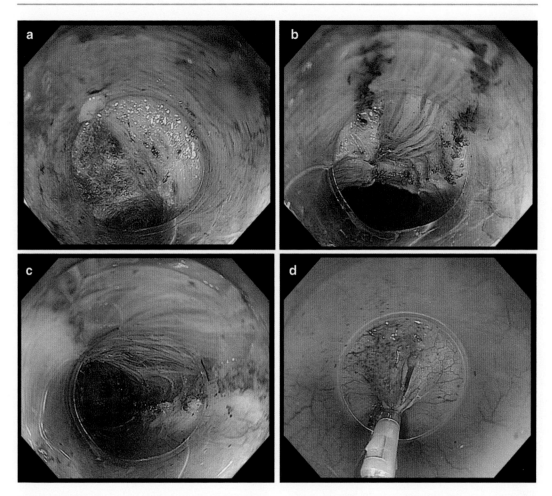

Fig. 21.2 Endoscopic images of POEM. (**a**) Submucosal tunnel. Submucosal dissection is made along the surface of the circular muscle layer. In this image, the top half is the muscle layer surface and the bottom half is the submucosal layer stained with indigocarmine. (**b**) Myotomy started. Myotomy begins at 2 cm distal from mucosal incision. Selective circular myotomy is intended in order to avoid mediastinal injury. (**c**) Completion of myotomy. Cut ends of circular muscle stay apart, resulting in good relaxation of the LES. (**d**) Closure of mucosal incision. Mucosal incision is closed with regular hemostatic clips. Complete closure of mucosal incision is confirmed by endoscopic vision

Coagulation Forceps

Monopolar coagulating forceps (Coagrasper, FD-411QR; Olympus) are used for hemostasis and coagulation of large vessels, when encountered during dissection. The preferred electrocautery setting is soft coagulation 80 W, effect 2.

POEM Procedure

The following technical details of the POEM procedure have consistency from original report [24–27] (Fig. 21.2).

Step 1: General Anesthesia and CO_2 Insufflation Through Endoscope

POEM is performed under general anesthesia with endotracheal intubation, keeping the patient in the supine position. CO_2 insufflation is absolutely mandatory to perform a safe POEM procedure. CO_2 insufflation theoretically avoids pneumomediastinum and air embolization. It is extremely important to check that the air feed button on the endoscopy unit remains closed, repeatedly throughout the entire procedure, even when the CO_2 insufflation switch is turned on. If air was insufflated, it could cause catastrophic complications. To prevent abdominal compartment syndrome, the upper abdomen is checked periodically during the procedure. When the abdomen is excessively distended, abdominal wall puncture will be performed using an injection needle so as not to develop into abdominal compartment syndrome.

Step 2: Submucosal Tunneling

After injection of normal saline with indigo carmine dye, a 2-cm longitudinal incision is created on the anterior wall. Submucosal tunnel is generally created at anterior wall with one-third circumferential dissection of the esophageal lumen.

Myotomy at 2 o'clock direction, continuing toward lesser curve of stomach, potentially avoids damage to the sling collar muscle that is the major component of His angle. His angle is considered a natural anatomical barrier to postoperative GERD. The estimated length of the submucosal tunnel, although individualized, becomes approximately 16 cm (from 29 to 45 cm from patient's teeth). If patients have abnormal contractions of the upper esophagus, myotomy is extended toward proximal side. The longest myotomy performed at Northern Yokohama Hospital was 25 cm.

Step 3: Endoscopic Myotomy

Dissection of the circular muscle bundle is usually started at the level of 2 cm distal to the mucosal entry point in submucosal tunnel. The standard length of myotomy is more than 10 cm (average 13 cm). A TT-knife permits selective dissection of the inner circular muscle layer, which potentially avoids incidental damage to the mediastinal critical organ. In other words, preserved longitudinal muscle layer is the safety margin of myotomy. All processes can be done with direct endoscopic visual control, and careful dissection is the simplest way to maintain safety. If during initial myotomy the thickness of the circular muscle cannot be predicted, it is advisable to begin myotomy by careful step-by-step dissection until the longitudinal muscle layer is identified at the bottom of the myotomy site. Even though the outer longitudinal muscle layer has been preserved, it is thin enough to split just by CO_2 insufflation or even subtle touch of endoscopy on it.

Circular muscle dissection advances from proximal to distal, maintaining the correct dissection plane. The myotomy is extended to a distance of 2 cm toward the stomach. Myotomy at the narrow gastroesophageal junction (GEJ) has a higher risk of incidental mucosal damage, though repeated submucosal injection may work as a cushion and potential way to avoid damage. Smooth passage of the endoscope through the GEJ at the end of myotomy provides immediate confirmation of complete myotomy. At the LES, particular attention should be paid to ensuring that all circular muscle bundles responsible for achalasia are completely cut.

In laparoscopic Heller myotomy, the surrounding structures (phrenoesophageal ligament) of distal esophagus need to be dissected to expose the abdominal esophagus. This dissection causes potential hiatal hernia resulting in severe postsurgical GERD. In order to prevent it, a partial antireflux procedure, such as Dor fundoplication, is routinely performed. In contrast, no antireflux procedure is added after the POEM procedure, because the original hiatal attachments and the acute angle of His are left untouched and the flap-valve mechanism is kept intact.

Another major advantage of POEM is the flexibility of myotomy length. In POEM, myotomy is routinely made more than 10 cm, with at least 1 cm cut to gastric side. In laparoscopic surgery, a limited length with a maximum of 10 cm is capable to be performed because there is limited exposure of the distal esophagus under laparoscopic vision. In cases with vigorous achalasia or diffuse esophageal spasm, long myotomy is recommended. In POEM, the direction of myotomy can also be flexibly set. In cases of previous surgical failure, posterior myotomy is recommended to avoid access to the scar site from previous surgical myotomy.

After completion of the myotomy, complete LES relaxation is confirmed upon retroflex view of the cardia.

Step 4: Closure of Mucosal Entry

Before closing mucosal entry, 10 cc of saline with 80 mg gentamycin is sprayed into the submucosal tunnel. The stomach should also be emptied of fluid and gas. The mucosal entry site,

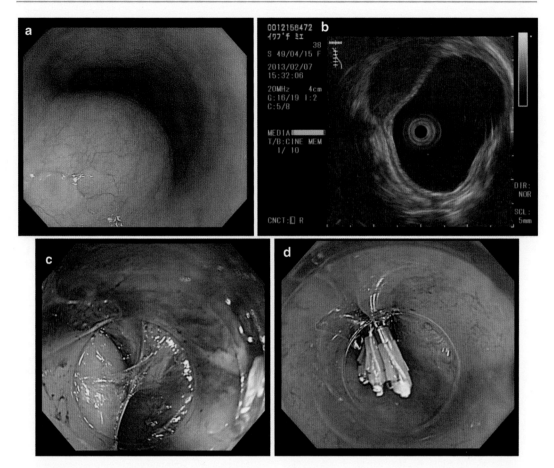

Fig. 21.3 Endoscopic images of POET. (**a**) Endoscopic view of SMT. SMT is observed at middle part of the esophagus. (**b**) Endoscopic ultrasonography (EUS). EUS-identified tumor is derived from the fourth muscle layer. (**c**) Tumor excision in submucosal tunnel. SMT was dissected in submucosal tunnel. (**d**) Closure of mucosal entry. Closure of mucosal entry was done by regular hemostatic clip after removal of submucosal tumor through this incision

which is usually 2–3 cm long, is closed with 5–10 endoscopic clips. The first clip should be placed at the distal end of the longitudinal opening to create a mucosal fold. This fold is used as a guide to place next clip. The span between two clips is about 3 mm. Successful closure of mucosal entry can be confirmed by endoscopic appearance. Even when mucosal entry is elongated over the myotomy site, tight mucosal closure with clips avoids leakage of esophageal contents into the mediastinum.

An Extension of POEM, POET (Per-oral Endoscopic Tumor Resection)

The clinical success of POEM encouraged another application of submucosal tunneling; per-oral endoscopic tumor resection (POET) [4] is an offshoot of POEM. At the same time, this technique was also reported as STER (submucosal tunneling endoscopic resection) [28]. Submucosal tumors such as leiomyomas and GISTs can be resected endoscopically through submucosal tunneling (Fig. 21.3). In these procedures, preserving the mucosal layer intact is a key to avoid mediastinal contamination, but even when mucosal tear may occur tight closure by endoscopic clipping device secures sealing of mediastinum from GI luminal content. A successful report of full layer resection of aberrant pancreas in the esophagus supports this concept [4].

References

1. Inoue H, Minami H, Kobayashi Y, et al. Peroral endoscopic myotomy (POEM) for esophageal achalasia. Endoscopy. 2010;42:265–71.
2. Kalloo AN, Singh VK, Jagannath SB, et al. Flexible transgastric peritoneoscopy: a novel approach to diagnostic and therapeutic interventions. Gastrointest Endosc. 2004;60:114–7.
3. Inoue H, Minami H, Satodate H, et al. First clinical experience of submucosal endoscopic myotomy for esophageal achalasia with no skin incision. Gastrointest Endosc. 2009;69:AB122.
4. Inoue H, Ikeda H, Hosoya T, et al. Submucosal endoscopic tumor resection for subepithelial tumors in the esophagus and cardia. Endoscopy. 2012;44:225–30.
5. Dehyle P, Largiader F, Jenny S. A method for endoscopic electroresection of sessile colonic polyps. Endoscopy. 1973;5:38–40.
6. Inoue H, Takeshita K, Hori H, et al. Endoscopic mucosal resection with a cap-fitted panendoscope for esophagus, stomach, and colon mucosal lesions. Gastrointest Endosc. 1993;39:58–62.
7. Stiegmann CV. Endoscopic ligation: now and the future. Gastrointest Endosc. 1993;39:203–5.
8. Chaves DM, Sakai P, Mester M, et al. A new endoscopic technique for the resection of flat polypoid lesions. Gastrointest Endosc. 1994;40:224–6.
9. Satodate H, Inoue H, Yoshida T et al. Circumferential EMR of carcinoma arising in Barrett's esophagus: case report. Gastrointest Endosc
10. Ell C, May A, Grossner L, et al. Endoscopic mucosal resection of early cancer and high-grade dysplasia in Barret's esophagus. Gastroenterology. 2000;118:670–7.
11. Ono H. Early gastric cancer: diagnosis, pathology, treatment techniques and treatment outcomes. Eur J Gastroenterol Hepatol. 2006;18:863–7.
12. Mikaeli J, Islami F, Malekzadeh R. Achalasia: a review of Western and Iranian experiences. World J Gastroenterol. 2009;15(40):5000–9.
13. Gockel HR, Schumacher J, Gockel I, Lang H, Haaf T, Nöthen MM. Achalasia: will genetic studies provide insights? Hum Genet. 2010;128(4):353–64.
14. Campos GM, Vittinghoff E, Rabl C, et al. Endoscopic and surgical treatments for achalasia: a systematic review and meta-analysis. Ann Surg. 2009;249:45–57.
15. Ahmed A. Achalasia: what is the best treatment? Ann Afr Med. 2008;7:141–8.
16. Allescher HD, Storr M, Seige M, et al. Treatment of achalasia: botulinum toxin injection vs pneumatic balloon dilation. A prospective study with long-term follow-up. Endoscopy. 2001;33:1007–17.
17. Carter JT, Nguyen D, Roll GR, et al. Predictors of long-term outcome after laparoscopic esophagomyotomy and Dor fundoplication for achalasia. Arch Surg. 2011;146:1024–8.
18. Francis DL, Katzka DA. Achalasia: update on the disease and its treatment. Gastroenterology. 2010;139:369–74.
19. Shimi S, Nathanson LK, Cuschieri A. Laparoscopic cardiomyotomy for achalasia. J R Coll Surg Edinb. 1991;36:152–4.
20. Ortega JA, Madureri V, Perez I. Endoscopic myotomy in the treatment of achalasia. Gastrointest Endosc. 1980;26:8–10.
21. Pasricha PJ, Hawari R, Ahmed I, et al. Submucosal endoscopic esophageal myotomy: a novel experimental approach for the treatment of achalasia. Endoscopy. 2007;39:761–4.
22. Sumiyama K, Gostout CJ, Rajan E, Bakken TA, Knipschield MA, Marler RJ. Submucosal endoscopy with mucosal flap safety valve. Gastrointest Endosc. 2007;65:688–94.
23. Perretta S, Dallemagne B, Donatelli G, Diemunsch P, Marescaux J. Transoral endoscopic esophageal myotomy based on esophageal function testing in a survival porcine model. Gastrointest Endosc. 2011;73:111–6.
24. Inoue H, Minami H, Satodate H, Kudo SE, et al. First clinical experience of submucosal endoscopic myotomy for esophageal achalasia with no skin incision. Gastrointest Endosc. 2009;69:122.
25. Inoue H, Minami H, Kobayashi Y, et al. Peroral endoscopic myotomy (POEM) for esophageal achalasia. Endoscopy. 2010;42:265–71.
26. Inoue H, Tianle KM, Ikeda H, et al. Peroral endoscopic myotomy for esophageal achalasia: technique, indication, and outcomes. Thorac Surg Clin. 2011;21:519–25.
27. Eleftheriadis N, Inoue H, Ikeda H, et al. Training in peroral endoscopic myotomy (POEM) for esophageal achalasia. Ther Clin Risk Manag. 2012;8:329–42.
28. Zhou PH. Application and evaluation of submucosal tunneling endoscopic resection of gastric submucosal tumors originating from the muscularis propria layer. Zhonghua Wei Chang Wai Ke Za Zhi. 2012;15:671–4.

ESD Expansion: NOTES—Eastern Perspective

22

Kazuhiro Yasuda, Hidefumi Shiroshita, Masafumi Inomata, and Seigo Kitano

Introduction

Natural orifice translumenal endoscopic surgery (NOTES) is an evolving, new, minimally invasive surgery technique that provides access to the peritoneal cavity through the mouth, vagina, colon, or urinary tract, thus avoiding abdominal incisions [1, 2]. This unique concept has garnered much attention from endoscopists and surgeons all over the world, and many experimental studies have been performed that have shown the technical feasibility of various surgical procedures using NOTES [3].

Ten years have passed since the introduction of the concept of NOTES when Kalloo et al. first published their results of transgastric peritoneoscopy in a porcine model in 2004 [4]. NOTES has moved from experimental studies in animals to clinical practice in humans. Although the number of human NOTES cases is still limited, several large NOTES case series in humans have demonstrated that hybrid techniques are feasible and safe alternatives to laparoscopic procedures [5–8].

K. Yasuda, M.D., Ph.D. (✉) • H. Shiroshita, M.D., Ph.D. • M. Inomata, M.D., Ph.D.
Department of Gastroenterological and Pediatric Surgery, Oita University Faculty of Medicine, 1-1 Idaigaoka, Yufu, Oita 879-5593, Japan
e-mail: kyasuda@oita-u.ac.jp

S. Kitano, M.D., Ph.D.
Oita University, Oita, Japan

Endoscopic submucosal dissection (ESD) was developed in Japan to remove gastrointestinal lesions en bloc that traditionally would have been treated surgically. This innovative endoscopic technique has contributed to the development of NOTES in Asia. Examples of NOTES procedures using techniques from ESD include transgastric peritoneoscopy, endoscopic full-thickness resection (EFTR), and peroral endoscopic myotomy (POEM).

This paper will review the clinical applications of NOTES in Asia, as well as summarize the activities of the Japan and the Asia Pacific NOTES working groups. Future directions of the development of NOTES in the East will also be discussed.

Clinical Applications in Asia

Published human NOTES experiences in Asia are summarized in Table 22.1 [9–30].

Cholecystectomy

The most reported NOTES procedure is cholecystectomy. Five different authors have published their experiences with transvaginal cholecystectomy [9–13]. The largest NOTES cholecystectomy series in Asia was reported by Niu et al. from China [13]. They retrospectively compared the clinical results of 43 transvaginal

Table 22.1 Published human NOTES studies in Asia

Procedure	Year	Author	Country	Route	Number	Operation time (min)	Complications	
Cholecystectomy	2008	Rao et al	India	Transvaginal	3	NA	None	
	2009	Palanivelu et al	India	Transvaginal	8	148	1 subhepatic collection	Combination of a flexible endoscope and a 3-mm trocar for retracting the gall bladder. Two conversions to laparoscopic cholecystectomy
	2009	Rudiman et al	Indonesia	Transvaginal	1	128	None	Transvaginal endoscope and two trocars (5 and 2 mm)
	2010	Sohn et al	Korea	Transvaginal	1	86	None	Use of a wound retractor with a glove for vaginal access
	2011	Niu et al	China	Transvaginal	43	87	None	Transvaginal endoscope and a 5-mm umbilical trocar
Appendectomy	2008	Rao et al	India	Transgastric	10	NA	1 ileus	Two conversions to laparoscopic appendectomy
	2008	Palanivelu et al	India	Transvaginal	6	103	None	Three conversions to laparoscopic appendectomy
	2010	Shin et al	Korea	Transvaginal	1	60	None	Transvaginal endoscope and a 5-mm umbilical trocar
Peritoneoscopy	2008	Kitano et al	Japan	Transgastric	1	NA	None	Transgastric submucosal endoscopy
	2013	Lee et al	Korea	Transgastric	5	33	None	Transgastric submucosal endoscopy
	2013	Chen et al	China	Transgastric	7	30	None	1-cm-long full-thickness gastric incision
Local resection of the stomach	2009	Nakajima et al	Japan	Transvaginal	2	365, 170	None	Transvaginal endoscope and two trocars
	2009	Abe et al	Japan	Transoral	4	201	None	Endoscopic full-thickness resection with laparoscopic assistance
	2011	Mori et al	Japan	Transoral	6	288	None	Endoscopic full-thickness resection with laparoscopic assistance
	2011	Cho et al	Korea	Transoral	14	143	1 gastric stasis	Endoscopic full-thickness resection with laparoscopic assistance and laparoscopic regional lymph node dissection. Five conversions to gastrectomy
	2013	Lee et al	Korea	Transgastric	5	33	None	Transgastric submucosal endoscopy

	Year	Author	Country	Route	n		Complications	Description
Peroral endoscopic myotomy	2010	Inoue et al	Japan	Transesophageal	17	126	None	Transesophageal submucosal endoscopy
	2013	Lee et al	Korea	Transesophageal	13	NA	None	Transesophageal submucosal endoscopy
	2013	Minami et al	Japan	Transesophageal	28	99	None	Transesophageal submucosal endoscopy
Specimen extraction after colectomy	2013	Li et al	China	Transesophageal	103 vs 131	41 vs 48	1 vs 1	Full-thickness myotomy vs circular muscle myotomy
	2008	Palanivelu et al	India	Transvaginal	7	222	1 ileus, 1 pouchitis, 1 deep vein thrombosis	Laparoscopic proctocolectomy
	2012	Cheung et al	China	Transrectal	1	NA	None	Laparoscopic right colectomy
Adrenalectomy	2011	Zou et al	China	Transvaginal	11	102	None	Transvaginal laparoscope and two trocars (10 and 5 mm). One conversion to open surgery
Thyroidectomy	2013	Nakajo et al	Japan	Transoral	8	208	8 sensory disorders around the chin, 1 laryngeal nerve palsy	Trans-oral video-assisted neck surgery

cholecystectomies with those of 48 conventional laparoscopic cholecystectomies. Transvaginal cholecystectomy was performed with a transvaginal flexible endoscope, a 5 mm laparoscopic grasper introduced through the vagina for retraction of the gallbladder, and a single umbilical trocar. The cystic duct and artery were clipped with laparoscopic clips through the umbilical trocar. Transvaginal cholecystectomies were successfully completed in all patients without conversion to conventional laparoscopic surgery, and there were no intra- or postoperative complications in any patients. The operation time for the NOTES cholecystectomies was longer than that of conventional laparoscopic cholecystectomies (87 vs. 60 min, $P < 0.05$). However, postoperative pain, hospital stay, and the cost of hospitalization with NOTES were less than those with the conventional laparoscopic operation. Sohn et al. from Korea applied a single-port access system with a wound retractor and a surgical glove at the vaginal port to improve operation efficiency [12]. Their mean operation time was 86 min.

All other series were performed in a hybrid fashion using laparoscopic assistance with one or two trocars, and no serious complications were reported. The additional trocar seems to be an optimal way to perform NOTES cholecystectomy safely and easily at the present time with the current lack of availability of NOTES-specific devices.

Appendectomy

Rao and Reddy from India were the first in the world to perform a transgastric appendectomy [9]. Appendectomies were completed using a double-channel endoscopes without laparoscopic assistance. Transgastric access was achieved with a needle knife and balloon dilation. The mesoappendix was dissected using a hot biopsy forceps with monopolar coagulation current. The appendix was secured with an endoloop and then transected using a polypectomy snare. The gastric access site was closed with multiple endoscopic clips. Two out of ten

cases required conversion to conventional laparoscopic operation. Postoperative ileus was noted in one patient and needle knife injury to the abdominal wall in one other.

Palanivelu et al. from India reported 6 attempts at pure NOTES appendectomy with two patients requiring laparoscopic assistance and three requiring conversion to conventional laparoscopic operation [14]. There were no complications, and the hospital stay averaged 1–2 days.

Peritoneoscopy

Kitano, Yasuda et al. performed transgastric peritoneoscopy for preoperative staging in a pancreatic cancer patient in 2008 [16]. This was the first case of NOTES performed in Japan. The submucosal tunneling technique was used in combination with ESD methods, after confirming the safety and feasibility of this technique in experimental studies [31–34]. After injection of normal saline solution into the gastric submucosal layer, a 2 cm incision of the mucosa into the submucosal cushion was created (Fig. 22.1a). Dissection of the submucosal layer was then carried out with an ESD knife to make a narrow longitudinal submucosal tunnel approximately 5 cm long (Fig. 22.1b). A small incision of the seromuscular layer was made at the end of the submucosal tunnel, and the opening was enlarged with an endoscopic dilation balloon. The endoscope was then advanced into the peritoneal cavity through the tunnel, which provided an excellent view. After we confirmed no hepatic or peritoneal metastasis, the patient underwent a standard open operation without complications. We have performed 14 cases of transgastric submucosal peritoneoscopy. In some cases, peritoneal or liver metastasis was able to be diagnosed with transgastric peritoneoscopy before operation (Fig. 22.1c–e).

Lee et al. from Korea performed five transgastric submucosal endoscopies with the same technique in patients under conscious sedation [17]. All peritoneoscopies were diagnostic, and there were no procedure-related complications. Chen et al. from China reported the outcome of transgastric peritoneoscopy in seven consecutive patients with

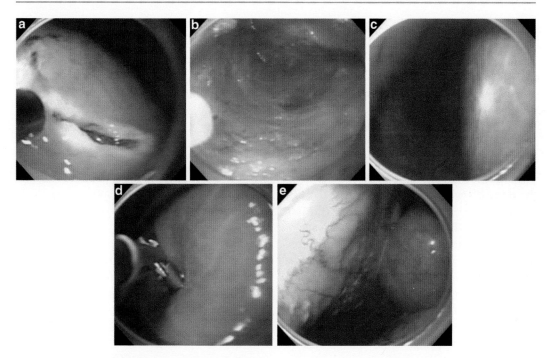

Fig. 22.1 Transgastric peritoneoscopy for preoperative staging of pancreatic cancer. (**a**) Initial mucosal incision with an ESD knife. (**b**) Creation of the longitudinal submucosal tunnel. (**c**) Peritoneoscopy revealed a liver metastasis. (**d**) Biopsy using endoscopy biopsy forceps during transgastric peritoneoscopy. (**e**) Peritoneoscopy revealed peritoneal metastatic nodules on the abdominal wall

suspected tuberculosis peritonitis [18]. They used the needle knife and balloon dilation technique for transgastric access. Suspicious peritoneal nodules were biopsied and confirmed pathologically as tuberculosis peritonitis, and no adverse events occurred.

Local Resection of the Stomach

Nakajima et al. from Japan reported two cases of transvaginal local resection of the stomach for gastric submucosal tumor [19]. They used a transvaginal flexible endoscope and two laparoscopic graspers for perigastric mobilization. After replacing the transvaginal endoscope with a digital stapling device, they were able to perform local resection of the stomach. Operation times were 365 and 170 min, respectively. Both patients reported no pain.

EFTR with laparoscopic assistance for gastric submucosal tumor or early gastric cancer was developed in Asia by applying the ESD technique. A total of 24 cases of EFTR were reported in the literature by Abe et al. [20], Mori et al. [21], and Cho et al. [22]. EFTR around the tumor was performed with an ESD knife under laparoscopic supervision, and the gastric-wall defect was closed laparoscopically. Although the mean operation times were long (ranging from 143 to 288 min), there were no complications besides gastric stasis in one patient. Lee et al. performed EFTR in five patients without any laparoscopic assistance [17]. After they created a longitudinal submucosal tunnel using the ESD technique, EFTR was performed with an insulation-tipped knife and a snare. The mucosal entry incision was closed with endoclips. En bloc and complete resections were achieved in all patients, and no procedure-related complications were reported.

POEM

There are now at least four different institutions in Asia publishing their results of POEM for esophageal achalasia [23–26]. Inoue et al. from Japan developed the procedure using the ESD technique [23]. After they created a longitudinal submucosal tunnel, the esophageal circular muscle layer was dissected from the midesophagus to the gastroesophageal junction at 2 cm distal to the mucosal entry site. They reported the first experience of 17 consecutive cases of POEM. In all patients, POEM reduced the dysphagia symptom score and improved the resting lower esophageal sphincter pressure. Li et al. from China compared the outcomes of 103 patients undergoing full-thickness myotomy with those of 131 patients undergoing circular muscle myotomy [26]. The treatment success rate was over 95 % for both methods, and one complication was reported for each of the two myotomy types.

Specimen Extraction

With the introduction of the NOTES concept, there has been renewed interest in using natural orifices for specimen retraction. This approach prevents wound-related complications by eliminating minilaparotomies for specimen extraction. Palanivelu et al. from India reported seven cases of laparoscopic proctocolectomy followed by transvaginal specimen retrieval [27]. There were no complications, and the vaginal wound healed completely with no complaints of dyspareunia. Cheung et al. from China reported a case of laparoscopic right hemicolectomy with transrectal extraction of the specimen using a transanal endoscopic microsurgery device [28]. The patient experienced an uneventful recovery.

Other Procedures

In 2011, Zou et al. from China first reported the outcome of 11 consecutive patients who underwent transvaginal hybrid NOTES adrenalectomy [29]. They used a transvaginal laparoscope and two umbilical trocars. The median operation time was 102 min, and there was one conversion to open surgery. Nakajo et al. from Japan reported eight cases of gasless transoral endoscopic thyroidectomy with a premandible approach [30]. Although the patients began oral intake on postoperative day 1, sensory disorder around the chin persisted more than 6 months after surgery in all eight patients.

Notes Activity in Asia

In Asia, several organizations, such as the Japan NOTES and Asia Pacific NOTES (APNOTES) working groups, were established, and their respective leaderships have contributed to the development of NOTES [35]. To encourage the responsible development and adoption of NOTES into clinical practice, the Japan Society for Endoscopic Surgery (JSES) and the Japan Gastroenterological Endoscopy Society (JGES) organized Japan NOTES in 2007, following the initiative of the Natural Orifice Surgery Consortium for Assessment and Research (NOSCAR). Japan NOTES published guidelines for NOTES research in Japan, including the nomenclature for NOTES in Japanese, guidelines for animal study, and a central IRB for NOTES studies. Japan NOTES also organizes annual meetings and research grants, and they have developed a registry system for clinical studies. The current list of procedures is outlined in Table 22.2, with a total of seven different procedures having been registered by July 2013. The most frequently performed procedure was POEM (76 %), followed by endoscopy-assisted laparoscopic local resection of the stomach (10 %). EFTR was performed in 34 patients (6 %), transgastric peritoneoscopy in 14 (3 %), transvaginal colectomy in 12 (2 %), transvaginal cholecystectomy in 5 (1 %), and transvaginal appendectomy in 2 (0.4 %).

The APNOTES working group was also established in 2007, and it too organizes yearly meetings. The members have discussed future potential activities and collaboration for the development of NOTES in Asia and have published several review papers on NOTES.

Table 22.2 Cases of human NOTES between February 2008 and July 2013 in the Japan NOTES registry

Procedures	No. of cases
Transgastric peritoneoscopy for cancer staging	14
Transvaginal cholecystectomy	5
Transvaginal appendectomy	2
Transvaginal colectomy	12
Endoscopic full-thickness resection with laparoscopic assistance	34
Endoscopy-assisted laparoscopic surgery	
Appendectomy	2
Cholecystectomy	1
Fundoplication	1
Local resection of the stomach	55
Peroral endoscopic submucosal myotomy	406
Total	532

NOTES is developing in a way that integrates advanced laparoscopic surgery with therapeutic endoscopy skills. Collaboration between surgeons and endoscopists is essential, and Japan NOTES and APNOTES play an important role as a bridge between the surgical and endoscopy societies in Asia.

Summary and Future Perspectives of Notes in Asia

The present number of human NOTES cases in Asia is limited; however, various types of NOTES procedures have been performed. Most of the cases have required laparoscopic assistance through abdominal trocars, but the complication rate has been low. The clinical application of NOTES has been introduced safely not only in Asia but also in other parts of the world.

Advanced therapeutic endoscopy techniques developed in Asia, such as ESD, have led to the development of the original NOTES procedures. These include transgastric submucosal peritoneoscopy, EFTR, and POEM. Several investigators in Asia have performed transgastric peritoneoscopy with the ESD submucosal tunnel technique. The main issue associated with NOTES is still the secure closure of the access site. The submucosal tunnel technique can provide safe closure of the gastric incision site with currently available devices. EFTR is the treatment of choice for selected patients with gastric submucosal tumors. This technique makes it possible to perform en bloc resection of the tumor that is as small as possible while maintaining an adequate surgical margin. The procedure was first applied to human clinical practice in Asia. Although laparoscopic assistance was required due to the limitations of current endoscopic devices, EFTR has been safely performed and has contributed to the prevention of deformity of the stomach after resection. POEM using the ESD technique is currently one of the most promising of the NOTES procedures and has garnered significant interest. A number of institutions in Asia have performed POEM and have reported excellent short-term outcomes.

Japan NOTES and the APNOTES working group have played an important role in developing procedures and technologies for NOTES. The continued study of NOTES will contribute to the advancement of minimally invasive surgery and therapeutic endoscopy for the benefit of many patients.

References

1. Hawes R. ASGE/SAGES working group on natural orifice translumenal endoscopic surgery. Gastrointest Endosc. 2006;63:199–203.
2. Rattner D, Kalloo A. The SAGES/ASGE working group on natural orifice translumenal endoscopic surgery. ASGE/SAGES working group on natural orifice translumenal endoscopic surgery. Surg Endosc. 2006;20:329–33.
3. Flora ED, Wilson TG, Martin IJ, et al. A review of natural orifice translumenal endoscopic surgery (NOTES) for intra-abdominal surgery: experimental models, techniques, and applicability to the clinical setting. Ann Surg. 2008;247:583–602.
4. Kalloo AN, Singh VK, Jagannath SB, et al. Flexible transgastric peritoneoscopy: a novel approach to diagnostic and therapeutic interventions in the peritoneal cavity. Gastrointest Endosc. 2004;60:114–7.
5. Lechmann KS, Ritz JP, Wibmer A, et al. The German registry for natural orifice translumenal endoscopic surgery: report of the first 551 patient. Ann Surg. 2010;252:263–70.
6. Khashab MA, Kalloo AN. NOTES: current status and new horizons. Gastroenterology. 2012;142:704–10.

7. Moris DN, Konstantinos JB, Mantonakis EI, et al. Surgery via natural orifices in human beings: yesterday, today, tomorrow. Am J Surg. 2012;204:93–102.

8. Arezzo A, Zornig C, Mofid H, et al. The EURO-NOTES clinical registry for natural orifice transluminal endoscopic surgery: a 2-year activity report. Surg Endosc. 2013;27(9):3073–84.

9. Rao GV, Reddy DN, Banerjee R. NOTES: human experience. Gastrointest Endosc Clin N Am. 2008;18: 361–70.

10. Palanivelu C, Rajan PS, Rangarajan M, et al. NOTES: transvaginal endoscopic cholecystectomy in humans – preliminary report of a case series. Am J Gastroenterol. 2009;104:843–7.

11. Rudiman R, Wiradisuria E. Initial experience with laparoscopic-assisted transvaginal cholecystectomy: a hybrid approach to natural orifice surgery. Int Surg. 2009;94:258–61.

12. Sohn BS, Kim SR, Park II Y, et al. Transvaginal laparoscopic cholecystectomy (hybrid NOTS cholecystectomy). J Laparoendosc Adv Surg Tech. 2010;20: 245–7.

13. Niu J, Song W, Yan M, et al. Transvaginal laparoscopically assisted endoscopic cholecystectomy: preliminary clinical results for a series of 43 cases in China. Surg Endosc. 2011;25:1281–6.

14. Palanivelu C, Rajan PS, Rangarajan M, et al. Transvaginal endoscopic appendectomy in humans: a unique approach to NOTES – world's first report. Surg Endosc. 2008;22:1343–7.

15. Shin EJ, Jeong GA, Jung JC, et al. Transvaginal endoscopic appendectomy. J Korean Soc Coloproctol. 2010;26:429–32.

16. Kitano S, Yasuda K, Shibata K, et al. Natural orifice translumenal endoscopic surgery for preoperative staging in a pancreatic cancer patient. Dig Endosc. 2008;20:198–202.

17. Lee SH, Kim SJ, Lee TH, et al. Human applications of submucosal endoscopy under conscious sedation for pure natural orifice transluminal endoscopic surgery. Surg Endosc. 2013;27:3016–20.

18. Chen YX, Zeng CY, Shu X, et al. Use of natural orifice translumenal endoscopic surgery in the diagnosis of suspected tuberculosis peritonitis: a retrospective case series of 7 patients. J Laparoendosc Adv Surg Tech. 2013;23:610–6.

19. Nakajima K, Nishida T, Takahashi T, et al. Partial gastrectomy using natural orifice translumenal endoscopic surgery (NOTES) for gastric submucosal tumors: early experience in humans. Surg Endosc. 2009;23:2650–5.

20. Abe N, Takeuchi H, Yanagida O, et al. Endoscopic full-thickness resection with laparoscopic assistance as hybrid NOTES for gastric submucosal tumor. Surg Endosc. 2009;23:1908–13.

21. Mori H, Kobara H, Kobayashi M, et al. Establishment of pure NOTES procedure using a conventional flexible endoscope: review of six cases of gastric gastrointestinal stromal tumors. Endoscopy. 2011;43:631–4.

22. Cho WY, Kim YJ, Cho JY, et al. Hybrid natural orifice transluminal endoscopic surgery: endoscopic full-thickness resection of early gastric cancer and laparoscopic regional lymph node dissection – 14 human cases. Endoscopy. 2011;43:134–9.

23. Inoue H, Minami H, Kobayashi Y, et al. Peroral endoscopic myotomy (POEM) for esophageal achalasia. Endoscopy. 2010;42:265–71.

24. Lee BH, Shim KY, Hong SJ, et al. Peroral endoscopic myotomy for treatment of achalasia: initial results of a Korean study. Clin Endosc. 2013;46:161–7.

25. Minami H, Isomoto H, Yamaguchi N, et al. Peroral endoscopic myotomy for esophageal achalasia: clinical impact of 28 cases. Dig Endosc. 2013;26:43–51.

26. Li QL, Chen WF, Zhou PH, et al. Peroral endoscopic myotomy for the treatment of achalasia: a clinical comparative study of endoscopic full-thickness and circular muscle myotomy. J Am Coll Surg. 2013;217: 442–51.

27. Palanivelu C, Rangarajan M, Jategaonkar PA, et al. An innovative technique for colorectal specimen retrieval: a new era of "natural orifice specimen extraction" (NOSE). Dis Colon Rect. 2008;51:1120–4.

28. Cheung TPP, Cheung HYS, Ng LWC, et al. Hybrid NOTES colectomy for right-sided colonic tumors. Asian J Endosc Surg. 2012;5:46–9.

29. Zou X, Zhang G, Xiao R, et al. Transvaginal natural orifice transluminal endoscopic surgery (NOTES)-assisted laparoscopic adrenalectomy: first clinical experience. Surg Endosc. 2011;25:3767–72.

30. Nakajo A, Arima H, Hirata M, et al. Trans-oral video-assisted neck surgery (TOVANS): a new transoral technique of endoscopic thyroidectomy with gasless premadible approach. Surg Endosc. 2013;27:1105–10.

31. Yoshizumi F, Yasuda K, Kawaguchi K, et al. Submucosal tunneling using endoscopic submucosal dissection for peritoneal access and closure in natural orifice transluminal endoscopic surgery: a porcine survival study. Endoscopy. 2009;41:707–11.

32. Yoshizumi F, Yasuda K, Suzuki K, et al. Feasibility of fibrin glue versus endoclips to close the transgastric peritoneal access site in NOTES in a survival porcine study. Asian J Endosc Surg. 2011;4:73–7.

33. Akagi T, Yasuda K, Kono Y, et al. Safety and efficacy of the submucosal tunnel without mucosal closure for the transgastric approach in a porcine survival model. Surg Innov. 2012;19:415–20.

34. Kono Y, Yasuda K, Hiroishi K, et al. Transrectal peritoneal access with the submucosal tunnel technique in NOTES: a porcine survival study. Surg Endosc. 2013;27:278–85.

35. Kitano S, Tajiri H, Yasuda K, et al. Current status and activity regarding natural orifice translumenal endoscopic surgery (NOTES) in Japan. Asian J Endosc Surg. 2008;1:7–10.

Chad Kawa and Amitabh Chak

Introduction

The movement toward minimally invasive surgery, with smaller incisions, began in 1987 when Dr. Philippe Mouret performed the first laparoscopic cholecystectomy. Since that time, laparoscopic surgeries have spread worldwide and have become routine. The laparoscopic cholecystectomy, in particular, has become a surgery familiar to most, if not all, surgeons and continues to be one of the most commonly performed operations [1]. At the same time, over the past few decades, endoscopic technology and innovation has also advanced at a rapid pace. The introduction of endoscopic ultrasound (EUS) in the 1980s had a major impact on clinical management of digestive diseases. Prior to the development of EUS, endoscopists were limited to the lumen, but the echoendoscope provided a diagnostic tool that allowed visualization of adjacent structures. Soon, endoscopists began to develop therapeutic applications that expanded the endoscopic armamentarium and included, but were not limited to, fine needle aspiration of tumors and nodes, endoscopic drainage of cystic lesions, and nerve blocks.

At the same time that EUS broadened endoscopic therapies beyond the lumen of the digestive tract, endoscopists and surgeons began exploring opportunities to take the endoscope itself beyond the lumen as well. Many of these ideas were derived from the initial concepts that helped conceive the laparoscopic cholecystectomy. At the same time that some endoscopists were looking through the gastrointestinal wall, others were investigating the layers of the wall itself. Mucosal resection and submucosal dissection (ESD) were initially popularized in the Far East, and endoscopists were becoming more comfortable working in the submucosal space. Familiarity with deeper planes of the gastrointestinal layers, improved technology for making endoscopic incisions, and endoscopic accessories for closing mucosal defects eventually led to endoscopists crossing the luminal barrier, and the concept of natural orifice transluminal endoscopic surgery (NOTES) was born.

In 2000, Kalloo and colleagues published the first report describing a transluminal endoscopic procedure [2]. This report truly was the birth of NOTES as an incisionless alternative to other commonly performed surgeries, plus an opportunity to develop novel applications. Since the fledgling reports of NOTES in the early 2000s, continued studies on animal models have led to the more widespread experimentation with NOTES. In 2002, a single transvaginal, as well as a series of hybrid (using a NOTES concept

C. Kawa, M.D. • A. Chak, M.D., F.A.S.G.E. (✉)
Department of Gastroenterology, University Hospitals Case Medical Center, 11100 Euclid Ave, Cleveland, OH 44106, USA
e-mail: Amitabh.Chak@UHhospitals.org

N. Fukami (ed.), *Endoscopic Submucosal Dissection: Principles and Practice*,
DOI 10.1007/978-1-4939-2041-9_23, © Springer Science+Business Media New York 2015

with a transabdominal port for air insufflation) transvaginal, nephrectomies in porcine models was reported [3]. In addition to transvaginal access to the abdominal cavity, access points that were proposed included the bladder, colon, esophagus, and stomach. Many efforts were devoted to the investigation of full-thickness resection and subsequent closure in the stomach, which could lead to developing stable access points for more extensive transluminal operations [4].

Not only is the merger of endoscopy and surgery pushing clinical advancement, but there is undoubtedly increasing pressure from the public and healthcare providers to provide more economical and less invasive ways to perform routine procedures and operations. Shorter hospital stays and postoperative recovery, less pain, and the cosmetic appeal of smaller scars have contributed to the demands for continued development of NOTES [5].

Despite an initial unprecedented enthusiasm for the potential of NOTES, significant obstacles have prevented its widespread application, similar to those experienced with early laparoscopic surgery. There are five major challenges in performing NOTES that have limited its adoption into mainstream surgical practice and training:

1. Controlled and safe incision through the gastrointestinal wall.
2. Thorough inspection of the peritoneal cavity.
3. Stable retraction of peritoneal structures.
4. Dissection of surgical tissue planes and resection of pathological tissues.
5. Secure closure of access port to prevent leak and infection.

Technique

Incision

The rapid development of ESD in Asia has led to advancements in the tools available for the endoscopist. Many of these tools are specifically designed for submucosal dissection, either by

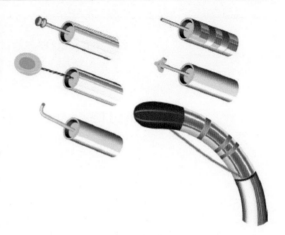

Fig. 23.1 Insulated tip knife, hook knife, flush knife, triangular tip knife, sphincterotome

enabling injection of water into the submucosal space with the dissection knife (Flush-knife, ERBE water jet) or by preventing full-thickness incisions (insulated tip knife) (Fig. 23.1). These cutting tools are also often used for the superficial incision around the planned resection. Some of these, and others, have been utilized in the incisions made during NOTES procedures. Though convenient because they are available and familiar to endoscopists who perform ESD, these tools are less than ideal for making a through and through incision through the bowel wall. Animal studies have described blind incision with a needle knife to gain access, followed by guidewire placement and completion of the incision with a sphincterotome and a snare [6]. Though no adverse effects such as bleeding or adjacent organ injury were reported in this small study, such concerns are warranted in NOTES. The ability to perform a suitable incision while visualizing the intraperitoneal surface of the GI tract may be a limiting factor in NOTES. During animal model experience, pneumoperitoneum must be considered, however it is worth noting that a full-thickness puncture with a needle knife results in an air leak. This may alleviate, at least, the concern for cautery injury to adjacent organs. EUS guidance of incision has also been suggested to increase safety but has not yet been validated or widely accepted.

Peritoneal Inspection

Control of pneumoperitoneum is a particular challenge in NOTES. Controlled insufflation through the endoscope is difficult and can result in wide variations of intraperitoneal pressures and potential for overinflation. Spatial orientation is also an issue, particularly for endoscopists who are not traditionally accustomed to intentionally visualizing the peritoneal cavity. This is likely overcome by familiarity with the procedure and development of controlled insufflation devices that can be used with the endoscope. During intraluminal endoscopy, a wide endoscopic viewing field and use of a distal cap have been utilized for improved visualization. Similar developments may aid inspection during NOTES.

Retraction

Retraction of abdominal organs in the peritoneal cavity is a challenging problem in NOTES. The flexibility of the endoscope complicates retraction. During intraluminal endoscopy the walls of the GI tract provide traction for the scope, which allows stabilization as well as deployment of endoscopic instruments through the scope. The instruments used during endoscopy are also too flexible to be utilized for retraction. The challenges of retraction were initially answered by using rigid equipment; this is an option in transvaginal, transcolonic, and transvesical NOTES. Additionally, utilization of a single transabdominal port has been attempted in what has been termed "hybrid NOTES."

Dissection

Endoscopic dissection is the most time-consuming aspect of ESD. The knives developed for ESD have been specifically designed for ease of dissection. Many of these knives have features that make dissection in the submucosal plane safe, by enabling injection of liquids into the submucosa (water jet function) or preventing full-thickness cautery injury (insulated tip knife).

Many of these knives have been used in NOTES, however similar dissecting challenges exist. In ESD, dissection along the submucosal plane is a challenge, as well as identification of submucosal vessels. With increased user experience, the risk of bleeding during ESD has been shown to decrease. Challenges in identifying vessels, nerves, lymphatics, and other structures are similar during NOTES.

Closure

Closure of the access site is the most studied aspect of NOTES; likely, current endoscopic practice could translate well. There are multiple closure devices on the market, for many different applications, that could work well for intentional closure of the viscera during NOTES, including conventional endoscopic clips, T-tags, T-bars, suturing devices, staplers, and over-the-scope clips (OTSC). These methods could likely all be used equally well, despite the point of access including the esophagus, stomach, colon, or nondigestive organs such as the vagina and bladder. Additionally, standard surgical closure techniques could be considered.

Post-procedure Considerations

There is concern by those investigating NOTES regarding sterilization of instruments and whether there is potential for infectious spillage of gastrointestinal flora through the access ports. Several methods have been proposed for sterilization of endoscopes to prepare them for NOTES. The quickest and cheapest method involves a 0.2 % peracetic acid solution. The longest and most expensive, though most stable, method involves ethylene oxide gas sterilization [7]. Precautions to decontaminate the GI tract have also been attempted, including 24-h preparations using a liquid formula diet, antibiotic irrigation, and systemic antibiotics [8]. Despite theoretical reduction in contamination from the access site by sterilization of the endoscopic tools or reducing flora, other reports have suggested that transgastric access may not result in postoperative infection any more than other procedures/surgeries [9].

Other factors that affect the effectiveness of the operator during NOTES include adequate air insufflation into the abdominal cavity and retraction of adjacent structures and organs. Not only do the instruments developed for NOTES procedures alter visualization, but familiarity with the procedures and adequate training are paramount.

Clinical Applications of Notes

Appendectomy and Cholecystectomy

The human experience with NOTES is somewhat limited; however, it continues to show promise. In 2003, the first NOTES procedure, a transgastric appendectomy, was performed on a human [10]. Multiple other procedures have been performed since that initial appendectomy. The first transluminal cholecystectomy was performed in France using a similar procedure, followed shortly thereafter in Italy and Brazil [11]. Transgastric rescue of a dislodged gastrostomy tube through the previous gastrostomy site was initially described in 2007 and continues to be used by those who initially described the procedure as an alternative to surgical rescue of prematurely dislodged gastrostomy tube [12]. Over 4,000 transvaginal NOTES have been reported, making the transvaginal approach the most commonly used for NOTES to date. Few complications have been reported and selected centers are commonly using a transvaginal approach as the standard procedure for cholecystectomy [13]. Limitations obviously include exclusive use in females and public concern regarding injury to adjacent structures.

In general, the inability to close NOTES incisions securely and challenges with organ retraction during surgery make procedures such as appendectomies and cholecystectomies difficult to perform. It is also not evident that a NOTES approach offers any advantage over a standard laparoscopic appendectomy or cholecystectomy. Thus, the initial enthusiasm for adopting NOTES has been tempered, and these procedures have not gained widespread acceptance. However, the NOTES movement, along with the development of ESD, has given rise to two procedures—per oral endoscopic myotomy (POEM) and endoscopic full thickness resection (EFTR)—that are beginning to gain clinical acceptance.

Per Oral Endoscopic Myotomy (POEM)

At the current time, the most common extraluminal procedure being both discussed and performed by endoscopists may be the peroral endoscopic myotomy (POEM). This technique most commonly uses a submucosal tunneling technique in the esophagus for the treatment of achalasia, which was previously only possible by surgical myotomy. Initially described in Japan, the procedure is now becoming more common in the United States as a minimally invasive alternative to the Heller myotomy.

Endoscopic Full-Thickness Resection (EFTR)

Full-thickness resection may be a reasonable treatment option to improve upon piecemeal resection. Pathologic assessment is vastly improved with full-thickness resection since the resection margin and depth of invasion are easily assessed. During the past decade, a large amount of research has been conducted on full-thickness resection. Such resection is performed by pulling the wall of the bowel toward the lumen, making the cut, and closing the defect. Many different techniques have been described. The wall can either be grasped or suctioned to provide traction. The incision can be made by a variety of instruments. Most of the cutting instruments have historically been designed for other applications, such as for ESD or sphincterotomy. A loop snare can also be used. Closure is typically performed by using a suture device or clips. Techniques for full-thickness resection will continue to improve and evolve as procedure-specific instruments are developed.

The increasing number of POEM procedures and EFTRs, as well as a growing body of data on other NOTES procedures, indicates that these procedures will quite possibly become common practice for endoscopists, both surgical and non-surgical alike. Despite the increasing number of procedures being performed, there continues to exist many limitations preventing more mainstream adoption of NOTES in clinical practice throughout the United States. Prevention of iatrogenic infection due to contamination, adequate control of air insufflation, development of dedicated NOTES instruments, and training of physicians remain significant limitations to more widespread dissemination of NOTES. Patient requests for less pain, less invasive surgery, and shorter postoperative stays are significant motivators for further development of NOTES. The rapid integration of laparoscopic surgery and the development of ESD are encouraging indicators that NOTES is a technique that will become a standard replacement for more invasive surgeries. Laparoscopic surgery has become a common procedure, taught to almost every surgical resident, and the rapid development of laparoscopic surgical tools have made the procedures safe and quick. Through skills obtained by endoscopists via ESD, including familiarity with the submucosal space, NOTES could become a less daunting undertaking for some endoscopists. It remains to be seen how quickly NOTES will enter into mainstream use for such surgeries as cholecystectomy or appendectomy, but the increasing volume of reports using NOTES and continued investigational studies indicate that NOTES will remain a possibility for endoscopists worldwide.

References

1. Spaner SJ, Warnock GL. A brief history of endoscopy, laparoscopy, and laparoscopic surgery. J Laparoendosc Adv Surg Tech A. 1997;7:369–73.
2. Kalloo AN, Kantsevoy SV, Singh VK, et al. Flexible transgastric peritoneoscopy: a novel approach to diagnostic and therapeutic interventions in the peritoneal cavity. Gastroenterology. 2000;118:A1039.
3. Gettman MT, Lotan Y, Napper CA, Cadeddu JA. Transvaginal laparoscopic nephrectomy development and feasibility in the porcine model. Urology. 2002;59:446–50.
4. Ikeda K, Fritscher-Ravens A, Mosse CA, Mills T, Tajiri H, Swain CP. Endoscopic full-thickness resection with sutured closure in a pig model. Gastrointest Endosc. 2005;62:122–9.
5. Moreira-Pinto J, Lima E, Correia-Pinto J, Rolanda C. Natural orifice transluminal endoscopy surgery: a review. World J Gastroenterol. 2011;17(33):3795–801.
6. Ikeda K, Mosse A, Park PO, Fristcher-Ravens A, Bergstrom M, Mills T, Tajiji H, Swain SP. Endoscopic full-thickness resection: circumferential cutting method. Gastrointest Endosc. 2006;41:82–9.
7. Spaun GO, Goers TA, Pierce RA, Cassera MA, Scovil S, Swanstrom LL. Use of flexible endoscopes for NOTES: sterilization or high-level disinfection? Surg Endosc. 2009;70:1137–45.
8. Shafi BM, Mery CM, Binyamin G, Dutta S. Natural orifice translumenal endoscopic surgery (NOTES). Semin Pediatr Surg. 2006;15:251–8.
9. Narula VK, Hazey JW, Renton DB, Reavis KM, Paul CM, Hinshaw KE, Needleman BJ, Mikami DJ, Ellison EC, Melvin WS. Transgastric instrumentation and bacterial contamination of the peritoneal cavity. Surg Endosc. 2008;22:605–11.
10. Rao GV, Reddy DN. Transgastric appendectomy in humans. Montreal: World Congress of Gastroenterology; 2006.
11. Marescaux J, Dallemagne B, Perretta S, Wattiez A, Mutter D, Coumaros D. Surgery without scars: report of transluminal cholecystectomy in a human being. Arch Surg. 2007;142:823–6.
12. Marks JM, Ponsky JL, Pearl JP, McGee MF. PEG "Rescue": a practical NOTES technique. Surg Endosc. 2007;21:816–9.
13. Khashab MA, Kalloo AN. NOTES: current status and new horizons. Gastroenterology. 2012;142:704–10.

Part VII

Dissemination of ESD

ESD Training in the East

24

Takuji Gotoda and Peter V. Draganov

Introduction

Endoscopic submucosal dissection (ESD) was developed in Japan in the late 1990s for endoscopic removal of early gastric cancers [1–5]. ESD yields a higher complete resection rate, regardless of size, as compared with standard endoscopic mucosal resection (EMR). In the West, EMR remains, of course, the most used approach for treating neoplastic lesions and early cancers [6–9]. While in Japan, ESD has become the standard therapeutic modality for superficial tumors in both the upper and lower gastrointestinal tract [3]. It has recently been considered that ESD has brought a renaissance of therapeutic endoscopy [10], as it is able to offer organ-sparing cures for patients with early gastrointestinal cancers [11].

ESD has been a significant advance in therapeutic endoscopy with its major advantages of being able to carry out higher en bloc resection allowing accurate histological evaluation and lower local recurrence rates [3, 12–14]. It is especially outstanding that ESD enables en bloc resection of previously unresectable lesions, such as large mucosal tumors, tumors with submucosal fibrosis, or recurrent and residual tumors [15, 16]. Despite its obvious advantages, ESD is one of the most complex endoscopic procedures, with a high level of technical difficulties and high complication rates, especially in the beginning of the learning curve [17–19]. The most frequent complications are bleeding and perforation [9, 20, 21].

Nowadays in Japan, ESD is routinely performed in many institutions, including local branch hospitals. On the other hand, in the West, ESD is still largely not available and is done only in a handful of centers by few advanced therapeutic endoscopy enthusiasts. The main obstacle for the wide availability of ESD in the West has been, and remains, the very flat learning curve and lack of training resources [22]. Recently, it became obvious that more endoscopists are and will be interested in acquiring this technique. It has been anticipated that the widespread adaptation of ESD for the treatment of superficial gastrointestinal neoplasia will require major shifts in training and practice culture [23]. Thus, the current state of training for ESD will be reviewed in this chapter. For the benefit of our patients, it is key to enhance trainee experience and to reduce the risks of procedure-related complications and inadequate treatment.

Takuji Gotoda provided the concept of the article, did the literature search and wrote the first draft of the manuscript. Peter V. Draganov provided critical review of the article.

T. Gotoda, M.D., Ph.D., F.A.S.G.E. (✉)
Department of Gastroenterology and Hepatology,
Tokyo Medical University, 6-7-1 Nishi-Shinjuku,
Shinjuku-ku, Tokyo 160-0023, Japan
e-mail: takujigotoda@yahoo.co.jp

P.V. Draganov, M.D., F.A.S.G.E.
Division of Gastroenterology, Hepatology and
Nutrition, University of Florida, Gainesville, FL, USA
e-mail: Peter.Draganov@medicine.ufl.edu

N. Fukami (ed.), *Endoscopic Submucosal Dissection: Principles and Practice*,
DOI 10.1007/978-1-4939-2041-9_24, © Springer Science+Business Media New York 2015

229

ESD Learning Curve for Gastric Lesions

Several reports have analyzed the learning curve for ESD in the stomach. Choi et al. investigated the learning curve for ESD and reported an increase in the en bloc resection rate from 45 to 85 % after experience of 40 cases [24]. They concluded that trainees need to perform 20–40 procedures to be able to use the technique effectively. Kakushima et al. estimated that a trainee could begin to treat lesions in the lower part of the stomach independently after performing about 30 supervised ESD procedures [11]. Gotoda et al. found that experience of at least 30 cases is required for a beginner to gain early proficiency in this technique [25].

In a more recent study, two out of three operators could not achieve a sufficient self-completion rate for submucosal dissection after 30 cases [26]. However, in this study, the trainees performed the ESD under the supervision of an experienced endoscopist but their training did not include hands-on training on animal models, which might have improved the learning curve. A study conducted by the same group, in 2012, showed that the trainees required approximately 40 and 80 cases for successful removal of early gastric lesions by ESD [27]. The procedural outcomes of ESD performed by preceptors who had experience in over 80 cases were similar to those by expert endoscopists. Thus, the minimal amount of training for achieving proficiency in ESD might require the performance of at least 80 procedures. Tsuji et al. concluded that the training system at their institution enabled trainees to perform gastric ESD without decline in clinical outcomes, although 30 procedures were not enough for them to perform all gastric ESDs independently without expert supervision, as expert assistance was still needed in 20 % of their ESD cases [28]. Oda et al. used procedure time as an indicator of ESD proficiency and determined that 30 cases was the learning curve point to acquire the basic technical skills of ESD in the lower third of the stomach [29]. In their estimation, performing at least 40 ESDs would be the minimum learning curve point before starting to perform ESD in the middle and upper thirds of the stomach.

ESD Learning Curve for Extra-gastric Lesions

Recent studies showed high cure rates in the esophagus and colon, with less complications, in ESDs performed by experienced endoscopists [30–33]. A meta-analysis indicates that ESD is the best minimally invasive endoscopic technique and an important alternative to surgery in the treatment of large (>2 cm) sessile and flat polyps, because it allows complete assessment of pathological staging in most patients [34].

Although most learning curve studies and training strategies have been studied and developed for gastric ESD, the increased use of ESD in extra-gastric sites created a demand for further studies [9, 35–42]. In Japan, endoscopists generally experience antrum ESD first, because of the high incidence of gastric neoplasms and the relative ease of ESD in this location [27]. These conditions allow for the opportunity to acquire sufficient manipulation while performing ESD. However, esophageal and colonic ESD present even more challenging difficulties and higher risk of severe complications. That is, the training for esophageal and colonic ESD is now a crucial issue even in Japan.

Dinis-Ribeiro et al. suggested that lesions located in proximal sites in the stomach, esophagus, and colon should be recommended only after performing 20–40 ESD procedures in the distal stomach [43]. Hotta et al. reported that performance of 40 procedures was sufficient to avoid causing perforation during the procedure on the learning curve for colonic ESD [44]. Sakamoto et al. proposed that trainees can perform colorectal ESD safely and independently after preparatory training and experience with more than 30 cases [45].

A small number of analyses conducted in an earlier Japanese multicenter study indicated a higher complication rate during colorectal ESD and that standardization of the colorectal ESD procedure would be difficult [46]. Despite greater risks of intra- and post-procedural complications, many endoscopists are making an effort to improve this novel technique in terms of its capability of large margin-free resection that will lower local recurrence rates.

Despite the significant efforts at establishment of a learning curve for acquiring ESD skills, in Japan, skills are still acquired in the traditional apprenticeship model of training in endoscopy: "see one, do one, teach one." There has been a recognized need for such a structured training system for ESD [11].

ESD Training Systems

Although no universally accepted algorithm for training in ESD has yet been established, a consensus on some key points has been considered. The minimal requirements and final attainments for trainees at each level must be established prior to the beginning of training [28].

As expected, most well-implemented training programs/algorithms are in Japan. These algorithms typically include two major stages of training: pre-procedural theoretic preparation and hands-on training [23, 26–29]. The first stage has two phases: phase 1—accumulation of basic knowledge and phase 2—observe experts in action. The second stage includes phase 3—assist experts performing the procedure, phase 4—work on simulator models, such as ex vivo and in vivo animal models, or synthetic models of the organ of interest, and phase 5—perform ESD procedures under expert supervision (Fig. 24.1).

One of the earliest proposed training algorithms by Yamamoto et al. in 2009 puts emphasis on the initial pre-procedural phase of the training [26]. Thus, the endoscopists who intended to start ESD must attend pre- and post-treatment conferences including gastroenterologists, surgeons, and pathologists, in order to learn how to diagnose the extent and depth of the tumor, establish the optimum treatment strategy, and manage the

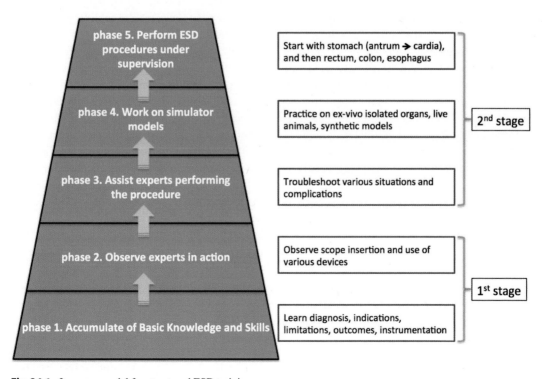

Fig. 24.1 Japanese model for structured ESD training

patients appropriately through the pathological staging. To improve R0 resection rates, that is by making marking dots correctly around the tumor boarder, the pre-procedural training to master detailed preoperative examination by magnifying endoscopy with narrow band imaging (NBI) is clinically essential [27]. A similar approach is proposed by Kaltenbach et al., where the trainees are assisted in developing crucial diagnostic skills to select appropriate lesions and in practicing specific management strategies for ESD cases [23].

The next phase is for trainees to observe various ESD procedures performed by expert endoscopists [29]. ESD is a technically demanding procedure, requiring a high level of endoscopic skill. Also, the trainees take part in actual ESD procedures for at least 1 year before beginning to do ESD. Trainees acquire the skills needed to troubleshoot various situations. Obtaining expertise in endoscopic hemostasis is especially key, since most of the difficulties surrounding the procedure are related to uncontrollable hemorrhage [26].

Consequently, in the second stage of training, the trainees start by assisting experts in performing ESD procedures. Next, the trainees are exposed to animal models to enhance their technical skills. Hands-on experience with ESD in the isolated porcine stomach or live porcine facilitates familiarity with the devices and techniques of ESD procedure. Trainees can appreciate the differences in technique depending on lesion size and location. Then, trainees typically start performing ESD in patients, initially removing small gastric lesions in the antrum (maybe on anterior wall or greater curve) or body (especially on lesser curve), under the supervision of experienced endoscopists who both offers suitable and valid advice and may have to rescue the remaining procedure, like a "closer," if necessary [23, 29]. Yamamoto et al. propose a system where the trainees do not use animal models but start as assistants in live patient cases and then continue with performing ESD on patients under expert supervision [26]. For this reason, they recommend that in this "supervision-only" training algorithm, one should start with small lesions in the lower third of the stomach (antrum). These lesions are relatively easy and less time-consuming to remove, so the trainees have the opportunity to learn the entire ESD procedure.

Ohata et al. propose a 7-step training system for learning colorectal ESD, which is very similar to the training algorithms used for gastric ESD, however impose complicated manipulations by performing the procedure in a narrower space and thinner wall [47]. One of the mandatory enrollment criteria is performance of at least 30 gastric ESDs. The results suggest that trainees with relatively little prior experience with gastric ESD could reach a stable level of technical competency in colorectal ESD after an average of 30 cases of the latter procedure. The study also found that, regardless of the gastric ESD experience, the mean procedure time of each trainee became less than 80 min after performing more than 30 cases.

The essential step of the training can be accomplished through independent effort, using printed and video materials to learn about the procedure, indication, and diagnosis. Then, the endoscopists attend live presentations and enroll in hands-on training courses to learn about the use of various devices and to practice on animal models. After accumulation of this theoretical and practical fund of knowledge, a visit to an expert center to observe the experts' technique is recommended. Most of these centers are, unfortunately, located in Japan. There are very few cases of early gastric cancer in other countries, therefore little opportunity for the trainee to start their training in locations that are considered easier, such as the gastric antrum. [26, 48, 49]. In addition, the choice of devices, endoscopes, and ancillary equipment for ESD that is available in the West is different compared with those available in Japan [50]. However, with more endoscopists learning this technique, it is anticipated that new training centers are already and will be conducted throughout the world. It is understood that not all endoscopists can spend long periods of time outside their practice; however, trainees are encouraged to spend at least 2–3 weeks visiting a high volume center, maybe in Japan. Upon return to their center, when working on human patients, the lesions located in the distal stomach or rectum, as these are relatively easier to remove and have a lower complication rate, might be good candidates. During the initial human cases, expert supervision by means of videoconference is encouraged if direct supervision is not possible.

Then, gradually, the endoscopists can expand to cases of increasing difficulty, such as treating larger lesions, or lesions located in the cardia, fundus, colon, or esophagus. Finally, as in any other field, we recommend continuous training, with attending/presenting at conferences, revisiting expert centers, reviewing literature, and participating in courses and live demonstrations.

In summary, in Japan, a consensus exists on the following issues: (phase 1) need for solid cognitive background regarding lesion evaluation, indications, contraindications, and technical aspects of ESD; (phase 2) need for observation of ESD as done by experts; (phase 3) need to assist experts and operate the ESD devices; (phase 4) need for hands-on training in humans under direct expert supervision; and (phase 5) starting hands-on training with easier lesions before progressing to more difficult ones.

Conclusions

ESD represents an evolutionary step as a new therapeutic concept in the endoscopic sphere, that is, ESD allows achievement of high rates of en bloc curative resection and has facilitated the development of new devices and peripherals. However, the learning process of this advanced endoscopic procedure requires a lengthy training period and considerable experience to become proficient. A well-structured training program that is safe, effective, and easily reproducible is essential for the trainee, because the outcome of ESD is highly dependent on the experience of the endoscopist. It is also recommended that training programs be tailored around specific needs based on culture and/or country, since the incidence of disease and working environment may be different.

References

1. Ono H, Kondo H, Gotoda T, Shirao K, Yamaguchi H, Saito D, Hosokawa K, Shimoda T, Yoshida S. Endoscopic mucosal resection for treatment of early gastric cancer. Gut. 2001;48:225–9 [PMID: 11156645].
2. Ohkuwa M, Hosokawa K, Boku N, Ohtu A, Tajiri H, Yoshida S. New endoscopic treatment for intramucosal gastric tumors using an insulated-tip diathermic knife. Endoscopy. 2001;33:221–6 [PMID: 11293753, doi:10.1055/s-2001-12805].
3. Tanaka M, Ono H, Hasuike N, Takizawa K. Endoscopic submucosal dissection of early gastric cancer. Digestion. 2008;77 Suppl 1:23–8 [PMID: 18204258, doi:10.1159/000111484].
4. Kato M, Nishida T, Tsutsui S, Komori M, Michida T, Yamamoto K, Kawai N, Kitamura S, Zushi S, Nishihara A, Nakanishi F, Kinoshita K, Yamada T, Iijima H, Tsujii M, Hayashi N. Endoscopic submucosal dissection as a treatment for gastric noninvasive neoplasia: a multicenter study by Osaka University ESD Study Group. J Gastroenterol. 2011;46:325–31 [PMID: 21107615, doi:10.1007/s00535-010-0350-1].
5. Gotoda T, Jung HY. Endoscopic resection (endoscopic mucosal resection/endoscopic submucosal dissection) for early gastric cancer. Dig Endosc. 2013;25 Suppl 1:55–63 [PMID: 23362925, doi:10.1111/den.12003].
6. Watanabe K, Ogata S, Kawazoe S, Watanabe K, Koyama T, Kajiwara T, Shimoda Y, Takase Y, Irie K, Mizuguchi M, Tsunada S, Iwakiri R, Fujimoto K. Clinical outcomes of EMR for gastric tumors: historical pilot evaluation between endoscopic submucosal dissection and conventional mucosal resection. Gastrointest Endosc. 2006;63:776–82 [PMID: 16650537, doi:10.1016/j.gie.2005.08.049].
7. Oka S, Tanaka S, Kaneko I, Mouri R, Hirata M, Kanao H, Kawamura T, Yoshida S, Yoshihara M, Chayama K. Endoscopic submucosal dissection for residual/local recurrence of early gastric cancer after endoscopic mucosal resection. Endoscopy. 2006;38:996–1000 [PMID: 17058164, doi:10.1055/s-2006-944780].
8. Saito Y, Uraoka T, Yamaguchi Y, Hotta K, Sakamoto N, Ikematsu H, Fukuzawa M, Kobayashi N, Nasu J, Michida T, Yoshida S, Ikehara H, Otake Y, Nakajima T, Matsuda T, Saito D. A prospective, multicenter study of 1111 colorectal endoscopic submucosal dissections (with video). Gastrointest Endosc. 2010;72:1217–25 [PMID: 21030017, doi:10.1016/j.gie.2010.08.004].
9. Kobayashi N, Yoshitake N, Hirahara Y, Konishi J, Saito Y, Matsuda T, Ishikawa T, Sekiguchi R, Fujimori T. Matched case-control study comparing endoscopic submucosal dissection and endoscopic mucosal resection for colorectal tumors. J Gastroenterol Hepatol. 2012;27:728–33 [PMID: 22004124, doi:10.1111/j.1440-1746.2011.06942.x].
10. Kwon CI. Endoscopic submucosal dissection (ESD) training and performing ESD with accurate and safe techniques. Clin Endosc. 2012;45:347–9 [PMID: 23251880, doi:10.5946/ce.2012.45.4.347].
11. Kakushima N, Fujishiro M, Kodashima S, Muraki Y, Tateishi A, Omata M. A learning curve for endoscopic submucosal dissection of gastric epithelial neoplasms. Endoscopy. 2006;38:991–5 [PMID: 17058163, doi:10.1055/s-2006-944808].
12. Uraoka T, Parra-Blanco A, Yahagi N. Colorectal endoscopic submucosal dissection in Japan and Western countries. Dig Endosc. 2012;24 Suppl 1:80–3 [PMID: 22533758, doi:10.1111/j.1443-1661.2012.01279.x].
13. Toyokawa T, Fujita I, Morikawa T, Okamoto A, Miyasaka R, Watanabe K, Horii J, Gobaru M, Terao M, Murakami T, Tomoda J. Clinical outcomes of ESD

for early gastric neoplasms in elderly patients. Eur J Clin Invest. 2011;41:474–8 [PMID: 21128933, doi:10.1111/j.1365-2362.2010.02428.x].

14. Cao Y, Liao C, Tan A, Gao Y, Mo Z, Gao F. Meta-analysis of endoscopic submucosal dissection versus endoscopic mucosal resection for tumors of the gastrointestinal tract. Endoscopy. 2009;41:751–7 [PMID: 19693750, doi:10.1055/s-0029-1215053].

15. Takeuchi Y, Uedo N, Iishi H, Yamamoto S, Yamamoto S, Yamada T, Higashino K, Ishihara R, Tatsuta M, Ishiguro S. Endoscopic submucosal dissection with insulated-tip knife for large mucosal early gastric cancer: a feasibility study (with videos). Gastrointest Endosc. 2007;66:186–93 [PMID: 17591498, doi:10.1016/j.gie.2007.03.1059].

16. Yokoi C, Gotoda T, Hamanaka H, Oda I. Endoscopic submucosal dissection allows curative resection of locally recurrent early gastric cancer after prior endoscopic mucosal resection. Gastrointest Endosc. 2006;64:212–8 [PMID: 16860071, doi:10.1016/j.gie.2005.10.038].

17. Oda I, Suzuki H, Nonaka S, Yoshinaga S. Complications of gastric endoscopic submucosal dissection. Dig Endosc. 2013;78:63–72 [PMID: 23368986, doi:10.1111/j.1443-1661.2012.01376.x].

18. Berr F, Ponchon T, Neureiter D, Kiesslich T, Haringsma J, Kaehler GF, Schmoll F, Messmann H, Yahagi N, Oyama T. Experimental endoscopic submucosal dissection training in a porcine model: learning experience of skilled Western endoscopists. Dig Endosc. 2011;23:281–9 [PMID: 21951087, doi:10.1111/j.1443-1661.2011.01129.x].

19. Toyonaga T, Man IM, East JE, Nishino E, Ono W, Hirooka T, Ueda C, Iwata Y, Sugiyama T, Dozaiku T, Hirooka T, Fujita T, Inokuchi H, Azuma T. 1,635 Endoscopic submucosal dissection cases in the esophagus, stomach, and colorectum: complication rates and long-term outcomes. Surg Endosc. 2013;27:1000–8 [PMID: 23052530, doi:10.1007/s00464-012-2555-2].

20. Oda I, Gotoda T, Hamanaka H, Eguchi T, Saito Y, Matsuda T, Bhandari P, Emura F, Saito D, Ono H. Endoscopic submucosal dissection for early gastric cancer: technical feasibility, operation time and complications from a large consecutive series. Dig Endosc. 2005;17:54–8 [doi:10.1111/j.1443-1661.2005.00459.x].

21. Sugimoto T, Okamoto M, Mitsuno Y, Kondo S, Ogura K, Ohmae T, Mizuno H, Yoshida S, Isomura Y, Yamaji Y, Kawabe T, Omata M, Koike K. Endoscopic submucosal dissection is an effective and safe therapy for early gastric neoplasms: a multicenter feasible study. J Clin Gastroenterol. 2012;46:124–9 [PMID: 21959325, doi:10.1097/MCG.0b013e31822f3988].

22. Deprez PH, Bergman JJ, Meisner S, Ponchon T, Repici A, Dinis-Ribeiro M, Haringsma J. Current practice with endoscopic submucosal dissection in Europe: position statement from a panel of experts. Endoscopy. 2010;42:853–8 [PMID: 20623442, doi:10.1055/s-0030-1255563].

23. Kaltenbach T, Soetikno R, Kusano C, Gotoda T. Development of expertise in endoscopic mucosal resection and endoscopic submucosal dissection. Tech Gastrointest Endosc. 2011;13:100–4 [doi:10.1016/j.tgie.2011.01.013].

24. Choi IJ, Kim CG, Chang HJ, Kim SG, Kook MC, Bae JM. The learning curve for EMR with circumferential mucosal incision in treating intramucosal gastric neoplasm. Gastrointest Endosc. 2005;62:860–5 [PMID: 16301026, doi:10.1016/j.gie.2005.04.033].

25. Gotoda T, Friedland S, Hamanaka H, Soetikno R. A learning curve for advanced endoscopic resection. Gastrointest Endosc. 2005;62:866–7 [PMID: 16301027, doi:10.1016/j.gie.2005.07.055].

26. Yamamoto S, Uedo N, Ishihara R, Kajimoto N, Ogiyama H, Fukushima Y, Yamamoto S, Takeuchi Y, Higashino K, Iishi H, Tatsuta M. Endoscopic submucosal dissection for early gastric cancer performed by supervised residents: assessment of feasibility and learning curve. Endoscopy. 2009;41:923–8 [PMID: 19802773, doi:10.1055/s-0029-1215129].

27. Yamamoto Y, Fujisaki J, Ishiyama A, Hirasawa T, Igarashi M. Current status of training for endoscopic submucosal dissection for gastric epithelial neoplasm at Cancer Institute Hospital, Japanese Foundation for Cancer Research, a famous Japanese hospital. Dig Endosc. 2012;24 Suppl 1:148–53 [PMID: 22533772, doi: 10.1111/j.1443-1661.2012.01278.x].

28. Tsuji Y, Ohata K, Sekiguchi M, Ito T, Chiba H, Gunji T, Yamamichi N, Fujishiro M, Matsuhashi N, Koike K. An effective training system for endoscopic submucosal dissection of gastric neoplasm. Endoscopy. 2011;43:1033–8 [PMID: 22135195, doi:10.1055/s-0031-1291383].

29. Oda I, Odagaki T, Suzuki H, Nonaka S, Yoshinaga S. Learning curve for endoscopic submucosal dissection of early gastric cancer based on trainee experience. Dig Endosc. 2012;24 Suppl 1:129–32 [PMID: 22533768, doi:10.1111/j.1443-1661.2012.01265.x].

30. Hurlstone DP, Atkinson R, Sanders DS, Thomson M, Cross SS, Brown S. Achieving R0 resection in the colorectum using endoscopic submucosal dissection. Br J Surg. 2007;94:1536–42 [PMID: 17948864, doi:10.1002/bjs.5720].

31. Honda K, Akiho H. Endoscopic submucosal dissection for superficial esophageal squamous cell neoplasms. World J Gastrointest Pathophysiol. 2012;3:44–50 [PMID: 22532931, doi:10.4291/wjgp.v3.i2.44].

32. Tamegai Y, Saito Y, Masaki N, Hinohara C, Oshima T, Kogure E, Liu Y, Uemura N, Saito K. Endoscopic submucosal dissection: a safe technique for colorectal tumors. Endoscopy. 2007;39:418–22 [PMID: 17516348, doi:10.1055/s-2007-966427].

33. Zhou PH, Yao LQ, Qin XY. Endoscopic submucosal dissection for colorectal epithelial neoplasm. Surg Endosc. 2009;23:1546–51 [PMID: 19263116, doi:10.1007/s00464-009-0395-5].

34. Puli SR, Kakugawa Y, Saito Y, Antillon D, Gotoda T, Antillon MR. Successful complete cure en bloc resection of large nonpedunculated colonic polyps by

endoscopic submucosal dissection: a meta-analysis and systematic review. Ann Surg Oncol. 2009;16:2147–51 [PMID: 19479308, doi:10.1245/s10434-009-0520-7].

35. Kobayashi N, Saito Y, Uraoka T, Matsuda T, Suzuki H, Fujii T. Treatment strategy for laterally spreading tumors in Japan: before and after the introduction of endoscopic submucosal dissection. J Gastroenterol Hepatol. 2009;24:1387–92 [PMID: 19702907, doi:10.1111/j.1440-1746.2009.05893.x].

36. Fujishiro M, Kodashima S, Goto O, Ono S, Niimi K, Yamamichi N, Oka M, Ichinose M, Omata M. Endoscopic submucosal dissection for esophageal squamous cell neoplasms. Dig Endosc. 2009;21:109–15[PMID:19691785,doi:10.1111/j.1443-1661.2009.00837.x].

37. Uraoka T, Saito Y, Matsuda T, Ikehara H, Gotoda T, Saito D, Fujii T. Endoscopic indications for endoscopic mucosal resection of laterally spreading tumours in the colorectum. Gut. 2006;55:1592–7 [PMID: 16682427, doi:10.1136/gut.2005.087452].

38. Uraoka T, Kawahara Y, Kato J, Saito Y, Yamamoto K. Endoscopic submucosal dissection in the colorectum: present status and future prospects. Dig Endosc. 2009;21 Suppl 1:S13–6 [PMID: 19691725, doi:10.1111/j.1443-1661.2009.00863.x].

39. Saito Y, Fukuzawa M, Matsuda T, Fukunaga S, Sakamoto T, Uraoka T, Nakajima T, Ikehara H, Fu KI, Itoi T, Fujii T. Clinical outcome of endoscopic submucosal dissection versus endoscopic mucosal resection of large colorectal tumors as determined by curative resection. Surg Endosc. 2010;24:343–52 [PMID: 19517168, doi:10.1007/s00464-009-0562-8].

40. Oyama T, Tomori A, Hotta K, Morita S, Kominato K, Tanaka M, Miyata Y. Endoscopic submucosal dissection of early esophageal cancer. Clin Gastroenterol Hepatol. 2005;3:S67–70 [PMID: 16013002].

41. Iacopini F, Bella A, Costamagna G, Gotoda T, Saito Y, Elisei W, Grossi C, Rigato P, Scozzarro A. Stepwise training in rectal and colonic endoscopic submucosal dissection with differentiated learning curves. Gastrointest Endosc. 2012;76:1188–96 [PMID: 23062760, doi:10.1016/j.gie.2012.08.024].

42. Repici A, Hassan C, De Pessoa Paula D, Pagano N, Arezzo A, Zullo A, Lorenzetti R, Marmo R. Efficacy and safety of endoscopic submucosal dissection for colorectal neoplasia: a systematic review. Endoscopy. 2012;44:137–50[PMID:22271024,doi:10.1055/s-0031-1291448].

43. Dinis-Ribeiro M, Pimentel-Nunes P, Afonso M, Costa N, Lopes C, Moreira-Dias L. A European case series of endoscopic submucosal dissection for gastric superficial lesions. Gastrointest Endosc. 2009;69:350–5 [doi:10.1016/j.gie.2008.08.035].

44. Hotta K, Oyama T, Shinohara T, Miyata Y, Takahashi A, Kitamura Y, Tomori A. Learning curve for endoscopic submucosal dissection of large colorectal tumors. Dig Endosc. 2010;22:302–6 [PMID: 21175483, doi:10.1111/j.1443-1661.2010.01005.x].

45. Sakamoto T, Saito Y, Fukunaga S, Nakajima T, Matsuda T. Learning curve associated with colorectal endoscopic submucosal dissection for endoscopists experienced in gastric endoscopic submucosal dissection. Dis Colon Rectum. 2011;54:1307–12 [PMID: 21904147, doi:10.1097/DCR.0b013e3182282ab0].

46. Taku K, Sano Y, Fu KI, Saito Y, Matsuda T, Uraoka T, Yoshino T, Yamaguchi Y, Fujita M, Hattori S, Ishikawa T, Saito D, Fujii T, Kaneko E, Yoshida S. Iatrogenic perforation associated with therapeutic colonoscopy: a multicenter study in Japan. J Gastroenterol Hepatol. 2007;22:1409–14[PMID:17593224,doi:10.1111/j.1440-1746.2007.05022.x].

47. Ohata K, Ito T, Chiba H, Tsuji Y, Matsuhashi N. Effective training system in colorectal endoscopic submucosal dissection. Dig Endosc. 2012;24 Suppl 1:84–9 [PMID: 22533759, doi:10.1111/j.1443-1661.2012.01272.x].

48. Bergman JJ. How to justify endoscopic submucosal dissection in the Western world. Endoscopy. 2009;41:988–90[PMID:19866397,doi:10.1055/s-0029-1215247].

49. Gotoda T, Yamamoto H, Soetikno RM. Endoscopic submucosal dissection of early gastric cancer. J Gastroenterol. 2006;41:929–42 [PMID: 17096062, doi:10.1007/s00535-006-1954-3].

50. Conlin A, Kaltenbach T, Kusano C, Matsuda T, Oda I, Gotoda T. Endoscopic resection of gastrointestinal lesions: advancement in the application of endoscopic submucosal dissection. J Gastroenterol Hepatol. 2009;25:1348–57 [doi:10.1111/j.1440-1746.2010.06402.x].

Endoscopic Submucosal Dissection Training in Western Countries

25

Adolfo Parra-Blanco, Vitor Arantes,
Nicolás González, Alberto Herreros de Tejada,
and Andrés Donoso

Introduction

This chapter has been included because there are major differences between Japan, and to a lesser extent South Korea, and western countries in the application of endoscopic submucosal dissection (ESD). Among the differences is the fact that for decades special consideration has been given in Japan to early flat neoplastic lesions in the digestive tract, which forms an important part of their macroscopic classifications. As well, endoscopic mucosal resection (EMR), only now considered standard in western countries, has been applied in Japan for many years (especially before the advent of ESD). Staining and digital chromoendoscopy, and magnification endoscopy for the detailed diagnosis of early neoplasms, are part of the basic knowledge of endoscopists in Japan, while in western countries even traditional chromoendoscopy has not yet been fully adopted. For example, while ESD was being developed in Japan, the importance of flat colorectal lesions was still debated in western countries and EMR was still not routinely performed in many endoscopy units. In effect, Japan and to a lesser extent South Korea are much more advanced than western countries in ESD and should be a reference in training endoscopists in this complex, exciting, and useful technique.

The Current State of ESD in Western Countries

The history of ESD is reviewed in another chapter of this book, but as a reminder, it began in western countries with the efforts of individual therapeutic endoscopists, most of whom had received training in Japan [1–4]. Knives designed for ESD became available in Europe around 2005, although with restricted access for endoscopists without ESD training. This was a sensible approach, given the ESD learning curve and the fact that complications occur most often when endoscopists are less experienced. ESD is one of the most technically challenging methods of endoscopy, and

A. Parra-Blanco, M.D., Ph.D. (✉)
Department of Gastroenterology, School of Medicine,
Pontificia Universidad Católica de Chile, 833-0024
Santiago, Chile
e-mail: parrablanco@gmail.com

V. Arantes, M.D., M.S., Ph.D.
Alfa Institute, School of Medicine, Minas Gerais
Federal University, Belo Horizonte, Brazil

N. González, M.D.
Department of Gastroenterology, Hospital de
Clínicas, Montevideo, Uruguay

A. Herreros de Tejada, M.D., Ph.D.
Department of Gastroenterology, IDIPHIM. Puerta de
Hierro University Hospital, Universidad Autónoma
de Madrid, Madrid, Spain

A. Donoso, M.D.
Department of Surgery, School of Medicine,
Pontificia Universidad Católica de Chile,
Santiago, Chile

only endoscopists with sufficient training in advanced therapeutic endoscopy took on the challenge of applying it to patients. Because of this expertise in advanced endoscopy, the initial results were generally acceptable in terms of safety and efficacy, although it soon became clear that the perforation rate for colorectal ESD was high (as high as 30 %) [5, 6]. It was also clear that endoscopists should not begin practicing their ESD skills on human patients. For example, an early report noted that six European experts in therapeutic endoscopy performed gastric ESD on porcine models before applying the technique with human patients with a special double-channel endoscope [1]. While there was a success rate of 82 % with the animal cases, but there were perforations, including microperforations, in 50 % of the human cases. Better results than these could not be expected at the beginning of the learning curve for most therapeutic endoscopists. Since that 2006 study, education resources for ESD for western endoscopists are much more abundant, and most live demonstration courses include ESD cases. Moreover, visits by Japanese experts to teach western endoscopists are now common, and hundreds of endoscopists have visited Japanese endoscopy units. In other words, there is now an ESD culture among western endoscopists that was absent a decade ago. This ongoing education is reflected in the improved results in recent series on ESD outside of Japan and Korea [7, 8].

Training started becoming available at hands-on courses, usually with the participation of Japanese experts. A consensus meeting was held in Rotterdam, with expert European and Japanese endoscopists that resulted in recommendations about training, record-keeping, and quality standards [9]. A European ESD survey published in 2010 revealed that only 20 of the surveyed institutions had any experience with human gastric ESD. The rate of major complications was 13 % [10]. A multicenter review by the French Society of Gastrointestinal Endoscopy found a mean load of six cases per center among 16 centers (range of cases: 1–43) [6]. Including upper and lower ESD, 18 % of cases involved perforations. Interestingly, the rates in the colon and rectum were higher, 54 % and 22 %, respectively.

These results clearly indicate that the approach to ESD in western countries should be conservative, starting with animal models, as will be dealt with later in this chapter. Ideally, less difficult cases should be considered initially. As well, cases should be registered prospectively.

There have been an increasing number of papers and presentations at meetings in western countries in recent years. Given that there are relatively few gastric neoplastic lesions, and that early lesions in Barrett's esophagus can be treated relatively easily with EMR and radiofrequency, the main application for ESD in western countries seems to be the colorectum. There are still few units performing colorectal ESD, although the number is increasing. Recent publications indicate that colorectal ESD is feasible with relatively little specific training [7]. Based on the literature, there are fewer than five endoscopy units in Europe and perhaps only one in the US with experience with more than 100 colorectal ESD cases. A survey in Latin America found that approximately 700 ESD cases have been performed by 25 endoscopists (62 % gastric, 15 % esophageal, 15 % rectal, 7 % colonic), with an average perforation rate of 4 % [unpublished observation; submitted material]. Arantes et al. reported their results with esophageal ESD using the tunnel technique on patients diagnosed as high risk (head and neck cancers) [11]. The difference in ESD performance in Latin America from that in the US and Europe may be due to the higher incidence of gastric cancer in several South American countries. If early lesion detection improves, and there are several initiatives in this area, endoscopists will have sufficient cases of early gastric lesions for ESD training.

In summary, although ESD is becoming part of the regular procedures in a growing number of endoscopy units in western countries, western endoscopy units must still be considered beginners compared to units in Japan where they have over a decade of experience and thousands ESDs have been performed. Training should be more readily available, and advanced endoscopes and accessories for ESD used in Japan should be introduced by manufacturing companies in western countries to facilitate the safe and effective practice of ESD.

Should We Offer ESD to Our Patients?

The answer to the question above will determine whether we make the effort to master ESD or simply continue performing EMR and sending patients with more complex lesions to surgery. It is not an easy question to answer since many factors have to be considered including the setting, the type of ESD, the degree of available expertise in advanced therapeutic endoscopy and minimally invasive surgery, as well as others.

ESD is a diagnostic and therapeutic technique for different types of lesions that should be considered separately, but for simplicity sake, the lesions can be divided into esophageal squamous, esophageal-cardial columnar neoplasms (often in Barrett's esophagus), and gastric and colonic neoplasms. Many of these types of lesions are being treated endoscopically, with excellent results by Asian experts. Their expertise in diagnostics, in particular the early detection of subtle and often non-invasive lesions and exact prediction of invasive depth, as well as in techniques of ESD itself, is well advanced. However, because of the significant differences between Asian and western endoscopists in terms of their levels of expertise in ESD, the results by western endoscopists might not be as good initially, and, therefore, consideration for the indications may be different (for instance, excluding more technically complex cases, in locations with greater risk of complications).

en bloc resection more often than EMR; the latter being an independent factor related to recurrence [14]. As an alternative, radiofrequency ablation has shown good results with superficial lesions, although a major drawback is the lack of specimens for histological study, which is certainly desirable with this type of lesion [15].

Endoscopic treatment with radiofrequency, with or without EMR (depending whether there are visible nodules), is the recommended treatment for high-grade dysplasia and intramucosal carcinoma in Barrett's esophagus [16]. There is ample clinical evidence that endoscopic treatment is appropriate and provides long-term cures for over 90 % of early neoplasm cases that are resected by EMR. Success rates are particularly high among well-selected cases. However, when patients with larger lesions are included, usually because of comorbidity, the cure rate drops slightly [17]. ESD has proven feasible for early Barrett's neoplasms in the hands of western experts. However, the R0 resection rate is modest, although still higher than with EMR, due to a field effect in the background mucosa in which there is often inconspicuous high-grade multifocal dysplasia [18, 19]. Complete en bloc ESD resection of the Barrett's epithelium offers the benefit of accurate histopathological diagnosis, but at the expense of technical complexity and very high risk of stricture. ESD is not yet generally accepted by most experts as a standard procedure for the treatment of early neoplasms in Barrett's esophagus [20], but if enough expertise in ESD is available, this is certainly an excellent choice.

Squamous Esophageal Neoplasms

There are well-known risk populations for squamous esophageal neoplasms that can be screened for the presence of relevant lesions using digital chromoendoscopy and/or iodine staining [12, 13]. It can be expected that large numbers of lesions will be detected with screenings, which can allow professionals with large institutions the opportunity to advance along the learning curve [11]. Moreover, it has been proven that ESD provides

Early Gastric Neoplasms

ESD is accepted in Japan as the gold standard for the treatment of early gastric neoplams. It has been clear for many years that piecemeal resections lead to recurrence, which can be difficult to treat successfully and may require surgery [21]. The stomach, in particular the antrum, is certainly the most simple and appropriate location to start training in this technique. Experts recommend that beginners should only start practicing on humans after training on animals with antral lesions, and after approximately 30 more cases should proximal lesions be attempted [22, 23]. It is advisable that endoscopists perform as many gastric procedures as possible before attempting esophageal and colonic procedures. Because it may be difficult to collect and perform 30 antral cases, it is likely that more proximal lesions will be attempted early in the learning curve of most institutions. Although the expanded indications proposed by Gotoda et al. are accepted, such lesions can be more technically challenging (large, ulceration, and/or scarring) [24]. Therefore the authors of this chapter propose that traditional indications be considered for the initial 20–30 cases, depending on the level of experience with animal models and the results. Moreover, subepithelial lesions are relatively common and can constitute an adequate indication for ESD, while small carcinoid tumors can be treated easily and successfully by band-ligation EMR.

However, recent reports suggest that ESD provides curative resection with negative margins for subepithelial lesions more often than does EMR [25, 26]. In general, small (<1 cm) gastric submucosal lesions are common findings in endoscopy units in tertiary centers. Many studies have shown that endoscopic resection is often the only way to reach a diagnosis. The traditional recommendation is to follow patients with undiagnosed lesions with endoscopy and endoscopic ultrasound, which can be costly and cumbersome for the patient. We believe that in the context of an institutionally approved protocol, ESD can be a sensitive diagnostic tool and curative method for small gastric subepithelial lesions.

The Duodenum

The duodenum is the most challenging location for ESD, with perforation rates as high as 50 % [6]. Considering that most lesions can be treated by EMR, and given the low number of cases for this location, ESD is not recommended. If for any reason it must be applied, it is strongly recommended that ESD be performed in an operating room.

Early Colorectal Neoplasms

With the advent of colorectal cancer screening in western countries, there is a large number of endoscopically treatable colorectal neoplasms in tertiary health care centers. Most lesions are certainly amenable to endoscopic mucosal resection, although the largest and/or most complex of them usually require resection in a piecemeal fashion [27]. Indications for colorectal ESD are discussed in Chap. 12. It is very important to determine the macroscopic lesion type, its size, and whether or not there are signs of depressions or invasion, which indicate risk of invasion. Lesions with a high likelihood (>10–15 %) of invasion should be resected en bloc to allow for adequate histopathological assessment.

Granular-type laterally spreading tumors (LST-G) of the mixed type (large and small nodules) over 3–4 cm, and non-granular laterally spreading tumors (LST-NG) over 2 cm are the most common indications for ESD in Japan [28]. LST-Gs in particular are commonly detected in western countries. LST-NGs are supposedly less common in western countries than in Japan. However, they are difficult to detect and an optimal bowel cleansing and withdrawal technique is recommended to optimize detection [29]. Other indications for ESD are large protruding lesions, recurring polyps (remnant tissue after polypectomies), and complex lesions with chronic inflammatory bowel disease [30]. Considering the technical complexity of this location for ESD and the endoscopic (EMR) and surgical alternatives (laparoscopic resection and transanal resection) for many lesions, ESD should only be performed by sufficiently experienced endoscopists. The rectum presents fewer risks, although this does not mean that the procedure is less technically challenging. The results from expert centers are certainly excellent, and should be used as a benchmark to maintain the quality of individual endoscopy units [31].

ESD Training in Western Countries and the Learning Curve

Gastric ESD

A large number of superficial gastrointestinal lesions are diagnosed and treated by ESD in Japan. Early in their training, endoscopists are motivated to acquire skills in detection and endoscopic resection of early tumors. The difficulties inherent to performing ESD, the long process of training with a steep learning curve, and the low frequency of superficial gastric lesions diagnosed in western countries are some of the reasons that few medical centers outside Japan have adopted ESD. Furthermore, access to learning and application of ESD is limited due to lack of Japanese experts in western institutions. Although a substantial number of articles have been published on the applications, results and outcome of ESD, there are few publications related to the learning process. As well, there is no universally accepted and standardized teaching program dedicated to developing ESD skills. Initial studies about training and the learning curve for ESD have focused on gastric lesions [32–34].

A few expert centers have proposed training programs for ESD usually involving theoretical education on the diagnosis and treatment of early cancers, followed by hands-on training with ex vivo or live animal models [35]. In addition to this basic program, trainees have the opportunity to observe and assist in a good number of human ESD procedures conducted by experts. The final step in the training is supervised hands-on practice with human patients, assisted by an expert that not only guides the strategy and the dissection maneuvers, but also takes over from the trainee and completes the procedure if any technical difficulty arises [34, 36]. Moreover, the Japanese trainee may start with easier cases in the gastric antrum before being exposed to more challenging ESD procedures in the gastric body, esophagus, or colorectal locations. Trainees at the National Cancer Center in Tokyo perform the first ten ESD procedures with direct hands-on support from highly qualified endoscopists, working with small lesions in the antrum without ulceration or fibrosis. After that they start performing ESD by themselves with oral guidance from expert endoscopists. As their ESD techniques improve, trainees are gradually assigned to perform ESD on larger lesions and lesions located in the middle and upper thirds of the stomach [23]. This is certainly an ideal way to learn ESD, but programs like this are hardly available other than in Japan, China, and South Korea. We will review some of the training programs in Asia or Western countries to provide Western endoscopists with sufficient information to develop strategies to implement ESD at their own centers.

Gotoda et al. emphasized the importance of using porcine models in the early stage of an ESD training program [37]. The authors suggest that these models are a way to rise rapidly along the ESD learning curve, and stated that at least 30 submucosal dissections of gastric lesions should be performed to achieve a certain degree of mastery, since at the beginning of the learning curve it is estimated that the perforation rate can reach 20 %.

Vásquez-Sequeiros et al. described a sequential ESD training program in Spain aimed at identifying an inexpensive, safe, efficient, and reproducible method for teaching and disseminating ESD [38]. According to the authors, such training can be conducted in four phases: (1) theoretical phase to impart basic knowledge about ESD and review the scientific literature; (2) training with ex vivo animal models; (3) training with in vivo animals supervised by an expert; and (4) application of the ESD technique with patients. In this study, four endoscopists performed a total of 12 gastric ESDs on porcine models (six ex vivo and six in vivo) and later a gastric ESD on a patient supervised by an expert.

Tanimoto et al. assessed the usefulness of an in vivo canine model for ESD practice [39]. They performed five esophageal dissections and five stomach dissections, completing all the procedures without complications. Although the number and size of the resected pieces were small, the authors recommended this in vivo model, which has the advantage of being more realistic.

Parra-Blanco et al. proposed an ESD learning strategy based on an ex vivo gastric porcine model and an in vivo porcine model [40]. After an initial learning period working with isolated animal stomachs supervised by an expert, an endoscopist performed a training procedure on the esophagus and stomach of in vivo porcine models. The learning period was divided into two phases with 11 ESDs in each phase. As the learning process progressed, dissection and operating time decreased, suggesting that practice on live models helps development of ESD skills. The authors did not assess the impact of training on animal on ESD performance in humans.

Gonzalez et al. studied an ESD learning process in Uruguay for an individual endoscopist. Training was divided into three phases: Phase 1: 28 gastric ESDs on ex vivo animals; Phase 2: two gastric ESDs on in vivo animals; and Phase 3: five gastric ESDs on patients [41]. Technical aspects, size of pieces, duration of the procedure, speed and complications were registered. The mean size of the pieces was 28.4 ± 1.2 mm, and the mean duration of the ESD was 41.7 ± 2.4 min. The duration of the ESD in the first 15 procedures was 43.0 ± 3.0 min, while in the next 15 procedures it was 40.3 ± 3.9 min ($P=0.588$). The speed in the first 15 ESDs was 1.25 ± 0.11 cm^2/min versus 2.12 ± 0.36 cm^2/min in the remaining 15, $P=0.028$. There were no complications. With patients, the five lesions were resected en bloc. The mean size of the pieces was 25.2 ± 5.1 mm and the time was 85.0 ± 25.6 min. Endoscopic and histological controls did not show evidence of residual neoplastic tissue. The authors concluded that the sequential ESD training program of an individual endoscopist, based on practice with porcine models, contributed to learning ESD and its subsequent application with humans, yielding good results in efficacy and safety.

Kato et al. also evaluated the influence of the number of ESDs performed on ex vivo models on effectiveness and safety in a western setting [42]. Two endoscopists with no previous experience in ESD and an expert in this technique performed a total of 150 resections on a modified ex vivo EASIE model (Erlangen Active Simulator for Interventional Endoscopy) following 6 h of didactic sessions about ESD. After 30 ESD cases, the novices completed all resections en bloc,

without any perforations, and the dissection time was significantly shorter than that of the first 30 cases, suggesting that 30 sessions with animal models is sufficient to gain expertise, as some experts have proposed [37].

When an operator is ready to undertake human ESD following extensive training with animal models, it is of paramount importance that they begin with a judiciously selected case. Hirasawa et al. reviewed recommendations regarding suitable lesions for ESD by novice operators, with emphasis on risk factors related to the resectability or curability of a variety of lesions [43]. Studies show that factors like tumor size, location in the stomach, and the presence of ulceration are closely related to resectability and curability. Because the combination of these factors results in a much higher risk than any single factor, the authors established a "risk assessment chart" to determine an individual's total risk of treatment failure for early gastric cancer. The findings indicated that small, non-ulcerated lesions located in the lower third of the stomach have a high rate of curative resection and are technically less challenging for ESD performed by trainees. It is recommended, at least in Japan, that the novice operator should gain ESD experience with such lesions before attempting more difficult lesions in the gastric body, cardia or fundus. However, one major difficulty for following this strategy in western countries is that early gastric tumors in the antrum are seldom detected.

Once endoscopists begin performing ESD on human patients, there is the question of how many procedures must be carried out before one can be considered proficient. Certainly, it takes hundreds of procedures on different organs to become a real expert operator. There have been very few studies that address the ESD learning curve. Choi et al. showed that for hybrid gastric ESD (circumferential incision followed by en bloc snaring), the procedure can be performed efficiently and safely after 40 cases, with a significant increase in the en bloc and curative resection rate from 45 % to 85 % [32]. In addition, the perforation rate decreased from 15 % in the first 20 procedures to 1.7 % for the following 60 cases. Oda et al. also assessed the learning curve of ESD trainees at the National Cancer Center (NCC) in Tokyo and noted that experience with 30 operations was needed to acquire the basic skills to successfully perform ESD in the distal stomach [23]. However this fairly low threshold should be viewed with caution by western endoscopists, given that the NCC is considered one of the most prominent ESD centers in Japan and likely the world, with a large number of operations performed on a daily basis, and all trainees involved in this study had an average of 5 years experience in basic diagnostic and therapeutic endoscopy.

A study from another leading Japanese institution, the Cancer Center Hospital, reviewed procedural outcomes of more than 1,500 gastric ESD cases performed by 13 supervised trainees [22]. The training period for the endoscopists was divided into cases 1–40 (Group A), 41–80 (Group B), and over 80 (Group C). Outcomes were compared to those of cases treated by experts in the same facility (Group D). Lesions were classified as "guideline-indication lesions" and "expanded-indication lesions." In the initial 40 cases, lesions were generally smaller, located in the lower body, and not associated with ulcers, and corresponded to the "guideline-indications." In spite of that, outcomes between groups A and B were similar. Group C lesions were more difficult to resect due to their size and location, but outcomes were similar to those with Group B. Interestingly, outcomes were not different between Groups C and D. The study suggests that beginners will be able to perform ESD with good results after 40 cases of guideline-indication lesions, after 80 cases of expanded-indication lesions, and obtain similar results to those of experts after 80 cases. Although the training conditions of this expert Japanese center are not available in western centers, these numbers should be taken into account when considering the types of lesions to be treated by ESD, according to the endoscopist's experience.

In conclusion, before performing ESD, it is important that endoscopists have already developed sufficient expertise in therapeutic endoscopy, particularly in advanced EMR (cap EMR,

piecemeal EMR for large flat lesions, etc.), and that they have become skillful in assessing neoplastic lesions to identify the endoscopic characteristics that predict the existence of deep submucosal invasions and increased risk of lymph node metastasis, as well as demarcating the borders of tumors. It is also critical that endoscopists also acquire extensive practice with animal models, either ex vivo or live, with at least 30 procedures performed, before operating on human patients. Ideally, the first several procedures should be mentored by an expert in ESD; however, this possibility is limited to a few western institutions, therefore a judicious selection of appropriate cases for novice ESD operators (small non-ulcerous lesions in the antrum or rectum) is very important in order to avoid serious complications such as perforation or uncontrollable hemorrhage. When the time comes to perform ESD on humans, it is recommended that this practice be ongoing for continuous improvement in technical skills and that excessively long intervals between procedures be avoided. This means that endoscopists interested in ESD should be recognized as experts specialized in managing early neoplasms, for both their own center and others. Finally, endoscopists need to be self-critical and know their limitations and the limitations of their institutions. They also need to receive ongoing feedback so that ESDs are carried out safely and efficiently. Given all of the above, it is still challenging to set up ESD centers in western countries.

Colorectal ESD

The first study on colorectal ESD training was by Hotta et al. in Japan [44], which described the principal author's learning curve for an initial 120 cases performed over 5 years, supervised initially by an expert in upper ESD. The authors found that after 40 cases, the operator had an adequate level of competence for en bloc and R0 resections (rate of 85 %), and after 80 cases the operator performed with an adequate level of safety (perforation rate 5 % vs. 12.5 % in the first 40 cases).

Sakamoto et al. [36] reported on the ESD training of two endoscopists at the NCC in Japan. The prerequisites for performing colorectal ESD at the NCC are a high level of skill in the non-loop insertion colonoscopy technique (more than ten cases of total colonoscopy completed within 5 min each without any abdominal discomfort), skills in conventional or piecemeal EMR techniques, experience with >20 gastric ESD cases, and assistance during >20 colorectal ESDs conducted by experienced endoscopists. The self-completion rate for the first, second, and third blocks of ten cases were: 45 %, 70 %, and 80 %, respectively, while it rose to 100 % in the fourth block. The perforation rate was <2 % (two cases; one in the first block and one in the fourth). The authors concluded that with proper supervision and training, colorectal ESD may be performed independently after 30 cases.

Can the results and methods for colorectal ESD training in Japan be directly exported to other countries? Obviously not, because of the inherent differences between them regarding ESD. There are few reports about training for colorectal ESD in western countries. The first experience was reported by Repici et al., using what is now called a hybrid EMR technique (circumferential cutting and complete resection with a snare) for lesions that were not considered amenable to endoscopic resection by conventional methods [45]. The endoscopists who performed the treatments were internationally recognized experts in advanced endoscopy. The results were modest in terms of the en bloc resection rate (55 %), but good in clinical terms given that the perforation rate was low (1/29, 3 %) and surgery was avoided with all but one patient. The first author had performed supervised ESD with animal models in Japan, where he visited an expert center and observed gastric and colorectal ESD. He then continued working with animal models without supervision, and since 2005, has been performing ESD on a regular basis, with a current annual volume of approximately 25 gastric, 50 colorectal and ten esophageal ESDs. While the perforation rate was as high as 20 % in the early days (mostly for colorectal cases), it is now well below 5 % [personal communication].

Two western studies specifically described the learning curve for colorectal ESD [2, 7]. Probst et al. reported the results for 82 rectosigmoid ESDs (86 % rectal) performed by two endoscopists over 7 years, representing approximately one case per endoscopist every 2 months [2]. Their results were compared in three consecutive periods, and a learning curve was evident, the en bloc resection rate being 66 %, 88 %, and 92 %, while mean procedure times were 200, 193, and 136, minutes respectively. A significant improvement in en bloc resection rate was achieved after 25 cases, and in procedural time after 50 cases. There was only one evident perforation, and four additional patients with pneumoperitoneum. This group had received training from Japanese endoscopists, although the initial 12 cases were performed previously by one of the authors.

Iacopini et al. evaluated the learning curve for a moderately experienced therapeutic endoscopist in a series that included 30 rectal and 30 colonic ESDs [7]. Competence was defined as an en bloc resection rate >80 %, and a statistically significant improvement in dissection speed per cm^2. The endoscopist only performed colonic ESD after having achieved competence in rectal ESD. Previous training in ESD included five cases of unsupervised gastric ESD with an isolated porcine model, 2 weeks stay at an expert Japanese center, a supervised isolated porcine ESD model, and a supervised human ESD on a patient. The results of this study are encouraging for western endoscopists. The en bloc resection rate for rectal ESD increased from 60 to 80 % after five procedures, while the rate for colonic ESD increased from 20 to 80 % after 20 procedures. The perforation rate was low (3/60, 5 %; two of which eventually required surgery). A rectal perforation took place in one of the first five cases, and two colonic perforations occurred among the first ten cases.

The studies show that colorectal ESD is feasible in western countries, that there is a learning curve, and that appropriate training is required. In 2012, Probst et al. concluded that colorectal ESD remains at the clinical research level in Europe and should be restricted to endoscopic centers until further studies are presented [2].

Esophageal ESD

Esophageal ESD is more technically challenging than gastric or rectal ESD because the esophageal wall is thinner and the lumenal space is more limited. Generally, it is not possible to work with a retroflex view and both heart beat and respiration can impair a stable condition for SM dissection [11]. In addition to experience in performing ESD in the stomach or rectum, it is advisable that the novice operator interested in mastering esophageal ESD has the opportunity to work with animal models before working with humans. Standardized training programs for esophageal ESD are still lacking in the West and there are few reports on this.

Tanimoto et al. described training circumferential esophageal ESD with canine models [46]. Perforations occurred in the first seven animals, and circumferential ESD was completed only in the last three animals, with a mean procedure time of 192 min (range: 140–235 min).

One of the barriers to developing ESD expertise experimentally is that ex vivo models for practice on the tubular esophagus are difficult to set up. Therefore, the most popular experimental model is with live animals, whether porcine or canine. In our experience, the live porcine model is appropriate for ESD training on the esophagus. The environment is very similar to that of a human patient, experiencing difficulties with heart pulsation, floatation of liquids in the operating field and a narrow space to maneuver the endoscope and knife. However the esophageal wall of the pig is thinner than the human, which makes esophageal ESD in pigs apparently more challenging than in humans, with a higher risk of perforation. Pigs do not survive even microperforations, with subsequent pneumomediastinum or pneumothorax and cardiorespiratory arrest. Therefore it seems prudent to use CO_2 insufflation during ESD with pigs, although there is no scientific evidence to support this recommendation.

Another drawback to incorporating esophageal ESD in endoscopy units is the lack of a standardized procedure. Different centers in Japan have developed expertise in ESD with a particular knife and a certain approach, and this lack of a standardized protocol can make teaching and learning ESD difficult. One author's group has developed experience in esophageal ESD with a standardized tunneling method [11]. The technique was learned through intensive clinical training provided by an expert in the procedure. The standardized procedure was mastered over several sessions of hands-on practice in an animal laboratory, followed by opportunities to assist in human procedures. Unsupervised traditional ESD procedures were first attempted in gastric and rectal tumors (25 cases), as part of the learning curve process. Afterwards, esophageal endoscopic submucosal tunnel dissection (ESTD) was introduced at the author's institution. The technique of esophageal ESTD is described in detail elsewhere [11]. Using this approach, the authors carried out ESTD with 25 lesions in 23 patients, with a mean duration of 85 min. En bloc resection was successfully accomplished in 23 lesions (92 %). There were complications in three procedures (12 %); two cases with mediastinal and subcutaneous emphysema and one perforation in the distal incision that was repaired with endoclips, which allowed the ESD to be completed. Conservative management was successful with these patients, consisting of broad-spectrum antibiotics, no food intake for 3 days, and clinical monitoring. The results of this series are comparable to others reported in the literature by Japanese experts, suggesting that a combination of hands-on practice with animal models associated with preliminary experience with gastric and rectal ESD is potentially sufficient to carry out esophageal ESD on humans with satisfactory outcomes.

Animal Models for ESD

Animal models are often used for ESD training, with the porcine model being the most widely used, given anatomical similarity between pig and human, the wide availability of pigs, and their relatively low cost. The anatomy of the porcine stomach is very similar to that of the human stomach; the main differences being a gastric diverticulum near the cardia and the fact that the pylorus (called the torus pyloricus) is stronger and protrudes into the stomach. There have also been reports of good results for esophageal and gastric ESD training with canine models.

When working with animal models, whether ex vivo or in vivo, it is ideal to use facilities solely for that purpose. The procedures should be conducted with a qualified veterinarian, using equipment intended exclusively for animal models. Prerequisites are adequate endoscopic training and advice on ethical and legal considerations. Experimenting with dogs, cats and non-human primates is not allowed in the European Union unless the animals have been bred for such purposes (Directive 2010/63/EU of the European Parliament), while the use of primates is banned. Similarly, in many Latin American countries, the use of dogs and non-human primates as experimental models is not allowed. Furthermore, in the earlier stages of learning, the use of ex vivo models is preferable. Training with live models should always have the approval of pertinent ethics committees for animal research, including applicable institutional review boards (IRBs), and be conducted according to all current guidelines.

Preparation of the Ex Vivo Esophageal-Gastric Porcine Model

The esophagus and stomach are used for this model. There are different ways to set up the model, from the most rudimentary manner, as was the case initially, to the most sophisticated, using plastic boxes with accessories to secure organs. The Erlangen Active Simulator for Interventional Endoscopy (EASIE) has been proven an effective model for ESD training [42]. The isolated esophageal-gastric model can be easily configured for practicing ESD.

The isolated ex vivo model involves using a plastic box approximately $45 \times 30 \times 20$ cm with an 18–20 mm hole on one end through which a plastic tube, such as an overtube, is inserted. When small organs (from 20 kg pigs) are used, the tube connected to the esophagus should have a smaller diameter, about 14 mm. One simple

option is to cut a 10 ml syringe, leaving only the cylinder. Plastic clamps can be used to prevent the esophagus from slipping into the tube with the movement of the endoscope and air leakage. The size of the overtube and the tightness of the clamps should be adequate to accommodate the endoscope with the distal attachment free.

To make the esophagus more stable and provide a more realistic simulation of the human esophagus, a more sophisticated model has been proposed in which a modified second overtube is used [47].

Organs can be purchased at slaughterhouses, usually requiring special permission for experimental work. If possible, the model should be prepared with fresh organs, although it may be more practical to keep organs frozen and use them as desired. In the latter case, care must be taken to maintain them at room temperature for long enough (usually >12 h) for the body to regain as much elasticity as possible. However, in our experience, pre-frozen bodies often remain rigid, preventing successful injection into the submucosa.

Organ size is another issue to be considered. Large pigs (>70 kg) offer large stomachs that permit multiple resections in different topographies. As well, resection in the lesser curvature is more feasible with a larger than smaller organ. However, smaller animal bodies have thinner walls, so the risk of perforation is higher. On the other hand, working with smaller stomachs presents more difficulty and can therefore facilitate the development of greater skills. Consequently, the authors recommend the use of small stomachs after initial practice on larger organs.

Another key point in the assembly of ex vivo models is cleaning the stomach to properly perform ESD procedures. The stomach not only contains abundant mucus but even large amounts of food. In the experience of the authors, there are two ways to clean the esophagus and stomach. One is to pour warm tap water into the proximal end of the esophagus while the distal end is closed with forceps. The liquid is removed after vigorous shaking and the procedure is repeated until all effluents are washed out. The mucolytic agent N-acetylcysteine or even a few drops of

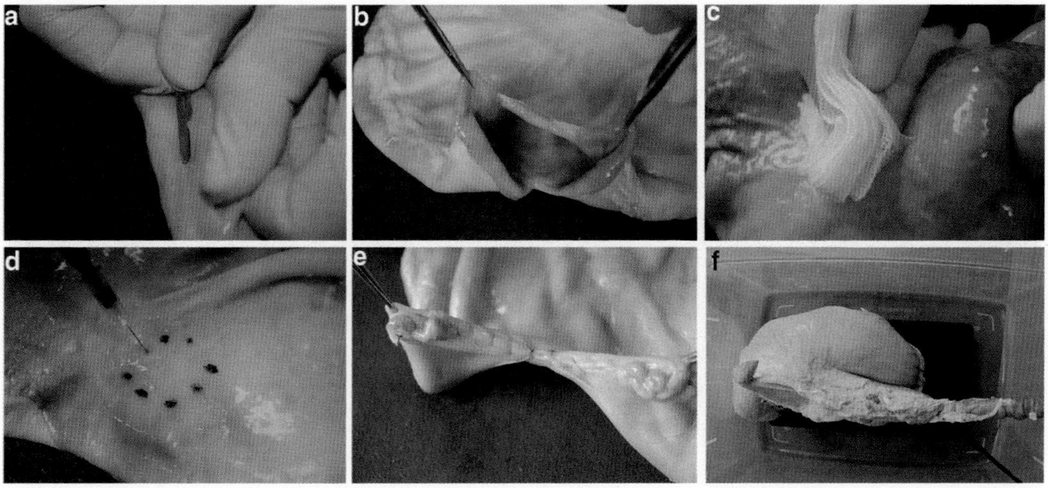

Fig. 25.1 Preparation of ex vivo porcine model. (**a**) Incision about 10 cm along the greater curvature with a scalpel; (**b**) Open porcine stomach greater curvature; (**c**) Gauze is applied to dry the tissue after profuse washing with water; (**d**) Tattooing artificial lesion with China ink; (**e**) Porcine stomach sutured with vicryl; (**f**) *Plastic box with cadaveric model*

liquid detergent can be added to the water. A second option is to make an opening with a scalpel about 10 cm along the greater curvature to facilitate washing, after which a brush can be used to gently remove mucus. Gauze is then applied to dry the tissue. Finally, the opening is closed with vicryl prolene sutures to prevent leakage of water or air during the procedure. Another advantage of the open stomach is the possibility of marking one or more artificial lesions of different diameters and different topographies by tattooing (Fig. 25.1). In this way, different degrees of difficulty can be established. Typically, the antrum is selected for the initial case, followed by the gastric body along the greater curvature, then the lesser curvature, and finally the subcardial region.

Preparation of the Ex Vivo Colonic Model

An ex vivo colonic porcine model was originally developed in the Endoscopy Unit of the Tokyo NCC for practicing ESD. This model, which is similar to the one developed for gastric ESD, has been successfully reproduced by others [48]. It is a simple model to prepare, low in cost, and, in this authors' experience, helpful for training colorectal ESD. Japanese experts also find the esophagus appropriate for training colorectal ESD. Fatty tissue is rather abundant in the porcine colon and rectum, which can hamper viewing the operation field because the lens is repeatedly stained by fat.

To assemble the model, a plastic box is used to mimic the abdomen, with a hole on one end to insert the endoscope. It is preferable to use a disposable laparoscopic port to dock with a plastic tube to simulate the anus, which helps to maintain a hermetic environment during the procedure. The distal end of the colon is attached to prevent air leakage and the other end is securely clamped to the plastic tube that houses the laparoscopic port.

Another way to build the ex vivo colon model is with a polyphony sheet that dynamically simulates the anatomy of the colon. The colon is inserted into the limited space and fixed in the same way as with model described above. A section of the colon can be wrapped in foil to increase electrical conductivity. The advantage of the model is its resemblance to human anatomy due to the presence of angles. As mentioned above, artificial lesions can be created by tattoos.

Yoshida et al. evaluated isolated bovine and porcine colon models, including blood flow to extend the training to hemostasis and make the procedure more realistic [49]. Research is needed to determine the best model for colorectal ESD training in this complex location.

Preparation of the Live Model

The in vivo porcine model has also proven suitable for endoscopic ESD training. The live model has the advantage of being more realistic because of the presence of peristalsis, intraluminal secretions, and bleeding, the latter representing a possible complication (although in the experience of the authors, bleeding during ESD in living models is less common and profuse than in humans). Another advantage of the live model is the possibility of assessing results in terms of survival rates.

We agree with the widely held view that in the first stage, basic ESD maneuvers and strategies can and should be learned with the ex vivo model and that there is no justification for using live pigs at that stage. Use of live pigs is more costly, requires more complex preparation and technical assistance, and, most importantly, would not be ethical.

The common domestic pig (*Sus Scrofa Domestica*) is used for training. It is generally recommended to use young pigs that weigh 30–40 kg. Notably, there is a small cul de sac at the caudal end of the pig pharynx called the pharyngeal pouch that can hinder endoscopic intubation.

Animals should be sedated and monitored by a veterinarian for any possible complications. The veterinarian must also be responsible for euthanizing the animals. Two strategies have been proposed for sedating pigs in in vivo models: (1) induction and maintenance with ketamine and midazolam or propofol, (2) intramuscular premedication with ketamine and maintenance with propofol and inhalation anesthesia (halothane, isoflurane or sevoflurane). Intravenous medication is administered by placing an easily accessible venous catheter in the ear. Occasionally, hyoscine butyl bromide may be necessary to decrease gastrointestinal motility.

The live model can be used for practicing not only gastric ESD but also with the esophagus and colon. In the latter case, one of the main limitations is the difficulty in cleaning the colon. Polyethylene glycol or sodium phosphate should be given orally for the preparation at least 2 days before the procedure. Bowel preparation can be completed by enemas after anesthetizing the animal. It is also important that the animal be kept away from food or objects that can be ingested. It is not unusual to find stomachs packed with ingested contents in live porcine models used in hands-on courses, which can undo the value of the activity. Given this, it is advisable to keep the pig on a liquid diet for 24 h and a complete fast for 8 h prior to the procedure.

Other limitations of the live model for practicing colonic ESD are: (1) the large amount of fat in the submucosal layer; (2) a thinner colon wall than that of humans; (3) differences in the structure of the pig colon from the human colon; and (4) the lack of abdominal fixations in the proximal colon (the large intestine only resembles that of humans in the rectosigmoid segment). These differences may limit the degree practice results in overcoming technical difficulties and the risk of making perforations.

The Gap Between Animal Models and Real Patients: The Western Perspective About Recommendations For ESD With Humans

The first approach to ESD procedures on real patients is always challenging. Even if training with animal models is exhaustive and well planned, there is a gap between ESD with animal models and with humans. In fact, in the animal models, only normal mucosa is resected, while with humans we are treating lesions. The most important factors in approaching the first human ESD with confidence is to have had sufficient training with animal models for both ESD and handling complications, and to have performed such procedures with the same seriousness and concentration as with procedures with human patients.

Although ESD procedures with animals are more relaxed and can even be undertaken with fun, we should remember that human ESD will not be so much fun when difficulties arise. As well, ESD should be elected when there are appropriate indications, because of which it is advisable to obtain expert (Japanese) consultation before electing to perform ESD. Experts confirm whether or not lesions show any signs of deep submucosal invasion, as well as providing guidance about the ESD strategy. Such advice can be invaluable during the procedure.

Another possibility with initial cases in the era of telemedicine is distance supervision via internet, ideally with high-quality transmission [50]. The first author attempted his first human ESD case with this form of supervision, provided by Dr. Oda and others at the National Cancer Center in Tokyo, which definitely was helpful.

The setting where the procedure is to be performed can be relevant. In Japan, ESD is almost always performed in the Endoscopy Unit. Recently the practice of sedating patients with propofol by non-anesthesiologists has been introduced in expert Japanese and Korean centers [5, 51]. We believe that in particular for upper GI ESD, having an anesthesiologist or a well-trained non-anesthesiologist present to handle sedation can be reassuring for the endoscopist, who can then concentrate exclusively on the endoscopic aspects of the procedure.

Continuous infusion of propofol and an opioid during gastric ESD is associated with a significantly higher rate of aspiration pneumonia than is the use of midazolam and intermittent propofol infusion (4.4 % vs. 1.5 %, $P = 0.002$) [53]. This is attributed to a decreased gag reflex with the former. On the other hand, general anesthesia with intubation is associated with significantly shorter procedural time for gastric ESD (nearly half, on average) than sedation with midazolam. As well, the complication rate is lower with anesthesia, although not significantly, and patient satisfaction is significantly higher. With these results, western endoscopists are recommended to perform upper ESD with general anesthesia, at least with the initial cases, until the procedure time can be reduced with experience. General anesthesia has the advantage of permitting the operator to work with less pressure, which can facilitate dealing with complications that may arise. The operator can feel as if they were working in the animal lab, where conditions are more relaxed, as opposed to the situation where the patient is only sedated, and especially if the operator is in charge of sedation.

Midazolam and pethidine or fentanyl are generally used in colorectal ESD in Japan. It is often necessary to change the patient's position several times during colorectal ESD to take advantage of gravity and avoid liquid accumulating in the target area. Deep sedation with propofol has the theoretical disadvantage that it makes changing the patient's position more complicated. However, in the authors' experience, Western patients tolerate colorectal ESD much worse, including when performed by Japanese experts, with deep sedation with propofol than with midazolam and an opiate.

Another step from the lab to the patient is that all the details related to the configuration of the procedure room, patient position, type of sedation, and the availability of experienced assistants have to be taken into account before the procedure, and are likely to be different from those in the animal lab. Even the equipment (endoscope, accessories, electrosurgical generator) may be different from those for training with animal models, although ideally similar equipment is used in both settings. Planning the configuration of the operating room is critical to ensure smooth and efficient procedure.

If the operator is a gastroenterologist that is unfamiliar with the operating room, it can seem an unknown territory. In this case, it is advisable that the operator visit the area in advance and discussing the best configuration for the procedure with the personnel. It is also advisable to discuss the case with a surgical team before the procedure, in case surgery is needed during or after the ESD.

Upper GI ESD (Fig. 25.2)

Patient Position

The patient has to be placed on his/her left side as in a regular endoscopy, but it is advisable to use a soft mattress to protect the patient against scarring

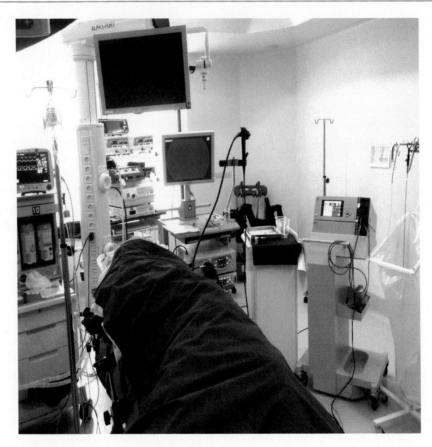

Fig. 25.2 Configuration of the operating room for upper ESD in a western center

since the procedure can last several hours. The skin at all the pressure areas has to be protected and the extremities need to be secured to the patient's body with soft pads so that they do not interfere with the procedure. The tracheal tube also has to be placed at the back of the patient's mouth so that front of the mouth is clear and the operator can move their hands without interference. It is also important to use a short overtube, so that the endoscope can be easily removed and reinserted during the procedure.

Operation Room Configuration

A recommended configuration for the operating room is to place the endoscopy tower at the top end of the patient's bed. This monitoring tower will be used by the operator and the assistant. However, if possible, a larger monitor should be placed behind the patient so that first the operator can work with it more comfortably. A small table

should be located to the right of the endoscopy tower from the operator's point of view on which are placed two 200–300 cc basins (one with the submucosal fluid cushion (SFC) solution and the other with saline) and three syringes (one of 20 ml for the SFC, another of 20 ml for saline, and finally one of 50 ml for a mixture of water and simethicone to wash the GI lumen). The electrosurgical generator is placed next to the table and is managed by the first assistant, who needs to have a complete knowledge of the energy source and how to change the settings whenever required. Needless to say, all the settings have to be selected and programmed into the electrosurgical unit before the procedure. Last but not least, an endoscopy rack is placed at the right of the energy source with all the devices ready to be used. This is very important, because during an ESD procedure it may be necessary to change endoknives quickly and frequently.

Independent of any preferences among endoknives, it is highly recommended to equip the ESD rack with a high flow injection needle, coagulation forceps, and at least two different types of knives. Among the knives we are most familiar with, the most advisable for a first procedure are an insulated-tip knife and a needle knife.

Lower GI ESD

Things are somewhat different in case of lower GI ESD. Even for western endoscopists still in the learning process, it is advisable to perform colorectal ESD under deep sedation using an endoscopy bed rather than an operating room bed. Endoscopy beds are wider than most operating room beds and allow the colonoscope loop (if it is the long type that are most commonly used in western endoscopy units) to rest comfortably on the bed. This simple detail can be a great help in a difficult colonic ESD cases. Moreover, the fact that the patient is under deep sedation supervised by an anesthesiologist, most often with propofol, makes it possible to change the patient's position with relative ease, as is often necessary with colonic ESD. Another advantage of performing colorectal ESD in the endoscopy unit is that it is likely that the patient can receive the agent for the bowel preparation according to a schedule that follows current recommendations (2–5 h before the examination), while patients sent to the surgical area are usually required to fast for at least 8 h. This results in poor preparation, representing a serious problem for the performance of ESD, including the treatment and prognosis of any complications, mainly perforations. Colonic ESD has the highest risk of perforation, so the surgical team must be familiar with the procedure should surgery be needed. Apart from patient position and the recommended bed, the configuration of the operation is the same as for gastric ESD.

Final Tips

A second assistant should ideally be next to the first to clean the devices when they are not being used. It is very useful to have a surgical blade and/or a toothbrush for this purpose because endoknives tend to accumulate debris that can interfere with their adequate functioning. The second assistant can also pass the operator other things needed during the procedure so that the operator can focus solely on the ESD.

Treatment of Complications as a Central Part of Training in ESD

During the ESD training process, developing the essential skills to successfully manage complications is of paramount importance. Perforation and bleeding are the main adverse events in ESD and the trainee must be aware and ready to handle them before attempting human cases [31, 54, 55]. As noted above, training with animal models should include dealing with ESD-related complications [40–56], initially with isolated organs, and after with live animals to develop skills in perforation closure and hemostasis of bleeding vessels.

Perforation

The trainee should take any opportunity after unintentional perforation during ESD to practice secure closure of the defect. If possible, the organ should be examined meticulously to confirm the quality of the closure (Fig. 25.3). Clipping is not always easy, in particular, with precise closure of target lesions in difficult locations. Skills in this area can make a substantial difference between a successful ESD and a frustrating failure with unpleasant results for the patient. However, ongoing training implies using many clips, which is not affordable for many centers. One alternative is the use of expired devices donated by manufacturing companies for training purposes.

Bleeding

Bleeding is a common complication during ESD procedures. Although some authors have reported setting artificial vessels in isolated harvested

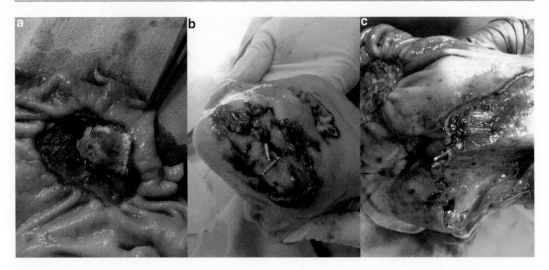

Fig. 25.3 Necropsy specimens of porcine stomach after ESD (*interior view*): (**a**) Closure of gastric perforation with OTSC clip; (**b**) Closure of gastric perforation with a Resolution clip®; (**c**) Demonstration of incomplete closure of perforation using surgical forceps

organs, only live animals can realistically reproduce the bleeding experienced with patients [49].

The trainee should anticipate and avoid bleeding with preventive coagulation based on adequate identification of vessels in the submucosal level [57]. It has been suggested that the deeper dissection level in the submucosal layer is associated with fewer vessels and less procedural hemorrhaging [58]. There are more details on this in Chap. 16.

Post-ESD Stenosis

This complication is usually related to radical, full circumferential ESD, either in the esophagus, the stomach, or the rectum. In animal model training we can only experience this in survival studies, where the animal undergoes endoscopy 2–4 weeks after the initial ESD.

Summary

In summary, intensive training for the successful management of complications is key for the ESD apprentice. Animal models provide an excellent opportunity to develop the required skills to deal with complications associated with ESD, especially perforation and bleeding. In our western environment, only through continuous practice will we have a good chance to obtain full competence in ESD.

Is More Training Required for ESD?

Most experts in the area argue that ESD is the final step in the training for early detection and treatment of GI neoplasias. Detection is the most important issue, since lesions undetected by endoscopists remain treated until they become symptomatic, while lesions that are detected are treated, whether by endoscopy or surgery.

Training for advanced diagnostic endoscopy is beyond the scope of this book, but the most advanced and experienced centers in diagnosis of early lesions are in Asia, and, if possible, training there is highly desirable.

The importance of an adequate endoscopic diagnosis before ESD cannot be overstated. The operator should understand perfectly the type of lesion to be treated, as well as its location and extension. To this end, diagnostic endoscopy should ideally be performed by the same operator who will perform ESD. Especially in the cases of squamous esophageal and gastric cancers, it can be impossible to trace the margins of the lesions with only white light endoscopy, even with high definition endoscopes. Digital or Lugol's iodine chromoendoscopy should be used for squamous lesions, while for flat-type early gastric cancers, indigo carmine, acetic acid-indigo carmine, or NBI with magnification can show the margins of most lesions. Although taking too many biopsies from lesions before ESD should be avoided to prevent the development of fibrosis, which can make ESD more challenging, biopsies should be taken to clarify the extension of the lesion and determine if there are synchronous lesions.

Technical Issues That May Help Western Endoscopists to Perform ESD

At least two technical issues should be considered by western endoscopists training in ESD. The first relates to performing more complex resections still using the snare, before moving to full ESD (transitional resections). Especially in the colon, small incision-assisted EMR is used for en bloc resection of lesions that cannot be easily trapped en bloc by the snare [59]. The technique consists of making a small slit with the tip of the snare in the normal mucosa at the oral margin (after injecting sufficient solution). The tip of the snare remains in the slit and

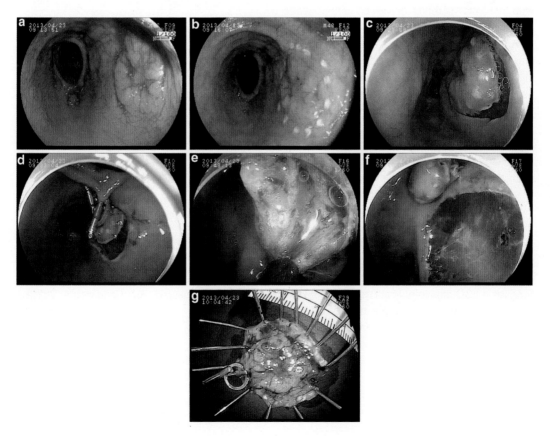

Fig. 25.4 (a) IIa+IIc lesion, 15 mm in diameter, located on the posterior wall of the antrum (with indigo carmine at 0.4 %); (b) Marking; (c) After circumferential cutting with an IT-Knife 2 (Olympus); (d) The clip-band system is applied; (e) Final step of the dissection; the dissection plane is well exposed thanks to the traction exerted by the clip-band system; (f) After ESD is completed, the specimen remains attached to the mucosa by the second clip; (g) The specimen is retrieved with a snare, pinned and measured

the snare is opened, preventing slippage of the snare distally and keeping it in an adequate position. The snare is then closed slowly.

The second technique is called hybrid EMR and represents an early application of ESD [60, 61]. In this technique, after having achieved the circumferential resection with an ESD knife, a snare is applied to complete the resection. The method can be applied as rescue therapy when it is difficult to complete ESD more conventionally, but can also be performed as a planned procedure. It is currently applied mainly with colonic lesions and has proven useful for lesions up to 3 cm in diameter. The method is an excellent way for operators to gain confidence with the use of the knives on humans, and in fact, some Japanese ESD experts have described their experience with the two methods described above while learning colorectal ESD [59].

Another technical issue that can facilitate the introduction and development of human ESD is the use of traction methods. It is well known that the dissection stage represents the most complex part of ESD, and the part where beginners are unable to complete the procedure by themselves [34]. Numerous methods have been proposed to apply traction (also called countertraction) from the resected mucosa upwards to facilitate observing the submucosal dissection plane. The available methods, which were recently reviewed [62, 63], can be classified as: double endoscope methods, traction tools attached to the endoscope, and traction tools independent of the endoscope. Most traction methods are indicated for gastric ESD, but colonic and esophageal ESD would also benefit by the application of efficient traction methods. Many of these devices are not commercially available or are very costly, and usually involve complex hand-made components. The first author developed a traction method using simple and available devices: two reopenable clips (Resolution, Boston Scientific) and a rubber band for orthodontic use (Fig. 25.4). The design is a simplified version of the S–O Clip (designed for colonic ESDs) [64]. In a randomized study comparing gastric ESD with live pigs with the hybrid knife (ERBE), with or without the clip-band traction method, the dissection

speed was faster when the clip was applied [65, 66]. The first author regularly uses this method for human gastric ESD with good results.

References

1. Neuhaus H, Costamagna G, Devière J, Fockens P, Ponchon T, Rösch T. Endoscopic submucosal dissection (ESD) of early neoplastic gastric lesions using a new double-channel endoscope (the "R-scope"). Endoscopy. 2006;38:1016–23.
2. Probst A, Golger D, Arnholdt H, Messmann H. Endoscopic submucosal dissection of early cancers, flat adenomas, and submucosal tumors in the gastrointestinal tract. Clin Gastroenterol Hepatol. 2009;7: 149–55.
3. Dinis-Ribeiro M, Pimentel-Nunes P, Afonso M, Costa N, Lopes C, Moreira-Dias L. A European case series of endoscopic submucosal dissection for gastric superficial lesions. Gastrointest Endosc. 2009;69:350–5.
4. Repici A, Hassan C, Carlino A, et al. Endoscopic submucosal dissection in patients with early esophageal squamous cell carcinoma: results from a prospective Western series. Gastrointest Endosc. 2010;71: 715–21.
5. Coda S, Trentino P, Antonellis F, et al. A Western single-center experience with endoscopic submucosal dissection for early gastrointestinal cancers. Gastric Cancer. 2010;13:258–63.
6. Farhat S, Chaussade S, Ponchon T, et al. Endoscopic submucosal dissection in a European setting. A multi-institutional report of a technique in development. Endoscopy. 2011;43:664–70.
7. Iacopini F, Bella A, Costamagna G, et al. Stepwise training in rectal and colonic endoscopic submucosal dissection with differentiated learning curves. Gastrointest Endosc. 2012;76:1188–96.
8. Chaves DM, Moura EG, Milhomem D. Initial experience of endoscopic submucosal dissection in Brazil to treat early gastric and esophagheal cancer: a multi-institutional analysis. Arq Gastroenterol. 2013;50: 148–52.
9. Deprez PH, Bergman JJ, Meisner S, et al. Current practice with endoscopic submucosal dissection in Europe: position statement from a panel of experts. Endoscopy. 2010;42:853–8.
10. Ribeiro-Mourão F, Pimentel-Nunes P, Dinis-Ribeiro M. Endoscopic submucosal dissection for gastric lesions: results of an European inquiry. Endoscopy. 2010;42:814–9.
11. Arantes V, Albuquerque W, Freitas Dias CA, Demas Alvares Cabral MM, Yamamoto H. Standardized endoscopic submucosal tunnel dissection for management of early esophageal tumors (with video). Gastrointest Endosc. 2013;78:946–52.
12. Yokoyama A, Ohmori T, Makuuchi H, et al. Successful screening for early esophageal cancer in alcoholics

using endoscopy and mucosa iodine staining. Cancer. 1995;76:928–34.

13. Muto M, Hironaka S, Nakane M, Boku N, Ohtsu A, Yoshida S. Association of multiple Lugol-voiding lesions with synchronous and metachronous esophageal squamous cell carcinoma in patients with head and neck cancer. Gastrointest Endosc. 2002;56:517–21.

14. Takahashi H, Arimura Y, Masao H. Endoscopic submucosal dissection is superior to conventional endoscopic resection as a curative treatment for early squamous cell carcinoma of the esophagus (with video). Gastrointest Endosc. 2010;72:255–64.

15. Bergman JJ, Zhang YM, He S, Weusten B, et al. Outcomes from a prospective trial of endoscopic radiofrequency ablation of early squamous cell neoplasia of the esophagus. Gastrointest Endosc. 2011;74:1181–90.

16. Bennett C, Vakil N, Bergman J, et al. Consensus statements for management of Barrett's dysplasia and early-stage esophageal adenocarcinoma, based on a Delphi process. Gastroenterology. 2012;143:336–46.

17. Ell C, May A, Gossner L, et al. Endoscopic mucosal resection of early cancer and high-grade dysplasia in Barrett's esophagus. Gastroenterology. 2000;118:670–7.

18. Neuhaus H, Terheggen G, Rutz EM, Vieth M, Schumacher B. Endoscopic submucosal dissection plus radiofrequency ablation of neoplastic Barrett's esophagus. Endoscopy. 2012;44:1105–13.

19. Deprez PH, Piessevaux H, Aouattah T, Yeung RC, Sempoux C, Jouret-Mourin A. ESD in Barrett's esophagus high grade dysplasia and mucosal cancer: prospective comparison with CAP mucosectomy. Gastrointest Endosc. 2010;71:126.

20. Bergman JJ. How to justify endoscopic submucosal dissection in the Western world. Endoscopy. 2009;41:988–90.

21. Kojima T, Parra-Blanco A, Takahashi H, Fujita R. Outcome of endoscopic mucosal resection for early gastric cancer: review of the Japanese literature. Gastrointest Endosc. 1998;48:550–4.

22. Yamamoto Y, Fujisaki J, Ishiyama A, Hirasawa T, Igarashi M. Current status of training for endoscopic submucosal dissection for gastric epithelial neoplasm at Cancer Institute Hospital, Japanese Foundation for Cancer Research, a famous Japanese hospital. Dig Endosc. 2012;24 Suppl 1:148–53.

23. Oda I, Odagaki T, Suzuki H, Nonaka S, Yoshinaga S. Learning curve for endoscopic submucosal dissection of early gastric cancer based on trainee experience. Dig Endosc. 2012;24 Suppl 1:129–32.

24. Gotoda T, Yanagisawa A, Sasako M, et al. Incidence of lymph node metastasis from early gastric cancer: estimation with a large number of cases at two large centers. Gastric Cancer. 2000;3:219–25.

25. Hopper AD, Bourke MJ, Hourigan LF, Tran K, Moss A, Swan MP. En bloc resection of multiple type 1 gastric carcinoid tumors by endoscopic multi-band mucosectomy. J Gastroenterol Hepatol. 2009;24:1516–21.

26. Sato Y, Takeuchi M, Hashimoto S, et al. Usefulness of endoscopic submucosal dissection for type I gastric carcinoid tumors compared with endoscopic mucosal resection. Hepatogastroenterology. 2013;60:1524–9.

27. Swan MP, Bourke MJ, Alexander S, Moss A, Williams SJ. Large refractory colonic polyps: is it time to change our practice? A prospective study of the clinical and economic impact of a tertiary referral colonic mucosal resection and polypectomy service (with videos). Gastrointest Endosc. 2009;70:1128–36.

28. Matsuda T, Gotoda T, Saito Y, Nakajima T, Conio M. Our perspective on endoscopic resection for colorectal neoplasms. Gastroenterol Clin Biol. 2010;34:367–70.

29. Bianco MA, Cipolletta L, Rotondano G, Buffoli F, Gizzi G, Tessari F, Flat Lesions Italian Network (FLIN). Prevalence of nonpolypoid colorectal neoplasia: an Italian multicenter observational study. Endoscopy. 2010;42:279–85.

30. Uraoka T, Parra-Blanco A, Yahagi N. Colorectal endoscopic submucosal dissection: is it suitable in western countries? J Gastroenterol Hepatol. 2013;28:406–14.

31. Saito Y, Uraoka T, Yamaguchi Y, et al. A prospective, multicenter study of 1111 colorectal endoscopic submucosal dissections (with video). Gastrointest Endosc. 2010;72:1217–25.

32. Choi IJ, Kim CG, Chang HJ, Kim SG, Kook MC, Bae JM. The learning curve for EMR with circumferential mucosal incision in treating intramucosal gastric neoplasm. Gastrointest Endosc. 2005;62:860–5.

33. Kakushima N, Fujishiro M, Kodashima S, Muraki Y, Tateishi A, Omata M. A learning curve for endoscopic submucosal dissection of gastric epithelial neoplasms. Endoscopy. 2006;38:991–5.

34. Yamamoto S, Uedo N, Ishihara R, et al. Endoscopic submucosal dissection for early gastric cancer performed by supervised residents: assessment of feasibility and learning curve. Endoscopy. 2009;41:923–8.

35. Draganov PV, Gotoda T, Chavalitdhamrong D, Wallace MB. Techniques of endoscopic submucosal dissection: application for the Western endoscopist? Gastrointest Endosc. 2013;78:677–88.

36. Sakamoto T, Saito Y, Fukunaga S, Nakajima T, Matsuda T. Learning curve associated with colorectal endoscopic submucosal dissection for endoscopists experienced in gastric endoscopic submucosal dissection. Dis Colon Rectum. 2011;54:1307–12.

37. Gotoda T, Friedland S, Hamanaka H, Soetikno R. A learning curve for advanced endoscopic resection. Gastrointest Endosc. 2005;62:866–7.

38. Vázquez-Sequeiros E, de Miquel DB, Olcina JR, et al. Training model for teaching endoscopic submucosal dissection of gastric tumors. Rev Esp Enferm Dig. 2009;101:546–52.

39. Tanimoto MA, Torres-Villalobos G, Fujita R, et al. Endoscopic submucosal dissection in dogs in a World Gastroenterology Organization training center. World J Gastroenterol. 2010;16:1759–64.

40. Parra-Blanco A, Arnau MR, Nicolás-Pérez D, et al. Endoscopic submucosal dissection training with pig models in a Western country. World J Gastroenterol. 2010;16:2895–900.

41. González N, Parra-Blanco A, Villa-Gómez M, et al. Gastric endoscopic submucosal dissection: from animal model to patient. World J Gastroenterol. 2013;19:8326–34.

42. Kato M, Gromski M, Jung Y, Chuttani R, Matthes K. The learning curve for endoscopic submucosal dissection in an established experimental setting. Surg Endosc. 2013;27:154–61.

43. Hirasawa K, Kokawa A, Kou R, Oka H, Maeda S, Tanaka K. Determining early gastric cancer lesions appropriate for endoscopic submucosal dissection trainees: a proposal related to curability. Dig Endosc. 2012;24 Suppl 1:143–7.

44. Hotta K, Oyama T, Shinohara T. Learning curve for endoscopic submucosal dissection of large colorectal tumors. Dig Endosc. 2010;22:302–6.

45. Repici A, Conio M, De Angelis C. Insulated-tip knife endoscopic mucosal resection of large colorectal polyps unsuitable for standard polypectomy. Am J Gastroenterol. 2007;102:1617–23.

46. Tanimoto MA, Torres-Villalobos G, Fujita R, et al. Learning curve in a Western training center of the circumferential en bloc esophageal endoscopic submucosal dissection in an in vivo animal model. Diagn Ther Endosc. 2011;2011:847831.

47. Tanaka S, Morita Y, Fujita T, et al. Ex vivo pig training model for esophageal endoscopic submucosal dissection (ESD) for endoscopists with experience in gastric ESD. Surg Endosc. 2012;26:1579–86.

48. Hon SS, Ng SS, Lee JF, Li JC, Lo AW. In vitro porcine training model for colonic endoscopic submucosal dissection: an inexpensive and safe way to acquire a complex endoscopic technique. Surg Endosc. 2010;24:2439–43.

49. Yoshida N, Yagi N, Inada Y, et al. Possibility of ex vivo animal training model for colorectal endoscopic submucosal dissection. Int J Colorectal Dis. 2013;28:49–56.

50. Kaltenbach T, Muto M, Soetikno R, et al. Teleteaching endoscopy: the feasibility of real-time, uncompressed video transmission by using advanced-network technologies. Gastrointest Endosc. 2009;70:1013–7.

51. Gotoda T, Kusano C, Nonaka M, et al. Nonanesthesiologist administrated propofol (NAAP) during endoscopic submucosal dissection for elderly patients with early gastric cancer. Gastric Cancer. 2014;17:686–691.

52. Chun SY, Kim KO, Park DS, et al. Safety and efficacy of deep sedation with propofol alone or combined with midazolam administrated by nonanesthesiologist for gastric endoscopic submucosal dissection. Gut Liver. 2012;6:464–70.

53. Park CH, Min JH, Yoo YC, et al. Sedation methods can determine performance of endoscopic submuco-

sal dissection in patients with gastric neoplasia. Surg Endosc. 2013;27:2760–7.

54. Probst A, Pommer B, Golger D, et al. Endoscopic submucosal dissection in gastric neoplasia—experience from a European center. Endoscopy. 2010;42:1037–44.

55. Toyokawa T, Inaba T, Omote S, et al. Risk factors for perforation and delayed bleeding associated with endoscopic submucosal dissection for early gastric neoplasms: analysis of 1123 lesions. J Gastroenterol Hepatol. 2012;27:907–12.

56. Teoh AY, Chiu PW, Wong SK, et al. Difficulties and outcomes in starting endoscopic submucosal dissection. Surg Endosc. 2010;24:1049–54.

57. Takizawa K, Oda I, Gotoda T, et al. Routine coagulation of visible vessels may prevent delayed bleeding after endoscopic submucosal dissection—an analysis of risk factors. Endoscopy. 2008;40:179–83.

58. Toyonaga T, Nishino E, Man IM, et al. Principles of quality controlled endoscopic submucosal dissection with appropriate dissection level and high quality resected specimen. Clin Endosc. 2012;45:362–74.

59. Toyonaga T, Man-I M, Morita Y, et al. The new resources of treatment for early stage colorectal tumors: EMR with small incision and simplified endoscopic submucosal dissection. Dig Endosc. 2009;21 Suppl 1:S31–7.

60. Moss A, Bourke MJ, Metz AJ, et al. Beyond the snare: technically accessible large en bloc colonic resection in the West: an animal study. Dig Endosc. 2012;24:21–9.

61. Sakamoto T, Matsuda T, Nakajima T, Saito Y. Efficacy of endoscopic mucosal resection with circumferential incision for patients with large colorectal tumors. Clin Gastroenterol Hepatol. 2012;10:22–6.

62. Sakurazawa N, Kato S, Fujita I, Kanazawa Y, Onodera H, Uchida E. Supportive techniques and devices for endoscopic submucosal dissection of gastric cancer. World J Gastrointest Endosc. 2012;4:231–5.

63. Fukami N. What we want for ESD is a second hand! Traction method. Gastrointest Endosc. 2013;78:274–6.

64. Sakamoto N, Osada T, Shibuya T, et al. The facilitation of a new traction device (S-O clip) assisting endoscopic submucosal dissection for superficial colorectal neoplasms. Endoscopy. 2008;40 Suppl 2:E94–5.

65. Parra-Blanco A, Nicolas D, Arnau MR, Gimeno-Garcia AZ, Rodrigo L, Quintero E. Gastric endoscopic submucosal dissection assisted by a new traction method: the clip-band technique. A feasibility study in a porcine model (with video). Gastrointest Endosc. 2011;74:1137–41.

66. Parra-Blanco A, Uraoka T, Ortiz Fernández-Sordo J, et al. Is a traction method (Clip-Band) useful to facilitate gastric endoscopic submucosal dissection? A prospective, randomized controlled trial in a live Porcine Model. Gastrointest Endosc. 2013;77:AB123.

Appendix: Commonly used ESD Knives

26

Norio Fukami

Electronic supplementary material Supplementary material is available in the online version of this chapter at 10.1007/978-1-4939-2041-9_26. Videos can also be accessed at http://www.springerimages.com/videos/978-1-4939-2040-2.

N. Fukami, M.D., A.G.A.F., F.A.C.G., F.A.S.G.E. (✉)
Division of Gastroenterology & Hepatology,
University of Colorado Anschutz Medical Campus,
Aurora, CO 80045, USA
e-mail: norio.Fukami@ucdenver.edu

Name	Company	Model number	
Needle knife (reusable by sterilization)	Olympus	KD-102-1	
IT knife	Olympus	KD-610L	
IT knife 2	Olympus	KD-611L	
IT knife nano	Olympus	KD-612L	

Name	Company	Model number	
Hook knife	Olympus	KD-620LR	
Dual knife	Olympus	KD-650L	
Triangle tip knife (TT Knife)	Olympus	KD-640L	
Hybrid knife, I-type (and T-type; photo)	ERBE	20150-060	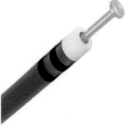

Name	Company	Model number	
Flush knife (and Flush knife BT, photo)	Fujinon	(Not available in the USA)	
Clutch cutter	Fujinon	(Not available in the USA)	
SB knife	Sumitomo Bakelite	(Not available in the USA)	

Index

N. Fukami (ed.), *Endoscopic Submucosal Dissection: Principles and Practice*,
DOI 10.1007/978-1-4939-2041-9, © Springer Science+Business Media New York 2015